Manual of
Neuroanesthesia

Manual of

Neuroanesthesia

Richard J. Sperry, M.D.

Assistant Professor of Anesthesiology
and Surgery (Neurosurgery)
Department of Anesthesiology
University of Utah Medical Center
Salt Lake City, Utah

Joseph A. Stirt, M.D.

Associate Professor of Anesthesiology
Department of Anesthesiology
University of Virginia Health Sciences Center
Charlottesville, Virginia

David J. Stone, M.D.

Assistant Professor of Anesthesiology
and Neurological Surgery
Department of Anesthesiology
University of Virginia Health Sciences Center
Charlottesville, Virginia

B.C. Decker Inc. • Toronto • Philadelphia

Publisher   **B.C. Decker Inc**   **B.C. Decker Inc**
                   3228 South Service Road   320 Walnut Street
                   Burlington, Ontario L7N 3H8 Suite 400
                                                Philadelphia, Pennsylvania 19106

Sales and Distribution

United States and Puerto Rico
The C.V. Mosby Company
11830 Westline Industrial Drive
Saint Louis, Missouri 63146

Canada
McAinsh & Co. Ltd.
2760 Old Leslie Street
Willowdale, Ontario M2K 2X5

Australia
McGraw-Hill Book Company Australia Pty. Ltd.
4 Barcoo Street
Roseville East 2069
New South Wales, Australia

Brazil
Editora McGraw-Hill do Brasil, Ltda.
rua Tabapua, 1.105, Itaim-Bibi
Sao Paulo, S.P. Brasil

Colombia
Interamericana/McGraw-Hill de Colombia, S.A.
Apartado Aereo 81078
Bogota, D.E. Colombia

Europe
McGraw-Hill Book Company GmbH
Lademannbogen 136
D-2000 Hamburg 63
West Germany

France
MEDSI/McGraw-Hill
6, avenue Daniel Lesueur
75007 Paris, France

Hong Kong and China
McGraw-Hill Book Company
Suite 618, Ocean Centre
5 Canton Road
Tsimshatsui, Kowloon
Hong Kong

India
Tata McGraw-Hill Publishing Company, Ltd.
12/4 Asaf Ali Road, 3rd Floor
New Delhi 110002, India

Indonesia
P.O. Box 122/JAT
Jakarta, 1300 Indonesia

Italy
McGraw-Hill Libri Italia, s.r.l.
Piazza Emilia, 5
I-20129 Milano MI
Italy

Japan
Igaku-Shoin Ltd.
Tokyo International P.O. Box 5063
1-28-36 Hongo, Bunkyo-ku,
Tokyo 113, Japan

Korea
C.P.O. Box 10583
Seoul, Korea

Malaysia
No. 8 Jalan SS 7/6B
Kelana Jaya
47301 Petaling Jaya
Selangor, Malaysia

Mexico
Interamericana/McGraw-Hill de Mexico, S.A. de C.V.
Cedro 512, Colonia Atlampa
(Apartado Postal 26370)
06450 Mexico, D.F., Mexico

New Zealand
McGraw-Hill Book Co. New Zealand Ltd.
5 Joval Place, Wiri
Manukau City, New Zealand

Panama
Editorial McGraw-Hill Latinoamericana, S.A.
Apartado Postal 2036
Zona Libre de Colon
Colon, Republica de Panama

Portugal
Editora McGraw-Hill de Portugal, Ltda.
Rua Rosa Damasceno 11A-B
1900 Lisboa, Portugal

South Africa
Libriger Book Distributors
Warehouse Number 8
''Die Ou Looiery''
Tannery Road
Hamilton, Bloemfontein 9300

Southeast Asia
McGraw-Hill Book Co.
348 Jalan Boon Lay
Jurong, Singapore 2261

Spain
McGraw-Hill/Interamericana de Espana, S.A.
Manuel Ferrero, 13
28020 Madrid, Spain

Taiwan
P.O. Box 87-601
Taipei, Taiwan

Thailand
632/5 Phaholyothin Road
Sapan Kwai
Bangkok 10400
Thailand

United Kingdom, Middle East and Africa
McGraw-Hill Book Company (U.K.) Ltd.
Shoppenhangers Road
Maidenhead, Berkshire
SL6 2QL England

Venezuela
McGraw-Hill/Interamericana, C.A.
2da. calle Bello Monte
(entre avenida Casanova y Sabana Grande)
Apartado Aereo 50785
Caracas 1050, Venezuela

Manual of Neuroanesthesia   ISBN 1-55664-105-2

Library of Congress catalog card number: 89-50931   10 9 8 7 6 5 4 3 2 1

Contributors

David L. Bogdonoff, M.D.
Assistant Professor of Anesthesiology
University of Virginia Health Sciences Center
Charlottesville, Virginia

Donald L. Boos, M.D.
Research Fellow in Neuroanesthesia
University of Virginia Health Sciences Center
Charlottesville, Virginia

William C. Broaddus, M.D., Ph.D.
Research Fellow in Neurological Surgery
University of Virginia Health Sciences Center
Charlottesville, Virginia

C. Morgan Cooper, M.D.
Research Fellow in Neuroanesthesia
University of Virginia Health Sciences Center
Charlottesville, Virginia

Johnny B. Delashaw, M.D.
Research Fellow in Neurological Surgery
University of Virginia Health Sciences Center
Charlottesville, Virginia

Adrian J. Hobbs, M.B.
Assistant Professor of Anesthesiology
University of Virginia Health Sciences Center
Charlottesville, Virginia

Bruce A. Mannes, M.D.
Chief Resident in Anesthesiology
University of Utah Medical Center
Salt Lake City, Utah

Scott L. Mears, M.D.
Fellow in Neuroanesthesia
University of Utah Medical Center
Salt Lake City, Utah

Hilary A. Noble, B.M., F.F.A.R.C.S.
Assistant Professor of Anesthesiology
University of Virginia Health Sciences Center
Charlottesville, Virginia

T. S. Park, M.D.
Professor of Neurological Surgery and Pediatrics
University of Virginia Health Sciences Center
Charlottesville, Virginia

Richard J. Sperry, M.D.
Assistant Professor of Anesthesiology and Surgery (Neurosurgery)
University of Utah Medical Center
Salt Lake City, Utah

Cary S. Sternick, M.D.
Chairman, Department of Neurology
Tomball Regional Hospital
Houston, Texas

Joseph A. Stirt, M.D.
Associate Professor of Anesthesiology
University of Virginia Health Sciences Center
Charlottesville, Virginia

David J. Stone, M.D.
Assistant Professor of Anesthesiology and Neurological Surgery
University of Virginia Health Sciences Center
Charlottesville, Virginia

Foreword

In the last three decades there have been enormous strides in neurosurgery. Many lesions which heretofore were beyond the realm of technical feasibility can now be boldly approached, and other challenging but somewhat more routine problems can be treated with considerably greater safety. A large component of the progress in technical neurosurgery is a direct result of the advances in neuroanesthesia.

This new *Manual of Neuroanesthesia* presents succinctly the state-of-the-art in practical terms that can be readily applied in the operating room. Written by three leaders in the field, this work promises to become an essential text for practitioners and teachers of neuroanesthesia, and for their students.

The emphasis of this text is clearly upon the basis of the clinical practice of neuroanesthesia. The authors are superb clinicians who have written a beautifully organized and interesting book. With the tremendous growth in neurosciences, it is refreshing to have a volume that relates the progress at the basic level to the actual giving of anesthetics to neurosurgical patients.

Neal F. Kassell, M.D.
John A. Jane, M.D., Ph.D.

To Robert M. Epstein, M.D., who made it possible

Preface

Why another neuroanesthesia book? While attempting to design and implement teaching programs in neuroanesthesia at our institutions, we quickly realized that none of the available texts met our needs. Although there are excellent books available in this field, we felt they did not emphasize the practical aspects of current neuroanesthesia practice in the United States. Too many times, a chapter could burst with facts yet leave the student with the uncomfortable question of "How do I actually do the anesthetic for a given neurosurgical procedure?"

The practice of neuroanesthesia depends heavily on the basic sciences of anatomy, physiology, and pharmacology, and we have not intended to downgrade the importance of these fields which lend a rationale to what we do and make it more enjoyable. However, we did not wish to shortchange clinical practice, leaving a brief piece on "how to do it" buried at the end of a long chapter. This book should be a useful guide for a resident undertaking a one-month rotation in neuroanesthesia, as well as a resource for the practicing CRNA or anesthesiologist who does not anesthetize neurosurgical patients with great frequency. The recovery phase and intensive care period have been covered in detail as well. Although not originally intended as such, the book should form a solid basis for review for both written and oral board exams in anesthesiology. Once the basic text has been absorbed, use of the references should allow those with a greater academic inclination to dig deeper into some of the current research in the field.

We believe that anesthesia for neurosurgery is especially gratifying, as our function interacts with that of the surgeon in a way not present in many other fields of anesthesia. Neuroanesthesia provides the practitioner with a real clinical test with challenging patients who require the physician's skill in *all* phases of anesthesia. We hope this book makes the practice of neuroanesthesia more rational, more accessible, and more fun.

Richard J. Sperry
Joseph A. Stirt
David J. Stone

Contents

William C. Broaddus, M.D., Ph.D., Johnny B. Delashaw, M.D., and
T. S. Park, M.D.

Anatomic, Physiologic, and Neurosurgical Considerations in Neuroanesthesia 1

The central nervous system (CNS) is unique in its vulnerability to both direct and indirect consequences of trauma, hypoxia, ischemia, and other pathophysiologic phenomena. Furthermore, it is unlike body systems in its relatively poor ability to recover from injury. For these reasons, several aspects of normal CNS anatomy and physiology play critical roles in the choices and effects of anesthesia. The wide range of pathologic conditions requiring neurosurgical treatment also frequently have mechanical or physiologic consequences that affect the choice of or response to anesthetic techniques.

Clearly, each patient represents a complex interplay of physiology, pathology, and the consequences of various interventions. The task of the surgical team is to develop a set of priorities by which to make decisions regarding the management of the individual patient. The purpose of this chapter is thus fourfold. First, selected aspects of CNS anatomy and physiology are briefly reviewed for their significance with respect to neuroanesthetic techniques. Second, a brief overview of mechanisms of CNS injury due to neurosurgical pathology is provided as a framework for discussion of surgical and medical treatment strategies undertaken by the neurosurgeon and neuroanesthesiologist. Third, a neurosurgical perspective of the significant issues in anesthetic management of patients is provided. Finally, we emphasize the importance of communication between neuroanesthesiologists and neurosurgeons prior to and during a procedure requiring anesthesia.

Anatomic and Physiologic Considerations

Central Nervous System Compartments

The craniospinal compartment is effectively a single contiguous space bounded by the calvaria and spinal canal. Although it is well suited for protecting the soft vulnerable neural tissue of the brain and spinal cord, its lack of distensibility is a major reason for the low compliance of the CNS. Brain parenchyma, cerebrospinal fluid, and intravascular fluid are the primary components contained within the intradural compartment. A pathologic increase in one of these compartments (e.g., tumor growth, hydrocephalus, or intraparenchymal bleeding) can result in compression and shift of surrounding structures. In addition, the increase in volume produces a rapid rise in intracranial pressure (ICP) and may result in deleterious consequences. The craniospinal space is anatomically separated into three intradural compartments: the supratentorial compartment, the posterior fossa, and the spinal intradural compartment (Fig. 1–1).

The Supratentorial Compartment

The supratentorial compartment comprises the largest component of the craniospinal space and is demarcated by the calvaria and the tentorium cerebelli. It is partially divided in the midline by the falx cerebri. The latter structure also divides the major contents of this compartment, the cerebral hemispheres. The importance of these structures in subserving higher aspects of function of the various sensory modalities, organized complex motor behaviors, and personality and intelligence is well known. Paradoxically, however, only relatively large lesions in this compartment are usually life-

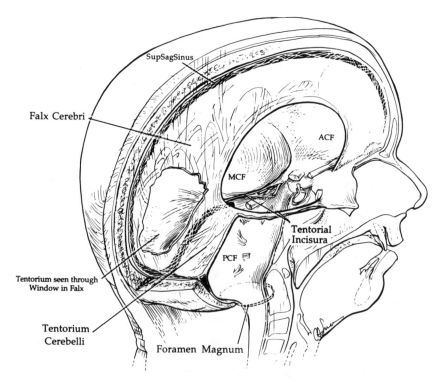

Figure 1-1 Illustration of the compartments of the craniospinal space in a drawing of the hemisected head. The dural structures, including falx cerebri and tentorium cerebelli, are left partially intact to illustrate how the cranial compartment is subdivided. Note that the supratentorial compartment is divided by the falx cerebri and is contributed to by the anterior cranial fossa (ACF) and middle cranial fossa (MCF). The supratentorial compartment communicates with the infratentorial compartment or posterior cranial fossa (PCF) via the opening of the tentorial incisura. The posterior cranial fossa in turn communicates with the intraspinal compartment by way of the foramen magnum.

threatening. Smaller lesions, which in the posterior fossa might be devastating to vital functions, may have only subtle consequences in the supratentorial compartment.

Both the inferior edge of the falx cerebri and the incisura of the tentorium are important sites for secondary injury to the CNS. When differential pressure develops as a result of a frontal lobe mass, subfalcial herniation can develop. This can lead to direct injury to the region of the cingulate gyrus, as well as cerebral ischemia by impingement of the anterior cerebral artery (Fig. 1-1 and Fig. 1-2)

Herniation through the tentorial incisura is of even greater clinical importance because of the other structures that are at risk of injury. In particular, these include brain stem structures which are important for maintenance of consciousness, the motor and sensory pathways within the cerebral peduncles, the oculomotor nerves (CN III), as well as the proximal portions of the posterior cerebral arteries (see Figs. 1-2 and 1-3).

Lateral masses cause downward and medial pressure on the temporal lobe resulting in herniation of the uncus (on the medial surface of the temporal lobe) over the edge of the tentorium. This results in ischemic injury to the cortex of the uncus and may result in pressure on the oculomotor nerve, posterior cerebral arteries, and cerebral peduncle (Fig. 1-3). The ominous consequences of these phenomena are well known:

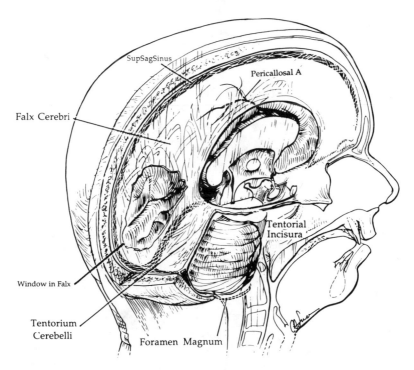

Figure 1-2 A view of the hemisected head similar to that in Figure 1-1 is shown with the cerebellum, caudal brain stem, and left cerebral hemisphere in place. This shows the important anatomic relationships of brain and vascular structures to the falx cerebri, tentorial incisura, and foramen magnum. Note that the pericallosal artery is an extension of the anterior cerebral artery and passes above the inferior edge of the falx as it courses posteriorly. Also note the potential for impaction of the cervicomedullary junction and cerebellar tonsils at the foramen magnum in the event of a downward shift of the brain.

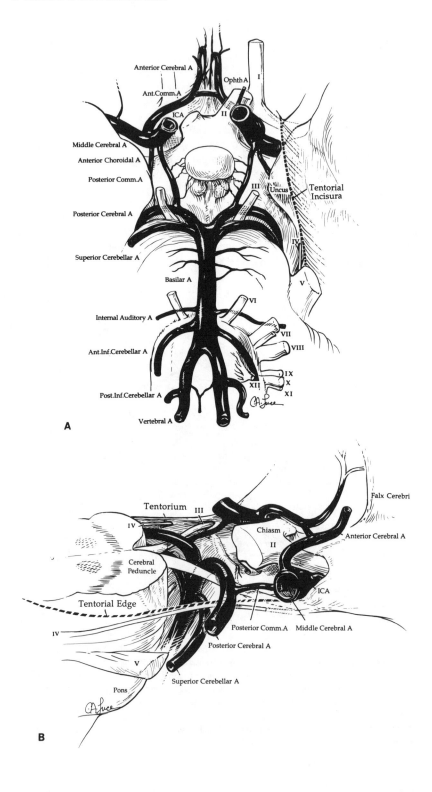

A

Anterior Cerebral A
Ant.Comm.A
Ophth A   I
ICA   II
Middle Cerebral A
Anterior Choroidal A
Posterior Comm.A
III Uncus
Tentorial Incisura
Posterior Cerebral A
IV
Superior Cerebellar A
V
Basilar A
VI
Internal Auditory A
VII
VIII
Ant.Inf.Cerebellar A
IX
X
XII XI
Post.Inf.Cerebellar A
Vertebral A

B

Tentorium   III
IV
Falx Cerebri
Chiasm
II
Anterior Cerebral A
Cerebral Peduncle
Tentorial Edge
ICA
IV
Posterior Comm.A   Middle Cerebral A
Posterior Cerebral A
V
Superior Cerebellar A
Pons

ipsilateral large irregular poorly reactive pupil, contralateral hemiplegia and posturing, and sometimes ipsilateral medial occipital lobe infarction. If the lateral to medial pressure is more diffuse, the contralateral-cerebral peduncle may be pressed against the medial edge of the contralateral portion of the tentorial incisura, resulting in Kernohan's notch phenomenon (ipsilateral hemiplegia). In fact, bilateral neurologic signs with predominance of one side over the other are more common than unilateral findings, and suggest a combination of the above described pathophysiologic phenomena.

Paramidline supratentorial masses can also result in herniation through the tentorial hiatus, and they may produce displacement of structures through the foramen magnum.

The Posterior Fossa

The posterior fossa is the portion of the cranial cavity below the tentorium, and it is notable for the vital structures contained within it. The compartment contains the cerebellum and caudal brain stem. The caudal brain stem lies ventrally along the clivus connecting with the rostral brain stem through the tentorial incisura and the cervical spinal cord through the foramen magnum. Relatively small mass lesions of the cerebellum and even smaller mass lesions adjacent to or within the caudal brain stem can have devastating consequences after presenting with only subtle symptoms. Injury to the reticular activating system frequently can result in a decreased level of consciousness, while injury to centers for respiratory and hemodynamic control can cause apnea and marked hemodynamic instability. In addition, lesions along the brain stem can result in impairment of function of the cranial nerves and ascending and descending pathways.

The tendency of large supratentorial masses to cause shifts of the brain through the tentorial incisura have been discussed. Central herniation caused by paramidline supratentorial masses, however, may also cause severe injuries by two other mechanisms. Differential movement of caudal brain stem structures caused by the relative immobility of the basilar artery as compared to the overlying pons may result in secondary pontine hemorrhages due to rupture of small perforating vessels. Second, the "pressure cone" phenomenon that occurs in herniation at the foramen magnum may result in impaction of the cerebellar tonsils on the cervicomedullary junction, frequently with fatal results (see Fig. 1-2 and Fig. 1-3)

The premonitory signs of impending herniation, particularly in the posterior fossa, may be relatively subtle and require a high index of suspicion for diagnosis. Computed tomography (CT) or magnetic resonance imaging (MRI) may be helpful in demonstrating asymmetric effacement of the ambient cisterns due to uncal herniation,

Figure 1-3 Vascular and neural anatomic relationships of the base of the brain are depicted from (A) a basal view and (B) a posterolateral view. Components of the anterior and posterior arterial circulations of the brain are shown. The anastomosis of these two circulations by way of the posterior communicating arteries bilaterally comprises the circle of Willis. Cranial nerves are labeled by Roman numerals, and the important relationship of the tentorial incisura and uncus of the temporal lobe are demonstrated. Abbreviations used are as follows: ICA = internal carotid artery; A = artery; Ophth A = ophthalmic artery; Ant. Comm. A = anterior communicating artery; Posterior Comm. A = posterior communicating artery; Ant. Inf. Cerebellar A = anterior inferior cerebellar artery; Post. Inf. Cerebellar A = posterior inferior cerebellar artery.

effacement of the fourth ventricle due to a cerebellar mass, or presence of cerebellar tonsils adjacent to the spinal cord in the foramen magnum. In the context of neuroanesthesiology, these signs should be used as indications for interventions that lower ICP, and protection against large increases in ICP during manipulations such as intubation or endotracheal suctioning.

The Spinal Intradural Compartment

The spinal intradural compartment represents a significant portion of the total volume of the craniospinal compartment. The spinal cord extends only down to the first lumbar segment, the lumbar and sacral subarachnoid space (L2 to S2) represents a cerebrospinal fluid (CSF) reservoir through which the lumbar and sacral nerve roots pass. Surrounding the dura within the spinal canal is the epidural venous plexus, which represents a displaceable extradural vascular volume. A slight distensibility of the spinal dura and the compressibility of the epidural venous plexus thus appear to underlie the ability of the spinal subarachnoid space to accommodate CSF displaced by the rapid expansion of an intracranial mass. This greater compliance of the spinal intradural compartment would also appear to be a significant factor in the pathogenesis of transforaminal herniation. With this in mind, it is obvious how further decompression of the spinal intradural compartment by lumbar puncture could precipitate a transforaminal herniation, with disastrous consequences. Conversely, it should be noted that a head CT scan frequently allows the clinician to proceed safely with lumbar puncture, even in the presence of a known intracranial mass, by demonstrating the lack of significant mass effect.

Structures of the Central Nervous System Parenchyma

The Cerebral Hemispheres

The cerebral hemispheres are responsible for cognitive function, personality, and meaningful sensory and motor function. Discrete neurologic deficits can result from direct destructive lesions. Although patients with lesions of the frontal lobes may present with subtle neurologic deficits, patients with lesions of the cerebral cortex adjacent to the Rolandic fissure, internal capsule, or basal ganglia may exhibit profound deficits in motor or sensory function. Furthermore, lesions that involve the speech areas in the dominant hemisphere, while not life-threatening, have the potential to render a patient unable to communicate with the outside world. Large lesions of the cerebral hemispheres have the potential for causing transtentorial or central herniation syndromes. Such patients are thus extremely vulnerable to otherwise insignificant changes in intracranial dynamics.

The Diencephalon

The diencephalon is the rostral portion of the brain stem that lies centrally within the supratentorial compartment. The diencephalon includes the thalamus, hypothalamus, and pineal gland, and encloses the third ventricle. These structures play an important role in relaying and integrating CNS function. The diencephalon is vulnerable to neoplastic involvement, ischemic injury due to impairment of blood flow in perforating arteries, and direct compression due to hemispheric mass effect.

The Cerebellum

The cerebellum is the largest structure occupying the posterior fossa and is involved in coordination of motor function. Although it is not vital for survival, midline or bilateral lesions may cause permanent disabling motor impairment. Unilateral lesions of the cerebellar hemispheres usually cause ipsilateral limb ataxia, which will partially resolve over time. Cerebellar lesions and associated edema can interfere with the vital functions of the brain stem by direct compression.

The Caudal Brain Stem

The caudal brain stem resides in the posterior fossa and is composed of the midbrain, the pons, and the medulla oblongata. This area of the brain stem serves as a conduit with significant processing functions of afferent and efferent activity between the brain and spinal cord. It serves similar functions for cranial nerves III through XII, and contains structures that are vital to maintenance of consciousness, equilibrium, and respiratory and hemodynamic control. These structures are vulnerable to injury by transtentorial, central, and transforaminal herniation, or by direct compression by posterior fossa lesions.

The Spinal Cord

The spinal cord extends from the cervicomedullary junction at the foramen magnum to the conus medullaris and cauda equina at the T12–L1 level. This structure is vulnerable to trauma, compression by intradural or extradural tumors, and occasionally vascular injury. The danger of such injuries to motor and sensory function below the segmental level of the injury is well known. In addition, certain important functions require intact innervation from specific segmental levels of the spinal cord. For instance, the ability of an individual to breathe independently requires intact phrenic nerve function as a minimum. The phrenic nerves, in turn, are formed by branches of the anterior nerve roots at the third to fifth cervical levels. For full respiratory function, thoracic spinal cord innervation of the muscles of respiration is also required. Thus, respiratory dysfunction is a concomitant of any spinal cord injury in the thoracic or cervical segments, with the degree of impairment related to the level of injury.

Another example of segmental dependence is the outflow of the sympathetic nervous system in the thoracic and lumbar nerve roots. Thus, lesions of the upper thoracic level or above will disrupt sympathetic tone. Practical consequences of such lesions include postural hypotension and bradycardia.

Intracranial Pressure

Determinants of Intracranial Pressure

The ICP can be expressed in terms of the volume of the contents of the craniospinal compartment and its compliance ($\Delta ICP = \Delta volume/compliance$). As previously discussed, the intracranial compartment has little if any compliance, while the spinal canal has a small degree of compliance related to distensibility of the spinal dura mater and surrounding epidural venous plexus. As a result, significant changes in total volume of the craniospinal contents are accompanied by large changes in ICP. In fact, significant changes in volume of any of the components occupying the craniospinal compartment are usually accompanied by passive changes in volume of the other components so that the change in total volume is minimal. The rise in ICP due to a given pathologic process is determined by the net increase in volume after primary pathologic changes and compensatory changes in volume of the other components are balanced.

There are three components that make up the craniospinal contents (Table 1-1). These are the brain and spinal cord parenchyma, the cerebral and spinal blood volume, and the CSF. Changes in the CNS parenchyma that may result in increased ICP include tumor growth and cerebral edema. The latter may be due to ischemic injury or trauma, or may be surrounding a hematoma, tumor, or inflammatory process such as an abscess.

Changes in the brain vascular compartment can have a major effect on ICP, particularly when involving venous blood volume. This is directly affected by systemic venous pressure as well as cerebral vascular tone related to autoregulatory functions. Both of these parameters are amenable to manipulation for amelioration of intracranial hypertension and, by the same token, are potential mechanisms by which existing intracranial hypertension may be exacerbated.

The CSF volume depends on a balance between production and disposition. The fact that production of CSF is poorly responsive to changes in ICP is responsible for the development of hydrocephalus in patients who develop problems in disposition of CSF. In the normal individual, the total CSF volume is approximately 140 ml, with daily production of about 500 to 600 ml. Since the majority of this production arises from the

Table 1-1 Determinants of ICP and Therapeutic Techniques to Lower Elevated ICP

Determinant	Therapeutic Intervention	Mechanism	Duration of Effectiveness
CSF volume	Ventricular or lumbar puncture	Volume reduction	Hours
	Ventriculostomy or lumbar drain	Volume reduction	Days
	Ventricular or lumbar shunt	Volume reduction	Indefinite
Cerebral blood volume	Hyperventilation	Cerebral vasoconstriction due to decreased Pco_2	Hours
	Barbiturates	Cerebral vasoconstriction	Hours to days
Volume of parenchyma	Mannitol infusion	Osmotic reduction of brain water content	Hours to days
	Corticosteroids	Reduction of peritumoral or peri-inflammatory edema	Days to weeks
	Excision of mass	Volume reduction	Indefinite
	Craniectomy	Increased craniospinal compliance	Indefinite

choroid plexus of the lateral and third ventricles, it is evident that acute obstruction of outflow at the cerebral aqueduct or fourth ventricle, or obstruction caused by acute shunt failure in a fully shunt-dependent individual, could be life-threatening within a matter of hours.

Consequences of Elevated Intracranial Pressure

ICP affects cerebral blood flow through its effect on cerebral perfusion pressure. Cerebral perfusion pressure is defined as the difference between mean arterial pressure (MAP) and intracranial pressure. Under normal conditions, as ICP rises, cerebral vascular resistance decreases to maintain a constant cerebral blood flow. However, as ICP approaches mean arterial pressure or when cerebral autoregulation is impaired (as in vasospasm or severe atherosclerosis), it is clear that cerebral blood flow will be more directly dependent on cerebral perfusion pressure. Differential pressures can also develop between different areas within the craniospinal compartment. Pressure differentials in turn cause shifts in brain parenchymal structures, and may result in one of the herniation syndromes discussed on pages 1 to 6.

Cerebral Blood Flow

General Considerations

The importance of blood flow to the brain is well known. Under normal conditions, permanent injury may begin to develop after only a few minutes of ischemia. This is particularly important in the case of global ischemia caused by severe systemic hypotension; hence the continued importance of the basic principles of life support to maintain adequate oxygenation and perfusion. Depending upon the rapidity of onset and location of the lesion, an extensive system of anastomoses can provide protection and may delay permanent injury when the loss of blood flow in a major cerebral vessel occurs. For example, it is not uncommon for a complete blockage of one of the major vessels proximal to the circle of Willis to go unnoticed clinically because of good collateral flow. Similarly, progressive occlusion of distal branches of the cerebral arterial vasculature may be fully compensated by development of collateral flow from overlapping distributions. As is discussed under Vascular Anatomy (pp. 11–12), however, the presence of vascular abnormalities frequently places the patient at special risk from otherwise innocuous manipulations of parameters that affect cerebral blood flow.

Determinants of Cerebral Blood Flow

As in more general cases, the cerebral blood flow (CBF) can be described as the driving force, or cerebral perfusion pressure (CPP), divided by the resistance of the system, or cerebrovascular resistance (CVR). Since the cerebral perfusion pressure is defined as the difference between the mean arterial pressure and the intracranial pressure, the cerebral blood flow can be defined as:

$$CBF = CPP/CVR = (MAP - ICP)/CVR.$$

In general then, changes in MAP, ICP, or CVR can significantly alter blood flow to the brain (Table 1–2).

Table 1-2 Determinants of CBF and Some Therapeutic Techniques to Increase CBF

Determinant	Therapeutic Intervention	Mechanism
Mean arterial pressure (MAP)	Normovolemia/ hypervolemia	Maintenance or elevation of cardiac output
	Pressors	Elevation of systemic vascular resistance
Intracranial pressure (ICP)	See Table 1-1	
Cerebrovascular resistance (CVR)	Hemodilution by hypervolemia (rarely by phlebotomy)	Reduction of resistance by decreasing blood viscosity (due to decreased hematocrit)
	Mannitol infusion	Reduction of resistance by decreasing blood viscosity (due to rheologic effect of mannitol)
	Revascularization	Restoration of flow beyond an area of occlusion or stenosis
	Angioplasty	Dilatation of focal arterial stenosis

In addition to ICP, localized elevations in tissue pressure are also thought to play a role in affecting regional blood flow. For instance, neurologic deficits following spinal cord contusion may primarily result from impaired blood flow rather than direct CNS parenchymal injury.

Factors that affect CVR are extremely important in neuroanesthesiology. Under normal circumstances, cerebral vascular autoregulation provides for relatively constant blood flow to a region commensurate with its oxygen demand over a wide range of perfusion pressures. Such regulation may be impaired or absent under pathologic conditions or pharmacologic manipulation (such as anesthesia), and increase the dependence of blood flow on perfusion pressure.

CVR is affected not only by vascular tone but also by rheologic characteristics of blood. Since blood viscosity increases with hematocrit, so does CVR. This provides a rationale for the use of hemodilution as a therapeutic technique under conditions of cerebral ischemia such as vasospasm. Mannitol in therapeutic doses is also known to decrease blood viscosity, which may help explain its apparent benefit in the treatment of vasospasm.

Regional Cerebral Blood Flow

In addition to the general importance of perfusion pressure and vascular resistance in control of CBF, it is important to remember that regional variations in these parameters result in regional variations in blood flow. Thus, while the primary considerations and therapeutic measures undertaken in a specific case may be directed to the control or alteration of global CBF, the possibility of various factors causing significant variations in regional blood flow must be kept in mind.

Impaired or absent autoregulation may develop in cerebral ischemia, brain tumors, and cerebral edema, or in vasospasm following subarachnoid hemorrhage. Atherosclerosis frequently causes focal areas of markedly increased vascular resistance due to luminal narrowing and may also impair vascular compliance. Thus, atherosclerosis can interfere with autoregulatory changes in vessel caliber. Vascular steal phenomena can develop in the setting of abnormalities such as arteriovenous malformations or carotid-cavernous fistulas. In such cases, regional blood flow is shunted through a low-resistance arteriovenous connection, resulting in ischemia of surrounding normal brain parenchyma. Finally, thromboembolic vascular occlusion can occur either spontaneously or as a consequence of vascular manipulation, such as aneurysm clipping or arterial catheterization.

Vascular Anatomy

Potential for Collateral Flow

The vascular anatomy of the brain and spinal cord is unique, and gives rise to several specific considerations with respect to neuroanesthesia. It is well known that the cerebral vasculature has a great potential for collateral blood supply. This depends first on the anastomoses of the primary arteries at the circle of Willis, and, second, on the potential redundancy of perfusion of most areas of the brain by different vascular supplies. Collateral flow by overlapping distribution of distal arteries develops slowly, however, so a sudden occlusion of a distal artery is likely to result in ischemic necrosis of an area of brain centered on its distribution. In contrast, sudden occlusion of a large feeding vessel such as an internal carotid artery may have no consequences because of good collateral flow by anastomotic vessels of the circle of Willis. Clearly, protection from such an event depends on the presence of a patent circle of Willis.

Adequate collateral blood supply for the cervical spinal cord is also usually provided by the anterior spinal artery and several additional major segmental arteries. The thoracic and lumbar portions of the spinal cord do not have as extensive a system of fully developed collateral blood supply. Two or three major radiculomedullary arteries usually perfuse this portion, with the major source of blood supply being the artery of Adamciewicz in the thoracolumbar region. As a consequence, the upper and midthoracic spinal cord (centered on T4) is at particular risk for ischemia because it represents the most distal region of vascular supply of cervical and thoracic segmental feeding arteries.

Like the cerebral arterial system, the venous system of the brain also has extensive anastomotic connections that provide for collateral venous drainage. Significant overlap exists in the drainage regions of the deep and superficial venous systems. Furthermore, the superficial venous system alone represents a kind of network of interconnected tributaries that coalesce in several directions into major draining veins. Loss of one of these major draining veins, such as may be required in the course of a neurosurgical procedure, usually has no neurologic consequences. As in the case of arterial anatomy, however, this depends on the presence of an adequate potential for collateral flow.

Anatomic Variations

Variations in the normal anatomy of the cerebral vasculature are common and may be acquired or developmental. Fully 28 percent of individuals lack at least one anastomotic component of the circle of Willis.

Portions of the cerebral vasculature may also become severely compromised or occluded by pathologic processes such as atherothrombotic events, embolic ischemia, cerebral aneurysms, or arteriovenous malformations. Such alterations in the "normal" cerebral vasculature are important, particularly in the neurovascular patient, for two reasons. First, these abnormalities can frequently be identified on diagnostic angiography prior to neuroanesthesia and surgery. Second, neurosurgical procedures frequently involve hemodynamic and vascular manipulation. Knowledge of any vascular abnormalities present is important in making decisions as to the extent and possible consequences of these manipulations.

Anatomic Relationships

The anatomic relationships of intracranial vascular structures are important under certain pathologic conditions. For instance, the posterior cerebral artery has its perimesencephalic course adjacent to the edge of the tentorial incisura and hooks around the oculomotor nerve in this same region. The artery is thereby at risk for impingement by herniation of the uncus, as described previously. The fact that it hooks over the oculomotor nerve is thought by some to be an explanation for the development of oculomotor palsy in patients with severe central herniation, as the posterior cerebral artery tends to be pulled downward, placing tension and compression on the nerve. The basilar artery is also thought to be less mobile than the pons during central herniation. Relatively greater downward movement of the pons is thought to place traction on perforating branches of the basilar artery. These perforating branches can be avulsed and produce secondary pontine hemorrhages with grave consequences.

The bony anatomy adjacent to vascular structures also becomes significant in the setting of trauma or degenerative joint disease. For instance, the petrous and intracavernous portions of the internal carotid arteries are vulnerable to traumatic injury from basilar skull fractures. Traumatic pseudoaneurysms and intimal dissection of the carotid arteries can result, as well as high-flow carotid-cavernous fistulas. The vertebral arteries are vulnerable to impingement in their passage through the foramina transversaria, particularly in patients with osteoarthritic changes. Such encroachment can be further exacerbated by turning the head on the shoulders to an extreme position. It is important to avoid such impingement of the vertebral artery when positioning patients for neurosurgery.

Vascular features of the meninges can also be important. The vulnerability of bridging veins between dura mater and cerebral cortex appears to be an important factor in the etiology of post-traumatic acute subdural hematomas. Meningeal arteries, such as the middle meningeal artery, can be lacerated by adjacent skull fractures and can result in acute epidural hematomas.

Mechanisms of Central Nervous System Injury and Treatment Strategies

Trauma

Direct Injury

Direct disruption of the brain parenchyma is the most obvious mechanism of traumatic injury to the CNS and commonly requires neurosurgical intervention. Penetrating injuries need to be debrided of foreign material, bone fragments, and hematomas. Blunt trauma may result in depressed skull fracture, with cerebral contusion or laceration that may require operative treatment.

Traumatic disruption of intracranial vascular structures is the common mechanism from which intracranial hematomas result. Rapid diagnostic evaluation and surgical treatment are extremely important in treating acute subdural or epidural hematomas and their associated CNS injuries.

Indirect Injury

Indirect injury to the brain by trauma occurs because of interaction of the traumatic force with the biomechanics of the skull and brain parenchyma. A high-speed penetrating projectile such as a bullet causes injury not only by direct destruction of CNS tissue in its path, but also by dissipation of its kinetic energy in a shock wave which extends the zone of destruction in relation to the energy of the projectile. Sudden linear deceleration of the skull, such as in a fall or a motor vehicle accident, frequently leads to direct injury of the brain near the point of impact, as well as indirect injury due to impact of the brain with the adjacent skull 180 degrees from the point of impact. This is the commonly described contrecoup injury. Angular acceleration or deceleration is a common component of motor vehicle accidents, but may also occur with blows to the head, such as in boxing. These rotational forces cause shear stresses within the brain parenchyma, which result in diffuse stretching and avulsion of neuronal processes. Such injuries are notable for the extensive neurologic dysfunction they can cause in spite of minimal evidence of damage to the brain parenchyma on head CT imaging.

Injury Due to Secondary Processes

Injuries due to secondary processes after trauma are also important, particularly since they may be treatable or preventable. Cerebral edema following a head injury is one example. Since this common sequela can lead to intracranial hypertension, impaired CBF, or herniation, aggressive treatment is indicated.

Another secondary process that may be important in the clinical consequences of head injury is transient respiratory arrest following the injury. Animal models suggest that this is a common sequela of head injury. The consequent cerebral hypoxia may have synergistic deleterious effects on the CNS.

Evidence is now accumulating that pathologic activation of specific neurophysiologic systems (such as cholinergic and glutaminergic systems) within the CNS may occur as a result of head trauma. This type of pathophysiologic response is thought to be responsible for neuronal injury over and above that which occurs as a direct result of the traumatic insult. These findings suggest that some of the consequences of head injury may be preventable if activation of these systems can be inhibited.

Mass Effect

Factors Determining Response to Mass Lesions

Mass lesions provide the most clear-cut need for neurosurgical intervention, whether the mass effect is due to spontaneous or traumatic hematomas or to an insidiously growing tumor that has reached a critical volume. Several factors determine the degree and type of neurologic injury resulting from mass lesions. The rapidity of development of the mass lesion is probably of greatest importance, since the CNS is surprisingly able to accommodate a growing mass if given sufficient time. Clearly, spontaneous and traumatic hematomas allow very little time for such accommodation. Shifts of venous blood to the extracranial circulation and CSF into the spinal subarachnoid space provide a degree of compensation, after which localized increased pressure or brain herniation may compromise the function of vital structures. At the other extreme, the brain is capable of accommodating the loss of a significant fraction of the intracranial volume to a very slow-growing tumor, such as a meningioma. Such patients may be surprisingly intact, without localized neurologic symptoms. However, since a heavy demand has already been placed on the compensatory mechanisms of their brain for accommodating such a mass, they are at great risk from otherwise innocuous elevations of their ICP. In the neurosurgical setting, this applies particularly to the potent elevation of ICP that occurs in response to endotracheal stimulation during intubation or suctioning.

Other etiologies of mass effect tend to be intermediate between the above cited examples with respect to the rapidity of their development and the danger of their consequences. Acute shunt failure causes a surprisingly rapid increase in ventricular volume in a shunt-dependent patient. Since the signs of acute hydrocephalus are frequently nonspecific, including headache and drowsiness, shunt failure in a shunt-dependent individual must be considered an emergent surgical problem. The edema which follows a large cerebral infarction is another type of subacute mass effect that progresses over several days and may result in problems due to mass effect well after the patient appears to have stabilized from the neurologic deficit of the infarction. Thus, a cerebral infarction from a proximal middle cerebral artery occlusion of the non-dominant hemisphere may present with hemiplegia, hemineglect, and homonymous hemianopsia. Several days after the ictus, the patient may become drowsy and then quickly show progression of signs of transtentorial herniation. This clinical situation can be extremely difficult to treat medically and may require surgical decompression.

The consequences of mass effect depend not only on the rapidity of its development but also on its location. The importance of the local effects of the developing mass will depend on the functions subserved by the parenchyma directly involved. The position of the developing mass with respect to structural components of the parenchyma and surrounding structures can also have a significant role in determining the consequences of the lesion. For instance, a mass lesion in the anterior temporal lobe is more likely to cause transtentorial herniation with early serious clinical consequences than a similar mass in the frontal pole. This particular distinction is frequently important in the setting of head injury, where both anterior frontal and temporal regions are prone to contusion and hematoma. A small-to-moderate-sized temporal contusion thus requires more careful monitoring of the patient to avoid sudden deterioration due to herniation.

Treatment for Mass Effect

Treatment of mass effect falls into three categories. First, removal of the mass is preferable in the majority of circumstances when it can be accomplished. It is mandatory when the mass has begun to cause serious consequences, such as progressive neurologic deficit or brain herniation. Mass effect that is expected to resolve spontaneously, however, such as cerebral edema due to head injury or cerebral infarction, or multiple metastatic foci that may respond to radiotherapy, may be successfully managed with temporizing measures.

Such temporizing measures comprise the second category of treatment for mass effect. These include long-lasting measures such as corticosteroid therapy to reduce the edema around tumors or brain abscesses and the use of barbiturates when a diffuse region of brain swelling causes otherwise uncontrollable elevations of the intracranial pressure.

The use of mannitol or other diuretics is another therapeutic modality that can be used to mitigate the effects of a developing mass lesion. Mannitol is a nonmetabolizable sugar alcohol that is thought to act primarily by osmotic reduction of brain water content and hence ICP. In addition, it is thought to improve rheologic properties of blood by reducing viscosity, and it may act as a free-radical scavenger. Both of these features may provide a basis for added protection against cerebral ischemia.

A more rapid but shorter-acting temporizing measure for the treatment of patients with acute symptoms of mass effect is the use of hyperventilation. This therapeutic maneuver rapidly reduces ICP by reducing the arterial Pco_2. The effect is mediated by reduction of intracranial vascular volume due to generalized cerebral vasoconstriction. At severe levels of hypocarbia (i.e., below Pco_2 of 25), however, cerebral arterial vasoconstriction becomes significant enough to impair adequate CBF, suggesting that aggressive hyperventilation should be avoided if possible. Furthermore, in spite of hypocarbia, the cerebral vasculature rapidly begins to accommodate with a return to baseline tone over 3 to 4 hours. After this time, the vasculature is even more sensitive to increases in Pco_2, so that attempts to return to baseline CO_2 levels are accompanied by even greater increases in ICP than the decreases seen on initial reduction of the Pco_2. For these reasons, hyperventilation is best viewed as a short-term temporizing measure, either for management of short-term elevations of ICP (which can occur in head-injury patients) or for rapid reduction of brain volume and ICP while preparing the patient for surgical decompression.

The third category of management strategies for mass effect consists of accommodating the mass by increasing the cranial or spinal compartment volume. For instance, in the case of a large right cerebral infarction with life-threatening cerebral edema, decompression of the cranial vault can avert herniation until after the cerebral edema has subsided.

Timing of neurosurgical treatment for consequences of mass effect is extremely important. It can be assumed that in patients whose mass has developed over minutes or hours, or who have signs of herniation, important parenchymal tissue is being lost by the minute. The importance of rapid hemodynamic and ventilatory stabilization of the patient and surgical decompression is obvious. On the other hand, patients with mass effect due to lesions that have developed insidiously over months, such as a meningioma or glioblastoma, often benefit from several days of corticosteroid therapy to reduce edema prior to surgical decompression.

Elevated Intracranial Pressure

Clinical Importance of Intracranial Pressure

The determinants of ICP and the mechanisms by which it can be pathologically elevated have been discussed in previous sections, as has the role of ICP in determining CPP. What is more difficult to define is the role of ICP in injury to the CNS and the relevance of raised ICP in clinical management. Clearly, very high ICP can interfere with cerebral perfusion and result in ischemia. The effects of more modest elevations of ICP may also be significant because of other aspects of the pathologic situation. For instance, under normal circumstances a moderate decrease in CPP would be compensated for by autoregulatory phenomena to maintain CBF. Pathologic conditions such as head injury, cerebral infarction, or vasospasm, however, may be associated with impaired autoregulation. Perfusion in these settings would thus be more directly sensitive to decreases in CPP due to increased ICP.

Mildly elevated ICP may also predict other consequences, such as localized cerebral compression or progression of adverse metabolic processes associated with underlying cerebral edema. Recent findings that more aggressive and earlier treatment of elevated ICP in head trauma patients is associated with better outcome appear to support such concepts and reinforce the need for vigorous treatment of intracranial hypertension after head injury.

Treatment of Elevated Intracranial Pressure

The principles of treating elevated ICP are similar to those discussed under Mass Effect (pp. 14–15). If a mass or specific pathologic process can be identified as the cause of intracranial hypertension, therapy should begin with appropriate treatment of these factors. Depending on the severity and expected duration of the process causing hypertension as well as the expected severity, temporizing pharmacologic and physiologic interventions that are designed to reduce the net volume of the intracranial contents may be indicated. Intravenous mannitol, intermittent hyperventilation for transient pressure spikes, and barbiturate therapy may be used. Corticosteroid therapy can be used in processes that are known to be responsive, such as peritumoral edema.

Occasionally, these therapeutic maneuvers are insufficient to maintain control of ICP and it becomes necessary to consider surgical decompression. If the elevated pressure is due primarily to a lateralized process, a hemicraniectomy procedure with duraplasty may be indicated. If the process is bilateral, the craniectomy may need to be extended across the midline in the frontal region with bilateral duraplasty.

Impaired Cerebral Blood Flow

Mechanisms of Ischemic Injury

Impaired CBF is an issue in a significant number of neurosurgical patients. It is of major importance in patients with cerebrovascular disease who are candidates for carotid endarterectomy and in patients with cerebral arterial vasospasm following subarachnoid hemorrhage. Research in the pathophysiology of ischemia has increased our understanding of the process and continues to suggest possible therapeutic interventions. In the absence of a direct clinical means for demonstrating lack of blood flow to an area of the CNS, we continue to assess ischemic injury, particularly in early phases, by the nature and magnitude of the neurologic deficit. It is now clear that ischemic areas may not be irreversibly damaged at the time the patient presents, thus providing hope of possible reversal of the apparent neurologic deficit that is seen in a patient during an ischemic process.

Neurosurgical and neuroanesthetic techniques for managing patients with subarachnoid hemorrhage have improved to such an extent in the last several decades that clinical efforts to prevent the syndrome of delayed ischemic deficit that correlates with the angiographic diagnosis of arterial vasospasm have increased. While constriction of the large conducting vessels is noted on angiography, it is generally thought that constriction of the much smaller "resistance" vessels is responsible for the ischemic sequelae of this phenomenon. Although the etiology of this poorly reversible process of vasospasm remains unknown, it seems clear that the causative process is related to escape of arterial blood into the subarachnoid space. This interpretation is strengthened by the correlation that has been demonstrated between the volume of subarachnoid blood with the likelihood and severity of vasospasm. Symptoms of vasospasm appear between 4 and 10 days after subarachnoid hemorrhage and may be insidious in development. Vasospasm is associated with impaired cerebral autoregulation. Although no specific treatment for the cause of vasospasm is yet available, it is well known that aggressive early therapeutic measures may halt and frequently reverse the neurologic deficit if instituted early enough.

Treatment Strategies for Impaired Cerebral Blood Flow

Treatment of cerebral ischemia in neurosurgical patients generally falls into two categories. The first category is one in which cerebral infarction has already occurred. Management should include aggressive care of all other body systems to avoid added complications, as well as basic measures to ensure optimal oxygen delivery to the CNS. Prevention of further ischemic events should also be a primary goal in patient management following infarction.

The second category deals with patients who show evidence of threatened or incipient cerebral ischemia, where intervention is intended to avert progression to significant cerebral infarction. This includes patients with carotid bifurcation disease with intermittent symptoms of ischemia and high-grade stenosis demonstrated by angiography. It is currently believed that this type of patient would benefit from surgical removal of the atheroma, although antithrombotic pharmacotherapy or physical dilatation of the stenosis by percutaneous techniques may prove to be effective alternatives in such a case.

Pharmacologic and physiologic manipulations that are calculated to optimize CBF are also important when treating ischemia (see Table 1-2). Basic techniques include maintenance of normal or slightly elevated blood pressure, arrangement of ventilatory parameters for optimal oxygenation, and optimization of CPP. The latter includes reducing the hydrostatic column between heart and brain by keeping the patient flat, as well as stringent avoidance of increased ICP. Mannitol infusion may also be added for its ICP, rheologic, and putative protective effects.

In the case of vasospasm following subarachnoid hemorrhage, where ischemia is due to constriction of vessels that are nevertheless patent, augmentation of the CPP by techniques designed to elevate cerebral arterial pressure are also commonly used. This includes infusion of colloid fluids to increase cardiac output by increasing vascular volume, as well as pressor agents to increase systemic arterial pressure. Fluid infusion frequently has the added benefit of reducing hematocrit, which in turn reduces blood viscosity. Because of the importance of oxygen-carrying capacity, red blood cell transfusion may also be necessary to maintain a hematocrit of 30 to 33. The latter figure has been calculated to be optimal for reduction of viscosity with maintenance of oxygen-carrying capacity. These aggressive techniques must clearly be tailored to the individual patient's physiologic status using invasive monitoring procedures. Although each of these interventions carries risks, the well-documented potential for reversing neurologic deficits due to vasospasm justifies them in the majority of cases.

Neurophysiologic and Neurochemical Responses to Injury

New Concepts in Central Nervous System Injury

Research efforts to understand the cellular pathophysiology underlying irreversible cell injury have been active for many years and have provided considerable information in understanding the evolution of injuries to the CNS. Recently, this work has begun to provide clues to important features of irreversible cell injury. On the biochemical level, the importance of intracellular pH, ionized calcium concentration, and cell membrane lipid peroxidation has become increasingly apparent. These three interrelated parameters of cellular physiology are potential targets for therapeutic intervention in CNS injury. Several reports have emerged reporting benefit from the use of an intracellular buffering agent in head injury patients. Protection of neurons against intracellular calcium accumulation may in part explain recent reports on the apparent benefit of calcium channel blockers in the setting of subarachnoid hemorrhage.

Several studies in animals have now demonstrated a benefit of treatments designed to reduce lipid peroxidation or free-radical formation in models of CNS injury. Agents such as α-tocopherol (vitamin E), superoxide dismutase, catalase, and the nonglucogenic 21-aminosteroids have been used. The promising clinical value of these agents remains to be determined in human trials, many of which have already begun.

The mechanisms producing irreversible ischemic injury in the CNS continue to receive extensive experimental attention. One current therapeutic practice that has grown out of these studies is the avoidance of hyperglycemia in the setting of ischemia. It is thought that anaerobic glycolytic metabolism may result in decreased cellular pH, thereby impairing other metabolic processes and promoting free-radical formation. By analogy with clinical studies of cardiac ischemia in myocardial infarction, the value of rapid intervention with powerful thrombolytic agents such as tissue plasminogen activator is also currently being explored.

Activation of Neural Systems as a Mechanism of Central Nervous System Injury

Evidence has accumulated in recent years that overactivation of certain receptor subtypes that are linked to calcium channels can cause irreversible cell injury and death. This has been well demonstrated by pharmacologic activation in various experimental systems, and theories have developed that such mechanisms may contribute to the deleterious effects of ischemia, trauma, and epilepsy. The muscarinic cholinergic antagonist scopolamine has been shown to improve outcome in an animal model of moderate head injury. Likewise, a calcium channel–receptor complex that is activated by excitatory amino acids such as N-methyl-D-aspartate (NMDA) has been implicated in the same head injury model. The NMDA receptor is also being studied in the pathogenesis of experimental epilepsy and the consequences of cerebral ischemia. The most exciting aspect of these theories is the concept that activating certain systems in the CNS may be responsible for part of the outcome of these difficult-to-treat processes. Interruption of these processes by pharmacologic agents may thus allow improvements in outcome.

Neurosurgical Considerations

General Considerations

Patient Positioning

Positioning of the neurosurgical patient is the subject of considerable discussion. Three principles should guide the position used for a given neurosurgical procedure. First is to obtain optimal access for the planned procedure. Optimal access involves consideration of surgical exposure, choice of a path to the surgical pathology that avoids important structures when possible, access of specialized instrumentation such as the operating microscope, and the ergonomics of the surgeon's operating position. Once the best operating position has been determined, the second principle is to adjust this position to maximize the patient's physiologic status and avoid adverse effects of the position. The third principle in patient positioning related to the goal of minimizing blood loss during the procedure and obtaining hemostasis when it is finished. Since the bulk of intraoperative bleeding and postoperative hematomas are venous in origin, venous pressure at the surgical site plays an important role in these considerations. An important factor in determining venous pressure is the relative position of the surgical site to that of the right atrium. Given the relatively low pressure in the venous system, minor changes in positioning, such as elevating the head, can potentially reduce the venous pressure at the operative site. This effect is so significant that it becomes a liability when the patient is placed in the sitting position due to the danger of air embolism entrained by the negative venous pressure.

In positioning patients prone for posterior fossa or spinal surgery, an additional hemostatic consideration becomes important. Because of the anastomotic connections between the spinal epidural venous plexus and the venous systems of the abdomen and thorax, it is important to avoid elevation of intrathoracic or intra-abdominal pressure. Thus, techniques that place the majority of the patient's weight on the shoulders and iliac spines or modified prone positions that accomplish the same thing, such as the kneeling position, tend to reduce the rate of blood loss in these procedures.

Hemostatic Considerations

The importance of hemostasis in neurosurgery is fundamentally different from that in most other surgical specialties for two reasons. First, obtaining hemostasis must depend primarily on bipolar coagulation and application of thrombogenic agents to activate natural hemostatic mechanisms. General surgical techniques such as ligation of large vessels or packing the wound are not commonly used in neurosurgery. Second, postoperative bleeding is more likely to have devastating consequences for the neurosurgery patient. It is thus critical to ensure that the patient's clotting mechanisms are adequate prior to surgery by history, appropriate laboratory studies, and transfusion of blood components when necessary. The importance of avoiding elevations of venous blood pressure by positioning techniques has been discussed in the preceding section. Likewise, avoiding drastic elevations in arterial blood pressure, except when the patient's clinical and physiologic condition demands it, should be pursued if possible during the intraoperative and postoperative periods. In the case of a patient with a recently ruptured intracranial aneurysm, this becomes paramount and demands specific preventive measures during positioning, induction, and endotracheal intubation.

In addition to the importance of adequate hemostatic mechanisms in successful neurosurgical management, it should be kept in mind that accumulating evidence suggests that the brain may affect homeostatic aspects of the clotting mechanism. The tendency of postoperative neurosurgical patients to develop deep venous thrombosis has been used as one piece of evidence in this regard. Stringent efforts to prevent this complication are important to all neurosurgical procedures. These include wrapping the lower extremities to avoid venous pooling and the use of intermittent inflating leg cuffs.

Brain Retraction for Surgical Access

Retraction of the brain is commonly required to gain access to deeper-seated structures. Retraction carries with it dangers of structural injury to the parenchyma, as well as possible local ischemia due to exertion of tissue pressures that are greater than local capillary perfusion pressure. Several strategies have evolved in attempts to avoid such complications. First, various designs and sizes of retraction instruments, including self-retaining systems, have been developed. The self-retaining systems have the advantage of being more stable and less likely to traumatize the retracted brain by motion. Occasional loosening of brain retractors may also help reduce adverse effects.

A second strategy that is utilized whenever possible is to allow gravity to retract the brain. This clearly involves an additional demand on positioning of the patient and is sometimes not feasible.

A third approach to minimizing the need for brain retraction is to reduce the volume of the brain that is in the way. Drainage of ventricular CSF either by ventricular catheter or by lumbar puncture is frequently used. Pharmacologic techniques such as osmotic diuresis with mannitol may also be used. Additional short-term reduction in brain volume can be obtained when needed by hyperventilation and additional diuresis with furosemide.

Other Medical Problems

In general, the presence of other medical problems in neurosurgical patients must dictate anesthetic management plans as in any other surgical setting. Plans for the neurosurgical procedure can then be tailored to these considerations, except where the need for the neurosurgical procedure overrides considerations of the patient's other medical problems.

On occasion, there may be situations in which the neurosurgical problem and the patient's other problems are in direct conflict with respect to specific management issues. For instance, a patient with coronary artery disease undergoing aneurysm surgery may be at risk for myocardial ischemia if induced hypotension is used during dissection of the aneurysm. Another potential conflict occurs in the trauma patient with signs of intracranial mass lesion and severe hemodynamic instability. Clearly, stabilization of the patient's hemodynamic status cannot be delayed, including laparotomy and/or thoracotomy if necessary. However, given the potentially fatal results of a traumatic intracranial hematoma, neurosurgical treatment should not be delayed while the patient is being stabilized. Such a situation may require modification of the usual approach, with bilateral diagnostic burr holes instead of head CT, followed by craniotomy on the appropriate side. Two things are needed to deal with such potential conflicts between the patient's general and neurosurgical needs. First is communication among the health-care professionals making therapeutic decisions, and second is rapid agreement on treatment priorities.

Age Considerations

Pediatric Patients

Pediatric neurosurgical patients differ from adults in the spectrum of pathology that they present and in their greater tendency to withstand injuries to the CNS. In addition, special considerations arise from their small size. First, their size makes it more difficult to establish and maintain reliable monitoring techniques. Second, their greater surface area-to-volume ratio increases the tendency for hypothermia with its attendant metabolic and anesthetic difficulties. Third, although children have a smaller blood volume, blood loss is not automatically reduced in a commensurate manner. This means that the danger of hypovolemia intraoperatively is much greater in pediatric patients than in adult patients, particularly with newborns and infants. Furthermore, if large scalp or skin flaps are used, the potential for significant blood loss by oozing in the postoperative period must be kept in mind. Solutions to this problem lie in meticulous attention to hemostasis during the procedure, careful attention to the often deceptive amount of blood loss during the procedure, and early institution of volume replacement with fluids or blood transfusion.

One fundamental difference between infants and adults is the unfused sutures of the cranial vault. Since the dura mater in neonates and infants is also more elastic and distensible than in older children and adults, the cranial cavity has considerably more compliance. This means that rapidly growing intracranial lesions in the pediatric patient can be accommodated with much less severe consequences. For instance, an intraventricular hematoma in a premature infant or rapidly expanding ventricles after an acute shunt failure may simply result in splitting of the sutures. Unlike the adult, the infant may present with signs of elevated ICP rather than brain herniation. More slowly growing lesions may have similar effects and may also result in asymmetric skull growth.

With regard to acute shunt failure, it must be remembered that ultimately the ability of the sutures to split will be lost, after which acute hydrocephalus can be a rapidly fatal problem. Thus, suspected shunt failure in children must be considered an emergency to be diagnosed and treated expeditiously.

Elderly Patients

The greater likelihood of other medical problems is one of the primary considerations in the neurosurgical management of elderly patients. Known problems are managed in the usual manner by establishing priorities between neurosurgical needs and the needs of other aspects of their medical status, weighing the risks and benefits of each potential intervention. The possibility of previously undiagnosed medical problems in elderly patients must also be considered and sometimes investigated with appropriate diagnostic procedures before making therapeutic decisions. For instance, the high association of coronary artery disease in patients with a symptomatic carotid artery lesion requires a careful evaluation for cardiac pathology, sometimes including coronary angiography.

It should also be noted that evidence has accumulated that brain injuries are less well tolerated by the older individual. For instance, poorer outcome by elderly patients in the head injury population cannot be explained solely on the basis of associated medical problems or medical complications developing following the injury. Thus, it appears that some intrinsic change in the aging CNS reduces its capacity to withstand an insult.

Neurosurgical Considerations in Trauma Patients

Acute Traumatic Intracranial Hematoma

Acute traumatic subdural hematoma is the most frequent indication for immediate surgery in trauma patients. Epidural hematomas are less common, but also demand immediate evacuation. Patients frequently have signs of herniation at the time of presentation, and the need for speed in evacuation cannot be stressed heavily enough. In the time intervening before definitive neurosurgical treatment, temporizing measures to reduce intracranial pressure are important. These include intubation with ICP precautions, hyperventilation, and diuresis with mannitol. The use of a short-acting barbiturate may also be considered after the patient has been examined. Acute subdural hematomas are also frequently associated with a significant degree of cerebral contusion in the underlying brain. Because of extensive swelling after evacuation of the subdural clot, the dura frequently must be left open with appropriate duraplastic material in place; leaving the bone flap out on a temporary basis may also need to be considered.

Early Repair of Traumatic Fractures

The primary indication for immediate repair of a traumatic skull fracture is the presence of an open depressed fracture. The purpose of the procedure is debridement and inspection of the dura to determine whether this covering has been penetrated. Controversy exists whether closed depressed fractures and facial fractures in the presence of significant head injury should be repaired immediately. Generally, markedly depressed fractures are often repaired primarily. The improved cosmetic results of immediate repair of facial fractures serves as an inducement to consider immediate repair of facial fractures. If the patient is stable with respect to head injury, such an approach may be safe using intraoperative ICP monitoring. As with any neurosurgical procedure, the need for immediate postoperative neurologic assessment is critical, and anesthetic management must be planned with this goal in mind.

Non-Neurosurgical Procedures in Head Injury Patients

It is not uncommon for head injury patients to require thoracic, abdominal, or orthopaedic surgery when no intracranial lesion requiring surgery is present. There are no absolute contraindications to procedures under general anesthesia in head injury patients, although those with moderate or severe head injuries should have intraoperative ICP monitoring. Patients who are not yet intubated should be considered to have decreased intracranial compliance as a precaution, and measures to prevent marked elevations of ICP on endotracheal intubation should be instituted. Again, anesthetic management should be geared to allow immediate postoperative neurologic assessment.

Neurosurgical Considerations in Cerebrovascular Patients

Intracranial Aneurysms or Arteriovenous Malformations

The key to satisfactory management of patients undergoing surgery for intracranial aneurysms or arteriovenous malformations is blood pressure control. In addition to the importance of the absolute level of mean arterial pressure in avoiding rupture of the aneurysm, it is also felt that rapid increases in arterial pressure may increase the likelihood of rupture as well. It is thus critical that the patient be adequately anesthetized prior to noxious stimuli such as placement of skull pins during positioning. It is preferable to lower the mean arterial pressure while the aneurysm is being dissected, but if it becomes necessary to place a temporary clip on the main vessel, a return of the blood pressure to normal levels may be desired. Finally, marked and precipitous elevations in blood pressure tend to occur when waking the patient and should be avoided.

Many of these patients have suffered a subarachnoid hemorrhage prior to the surgical procedure and may be at risk of developing vasospasm in the postoperative period. Because of the importance of maintaining and augmenting intravascular volume in the management of vasospasm (see Table 1–2), careful attention to fluid balance during the operative procedure is important. To assist in brain retraction and dissection of the vascular anomaly, hyperventilation, mannitol diuresis, and CSF drainage are commonly employed. The large volumes of fluid in and out thus make careful monitoring of fluid balance critical.

Management of patients who develop vasospasm with delayed ischemic deficit and measures to prevent or reduce vasospasm are rapidly evolving at the present time. The techniques are oriented to maximizing oxygen delivery to the brain. This includes hypertensive hypervolemic therapy with invasive monitoring to maximize cardiac output, reduction of blood viscosity by mannitol therapy, and optimizing oxygen content with supplemental inspired oxygen and hemodilution. The importance of avoiding hyperglycemia in ischemic brain has been discussed, and initial clinical trials suggest that calcium channel blockers may improve the outcome of patients suffering from vasospasm. Another therapeutic technique that appears to hold promise for selected patients with severe focal vasospasm is the use of percutaneous angiographic techniques to mechanically dilate the spastic arterial segment.

Carotid Artery Disease

The important considerations in patients undergoing carotid endarterectomy relate both to the underlying pathologic problem and to the procedure itself. In order for the carotid bifurcation to be opened and atherosclerotic plaque removed, the common carotid artery must be occluded for a period of time ranging from 20 to 40 minutes. The primary issue then is whether adequate perfusion of the brain is present during this time. Although preoperative assessment of the collateral circulation by angiography may be helpful, it frequently fails to show collateral flow when collateral flow is possible. Controversy exists as to whether an intravascular shunt should be used to allow for common carotid to internal carotid flow during removal of the plaque. Intraoperative electroencephalographic monitoring is also controversial. Aside from these considerations, maintenance of normal or slightly elevated blood pressure is important to optimize cerebral perfusion during the procedure. Furthermore, maneuvers that may tend to decrease CBF, such as hyperventilation, should be avoided.

Patients are heparinized prior to occlusion of the common carotid artery, and are frequently not reversed at the end of the procedure. Hence, the carotid endarterectomy patient not only has an arteriotomy of the carotid bifurcation and a fresh neck wound but is also anticoagulated. For these reasons, stringent avoidance of elevated arterial pressure is needed, particularly during reversal and extubation. The life-threatening danger of a rapidly growing hematoma in the carotid sheath adjacent to the trachea, and the suddenness with which airway obstruction can develop in these patients, should be emphasized.

Neurosurgical Considerations in Patients with Intracranial Tumors

Mass Effect

Patients requiring neurosurgical procedures for tumors frequently have significant mass effect from their neoplasms. If the tumor is large or situated in the temporal lobe, manipulations that tend to cause large increases in ICP should be carefully avoided.

These include endotracheal intubation without adequate precautions to prevent normal ICP response, as well as the casual use of anesthetic agents that tend to cause increased ICP by vascular dilatation. Placement of an ICP monitor under local anesthesia prior to induction may be helpful in managing these patients.

Tumor Location

The location of a tumor is important with respect to the functions subserved by the parenchyma that has been displaced. Tumor location dictates both the planned route of attack and the aggressiveness of resection of the mass. This is particularly true in the case of invasive tumors such as gliomas in which the demarcation between tumor and surrounding brain is difficult or impossible to distinguish.

When the tumor is located in a sensitive area, functional testing may be helpful both preoperatively and intraoperatively. The Wada test involves intravascular injection of sodium amytal while testing language to determine hemispheric dominance, and can be done in conjunction with angiography of a tumor. Intraoperative functional testing may involve motor cortex mapping using bipolar electrode stimulation, a similar approach to sensory testing, and testing of higher functions such as language by similar techniques. Sensory and language testing require the patient to be awake and the procedure to be done under local anesthesia, while motor mapping can be done under general anesthesia, provided the patient is not paralyzed.

Neurosurgical Considerations in Spine and Spinal Cord Surgery

Intubation and Positioning

The prone position is commonly used for spine surgery, and has been discussed in a previous section. Avoidance of elevated intrathoracic or intra-abdominal pressure in this position is important because of its tendency to increase epidural venous pressure by segmental anastomoses. The need to reduce venous pooling in the lower extremities of these patients by leg wraps or intermittent inflation cuffs has also been emphasized.

Patients with unstable spines or with critical encroachment on the spinal cord due to pathologic processes carry with them additional considerations. First, cervical instability or stenosis places the patient at risk of spinal cord injury if standard intubation techniques are employed. For this reason, techniques that do not require significant extension of the neck, such as intubation over a fiberoptic endoscope, are preferred. In addition, intubating the awake patient so that spinal cord function can be continuously monitored may also be considered.

After intubation, patients frequently need to be turned to the prone position on the operating table prior to the procedure. Again, if instability or spinal cord encroachment are present, this maneuver carries significant risk and must be carried out with extreme care. Doing this with the patient awake, or awakening the patient after positioning in order to check neurologic function may be helpful.

Intraoperative Functional Monitoring

It is frequently helpful to employ functional monitoring or testing during spine procedures. A simple approach to this is the "wake up test," in which the patient is allowed to emerge from anesthesia enough to follow simple commands with his extremities to demonstrate functional capabilities. More sophisticated monitoring techniques are also available, including spinal somatosensory potentials, electroproctography, and electromyography. Clearly, for motor testing, muscle relaxants must be avoided or temporarily antagonized.

Finally, a case can be made for avoiding relaxants altogether in spine surgery, except perhaps during intubation. This is because the motor response that frequently occurs on manipulation of a nerve root can be helpful in confirming the identity of this structure.

Conclusion

In this chapter, an attempt has been made to provide the anatomic and physiologic bases for neuroanesthetic decision making from a neurosurgical perspective. It should be clear that much of the information needed to make such decisions is not contained in the preoperative posting of diagnosis and planned procedure, nor may it be easily found simply by reading the patient's chart. It is for this reason that communication between neurosurgeon and neuroanesthesiologist is paramount. A few minutes of discussion would ideally allow a dialogue on the salient issues of a particular case and allow agreement on priorities for intraoperative management of the patient.

Finally, we would argue that neurosurgical patients tend to gain much from successful practice of the "art" of neuroanesthesia. By this we mean that the consistent ability to conduct neurosurgical patients through a smooth induction, operative course, and recovery benefits the patient both by preventing many of the pitfalls we have described and by avoiding unnecessary distraction of the surgical team. Thus, the seeming uneventfulness of a successful neuroanesthetic course is like a work of art, whose simplicity belies the energy, concentration, and experience that created it.

Richard J. Sperry, M.D.

Clinical Physiology of the Central Nervous System   2

Many aspects of intracranial physiology directly affect the anesthetic management of neurosurgical patients. This chapter highlights the salient features of cerebral metabolism and cerebral blood flow. These topics occupy a central position in neuroanesthesia and neurologic intensive care. A thorough understanding of the concepts presented in this chapter is essential to the administration of competent medical care to the patient with pathology of the central nervous system.

Cerebral Metabolism

Brain tissue has an unusually high energy requirement. The cerebral metabolic oxygen consumption ($CMRO_2$) is approximately 3.5 ml O_2/100 g brain tissue. This equals 50 ml/min for the typical 1,400-g brain, or roughly 20 percent of the whole body O_2 consumption. The main substrate for energy production in the brain is glucose. In an awake young adult male, the measured glucose consumption (CMRg) is 31 μm (5 mg)/ 100 g brain tissue/min.

 Although the global resting brain metabolic rate is fairly constant, there is a heterogeneity in brain metabolism. This heterogeneity reflects a different basal metabolic rate for different brain structures. Also, since neural activity results in an increased metabolic rate, patient stimulation results in a variable pattern of neuronal activation enhancing this heterogeneity.

 Michenfelder and Theye have suggested that brain oxygen consumption may be thought of as supporting two major functions: (1) basic cellular maintenance (45% of total) and (2) nerve impulse generation and transmission (55% of total). A basic assumption in their model is that a neuron will cease to propagate impulses in favor of cell integrity. Hence, when energy substrate delivery falls, there first is a loss of function with preserved cell viability. Cell viability is threatened only if substrate delivery falls further.

Cerebral Blood Flow

There are several techniques for measuring cerebral blood flow (CBF), but only a few are applicable to humans. The most common method in humans uses a diffusible indicator and the Fick principle. This technique, described by Kety and Schmidt in 1945, requires a 10- to 15-minute period of breathing an inert gas such as ^{85}Kr, ^{133}Xe, or N_2O, and a collection of arterial and venous blood samples. This technique yields a global value for CBF.

An important modification of the Kety-Schmidt technique is the use of scintillation detectors to monitor the washout of ^{133}Xe. The washout curves of the inert gas can be related to blood flow. If a series of small, focused scintillation counters is employed, flow to discrete areas of the brain (regional CBF) can be determined. However, it is important to realize that this technique only measures blood flow in the outer layer of the cerebral cortex.

Another technique that can be used with humans involves positron emission tomography (PET) scanning. PET scanners are not yet widely available, but this technique has great promise for the future.

Other techniques are commonly used in experimental animals and are reported in the literature of many disciplines. They include autoradiography, radioactive microspheres, hydrogen clearance, direct observation of pial vessels, and the measurement of cerebral arterial inflow or venous outflow.

Each technique for measuring CBF has certain advantages and disadvantages. In the intact animal and human, values for global cerebral blood flow represent an average of *all* brain structures, and values for regional blood flow represent only a sample of values from several distinct areas of thin, outer cerebral cortex. True regional blood flow, that is, flow to all substructures of the brain, is not measured in humans. Since cerebral blood flow can vary dramatically among different structures of the brain, a variance that can be greatly altered under pathologic conditions, it is important to remember the average nature of CBF measurements.

Normal CBF is approximately 50 ml/100 g perfused brain/min. Because most cell metabolism occurs in the cell body, gray matter has a greater average blood flow (75 to 80 ml/100 g/min) than white matter (20 to 30 ml/100 g/min).

Control of Cerebral Blood Flow

Many factors interact to regulate CBF. Brain metabolism, blood pressure, arterial oxygen and carbon dioxide tensions, and drugs all interact to produce the overall value of cerebral blood flow in a given region of the brain. A pathologic state within the central nervous system can also affect the global or regional value of cerebral blood flow. Although the various mechanisms of CBF control are presented independently, all these mechanisms may interact to produce a very complex picture of cerebral blood flow. A good approach to patient care, however, is to dissect the control of CBF into its various parts and then to devise a treatment scheme based upon this dissection.

Metabolic Regulation of Cerebral Blood Flow

The normal functioning brain has a fairly constant global metabolic rate and a fairly stable value of global cerebral blood flow. This global constancy, however, can be very misleading since regional metabolism and blood flow are not homogeneous. The heterogeneity of cerebral metabolism and blood flow is due to two factors. First, various substructures of the brain (e.g., cortex, thalamus, and medulla) have different basal metabolic rates. Second, a given substructure of the brain has a variable pattern of neuronal activation depending upon the activities of a patient. More neuronal work requires greater oxygen and glucose delivery.

Blood flow and metabolism are tightly coupled in the normal brain. For example, during voluntary movement of the hand, both CBF and cerebral metabolism (as measured by oxygen uptake) increase significantly within seconds in the contralateral brain area representing the hand. Pain, anxiety, and seizure activity can also cause a significant increase in brain metabolism and blood flow. Thus, the brain is very much a dynamic organ with metabolism regulating an ever-changing CBF pattern.

Despite active research, the mechanisms for metabolic regulation have not yet been determined. One theory is that the concentration in extracellular fluid of mediators such as H^+ and K^+ ions or metabolic products such as adenosine may act as local vasodilators to couple local blood flow to local metabolism.

Autoregulation

Autoregulation maintains CBF at a constant value over a wide range of cerebral perfusion pressure (Fig. 2–1). Cerebral perfusion pressure is defined as the difference between mean arterial pressure and intracranial pressure.

Autoregulation is accomplished by active arteriolar constriction when the distending pressure increases and by arteriolar dilation when the distending pressure decreases. Autoregulatory adjustments may take up to 2 minutes to become effective. Autoregulation has a lower limit and an upper limit. The lower limit for autoregulation is 50 to 60 mm Hg. Below this limit CBF decreases, following perfusion pressure in a linear fashion. The upper limit for autoregulation is 130 to 150 mm Hg. At the upper autoregulatory limit, arteriolar constriction is maximum; a greater pressure cannot be contained. This results in forced dilation of brain arterioles allowing blood flow to increase and pressure to be transmitted to the more fragile downstream blood vessels.

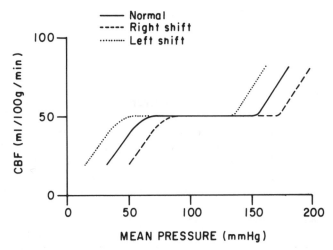

Figure 2-1 The normal autoregulatory curve with right and left shift depicted.

The blood-brain barrier may subsequently be disrupted, leading to focal plasma leakage, hemorrhage, and cerebral edema.

The limits of autoregulation are not well defined in children. Autoregulatory limits for spinal cord blood flow are roughly the same as for CBF.

The mechanism by which autoregulation occurs is uncertain. A myogenic hypothesis states that autoregulation is an intrinsic property of the smooth muscle cells in the arteriolar wall. A stretching of the smooth muscle cell by an increased arterial pressure leads to active constriction; a decreased distending pressure leads to smooth muscle relaxation.

A metabolic hypothesis states that arteriolar dilation is regulated by tissue oxygen and glucose requirements. A decrease in perfusion pressure decreases blood flow and oxygen delivery to a value lower than that required for tissue demands. This decrease in substrate delivery leads to a reflex arteriolar dilation.

The autoregulatory curve may be shifted in either direction. A shift to the right, increasing the lower and upper limits of autoregulation (see Fig. 2-1), occurs with chronic hypertension and with sympathetic activation (e.g., shock or stress). With a right-shifted curve, a greater perfusion pressure is required to maintain CBF. A right-shifted curve also allows for a greater perfusion pressure to be contained before autoregulatory breakthrough and disruption of the blood-brain barrier occurs.

A left-shifted autoregulatory curve is produced by hypoxia, hypercarbia, and vasodilators (see Fig. 2-1). A left-shifted curve allows CBF to be maintained at a lower than normal perfusion pressure.

Two major concepts should be emphasized here:

1. Pressure containment protects the chronically hypertensive patient from disruption of the blood-brain barrier. However, the chronically hypertensive patient will suffer a dangerous decrease in CBF at a greater arterial blood pressure than a normotensive patient. A gentle and sustained blood pressure reduction in a chronic hypertensive may shift the autoregulatory curve back toward normal.
2. Since hypovolemic hypotension is associated with sympathetic activation and a right-shifted autoregulatory curve, CBF will be better maintained with pharmacologic than with hypovolemic hypotension.

Blood Gases

Alterations in arterial Po_2 and Pco_2 can have a profound effect on CBF.

Oxygen. Cerebral blood flow changes with arterial oxygen content to maintain the appropriate tissue oxygen tension for cerebral metabolism. The actual chemical mediator for this response to oxygen is not known. However, a metabolic product, adenosine, is thought to play an important part in this response. Cerebral blood flow is not affected until the PaO_2 decreases below 50 mm Hg. At this point cerebral vasodilation begins, and CBF increases. At a PaO_2 of 35 mm Hg, CBF is increased 32%; at 15 mm Hg, it is four times normal (Fig. 2-2). However, this increase in CBF requires a normal blood pressure.

Carbon Dioxide. The relationship of CBF to arterial carbon dioxide tension is linear between a $PaCO_2$ of 25 mm Hg and 75 mm Hg. As the $PaCO_2$ increases, so does CBF. A decrease in the $PaCO_2$ will decrease CBF. Cerebral blood flow changes 4% (2 ml/100 g/min) for each 1 mm Hg change in $PaCO_2$. A good approximation is that a $PaCO_2$ of two

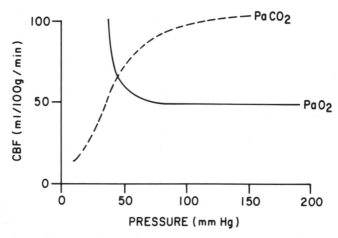

Figure 2-2 The relationship between oxygen and carbon dioxide tensions and cerebral blood flow.

times normal (80 mm Hg) will double CBF, and a $PaCO_2$ of one-half normal (20 mm Hg) will decrease CBF by one-half (see Fig. 2–2).

The effects of carbon dioxide on CBF are mediated by the pH of cerebrospinal fluid (CSF). As the arterial $PaCO_2$ increases, more CO_2 diffuses freely across the blood-brain barrier into the CSF. Bicarbonate ion, the major buffer in the CSF, does not cross the blood-brain barrier. Hence, as CO_2 enters or leaves the CSF, the pH will change in a manner predictable by the Henderson-Hasselbalch equation. An increase in CO_2 will decrease the pH, and a decrease in CO_2 will increase the pH. Eventually the bircarbonate ion concentration is adjusted, and the pH returns to normal. This adjustment has a half-life of approximately 6 hours. More information about CO_2 and CBF can be found in the discussion on treatment of increased intracranial pressure (see Chapter 7).

The effect of CO_2 on the magnitude of blood flow change in the spinal cord is approximately one-half the effect on CBF. The response of the vasculature takes 20 to 30 seconds.

The maximal increase in CBF from hypercapnia and hypoxemia is the same. At submaximal levels of change the effects of hypercapnia and hypoxemia are additive. Thus, a poorly ventilated and marginally oxygenated patient will have a dramatic increase in CBF.

Drugs and Cerebral Blood Flow. The CBF-drug story can be confusing. In most clinical and laboratory studies, the measured variable has historically been CBF; many anesthetic agents cause an increase in CBF. Superficial reading of these studies may lead one to conclude that an increase in CBF is harmful in patients with intracranial pathology. It is not the increase in CBF per se that is harmful, but rather the increase in cerebral blood volume (CBV) that may follow an increase in CBF. An increase in CBV can cause an increase in intracranial pressure and subsequent ischemia and brain tissue shifts (herniation). To the extent that CBV and CBF track together in both direction and magnitude, it makes sense to focus on the most conveniently measured variable, CBF. Measurements of CBV are technically more difficult to perform. However, making assumptions about CBV from CBF can be misleading. For example, high concentrations of any volatile anesthetic will significantly increase both CBF and CBV at normal blood pressure. Because the volatile anesthetic agents blunt autoregulation, CBF will fall if the blood pressure is reduced. The CBF value could, therefore, be reduced to normal, or even subnormal, by lowering the blood pressure. However, CBV would not be expected to decrease much, if at all, as the blood pressure is reduced. This is a possible clinical situation in which CBF and CBV will lie in opposite directions from the control values. Also, many drugs have different effects upon capacitance and resistance vessels in the peripheral circulation. It is reasonable to presume that this is true also for the cerebral circulation. Thus, alterations in CBF and CBV should not be conceived of as interchangeable values. Figure 2–3 shows the usual changes in CBF accompanying the administration of various drugs. Although CBF data have been generated for the indicated drugs, CBV and intracranial pressure data have not been published for most of the drugs. A further discussion on the pharmacology of these drugs can be found in Chapter 3.

Pathologic States.   Blood flow in and around areas of tumor, infarction, and trauma may be abnormal. Vasomotor paralysis, blood vessels which have lost the ability to actively control their own resistance, occurs in these areas. Hence, blood pressure autoregulation and response to CO_2 and drugs are lost. In this state of vasomotor paralysis, CBF becomes pressure dependent, rendering this area of brain more susceptible to ischemia at lower blood pressures and more likely to sustain injury at higher pressures.

Also, as the $PaCO_2$ increases and normal blood vessels dilate, blood is shunted away from the abnormal parts of the brain which do not respond to CO_2. This is called *steal*. An inverse steal occurs when the $PaCO_2$ is reduced, and the normal parts of the brain vasoconstrict, shunting blood to the abnormal brain, which does not vasoconstrict. This inverse steal phenomenon can also occur when drugs such as the barbiturates (which cause cerebral vasoconstriction) are administered.

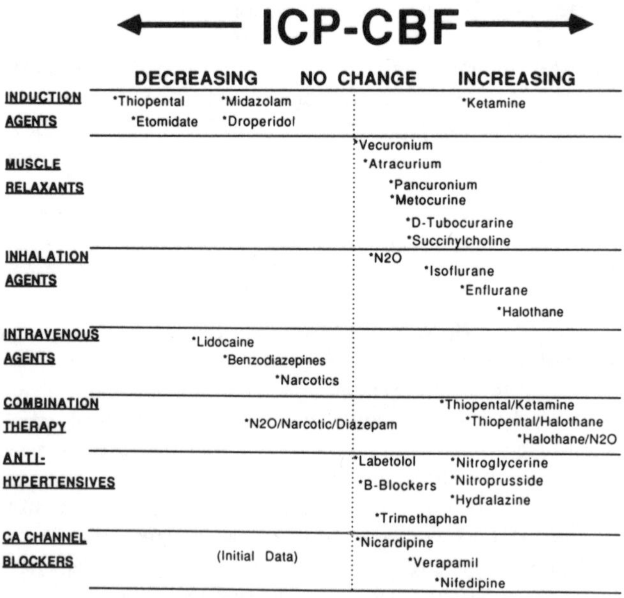

←——— ICP-CBF ———→

	DECREASING		NO CHANGE	INCREASING
INDUCTION AGENTS	*Thiopental *Etomidate	*Midazolam *Droperidol		*Ketamine
MUSCLE RELAXANTS			*Vecuronium *Atracurium *Pancuronium *Metocurine *D-Tubocurarine *Succinylcholine	
INHALATION AGENTS			*N2O *Isoflurane *Enflurane *Halothane	
INTRAVENOUS AGENTS	*Lidocaine *Benzodiazepines *Narcotics			
COMBINATION THERAPY		*N2O/Narcotic/Diazepam		*Thiopental/Ketamine *Thiopental/Halothane *Halothane/N2O
ANTI-HYPERTENSIVES			*Labetolol *B-Blockers *Trimethaphan	*Nitroglycerine *Nitroprusside *Hydralazine
CA CHANNEL BLOCKERS		(Initial Data)	*Nicardipine *Verapamil *Nifedipine	

Figure 2-3   The effects of various drugs and drug combinations on intracranial pressure (ICP) and cerebral blood flow (CBF).

Summary of Cerebral Blood Flow Control

Figure 2-4 demonstrates the clinically important variables that control CBF. With the exception of the $PaCO_2$ curve, all these curves change at a pressure of about 50 mm Hg. Also the average normal CBF is 50 ml/100 g/min, and the normal total brain oxygen consumption is 50 ml/min. The number 50 is a good one to keep in mind.

Cerebral Ischemia and Brain Protection

Cerebral perfusion pressure (CPP) is the driving force for substrate (oxygen, glucose) delivery to the brain. Cerebral perfusion pressure is defined as mean arterial pressure minus intracranial pressure. Both mean arterial pressure and intracranial pressure should be measured at the level of the brain. A good external landmark for the circle of Willis is the external auditory meatus.

Cerebral blood flow can be used to calculate oxygen delivery to the brain. A standard formula is used: Delivered oxygen (Do_2) equals arterial O_2 content (CaO_2) times CBF, or

$$Do_2 = CaO_2 \times CBF.$$

Normal CaO_2 is 16 to 20 ml O_2/100 ml arterial blood. CaO_2 is dependent upon hemoglobin content and PaO_2. Normal Do_2 is (16 to 20 ml O_2/100 ml) $\times$ 50 ml/100 g/min = 8 to 10 ml O_2/100 g/min. Since normal oxygen consumption (Vo_2) is 3.5 to 5 ml O_2/100 g min, there is a safety factor of 1.5 to 2 in delivered oxygen to consumed oxygen. These figures are a global average, and it is vital to keep in mind that the brain is a very heterogenous organ. Local areas of the brain may have a different ratio of Do_2 to Vo_2 secondary to a pathologic CBF or an altered metabolic rate.

Brain ischemic symptoms are seen when CBF falls to about 20 ml/100 g/min (Do_2 4 ml O_2/100 g/min). Electroencephalographic silence occurs at a CBF of 15 ml/100 g/min (Do_2 3 ml O_2/100 g/min; CPP 30 to 40 mm Hg). Cellular ion leakage and eventual cell death occurs at a CBF of 8 to 12 ml/100 g/min (Do_2 2 ml O_2/100 g/min)

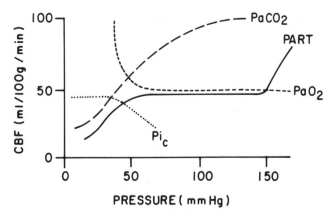

Figure 2-4 Summary of cerebral blood flow control. Pi_c represents intracranial pressure.

(Fig. 2–5). Although the effects on cerebral function and the electroencephalogram occur rather rapidly and reversibly, the irreversible effects on cell viability occur as a function of time and the level of Do_2.

At the tissue level, hypoxia can be defined as a reduction in oxygen availability to a level insufficient for tissue demands. Tissue hypoxia can be caused by either hypoxemia (low PaO_2) or ischemia (low CBF). The effects of these two insults are not equivalent. Hypoxemia with a PaO_2 of 50 mm Hg causes an increase in brain lactate; hypoxemia with a PaO_2 of 35 mm Hg will additionally cause a decrease in phosphocreatine. However, if arterial pressure does not drop significantly, brain ATP stores are not decreased. Therefore, neuronal survival is not threatened until the PaO_2 is less than 25 mm Hg. This defense of ATP levels occurs because hypoxemia induces a compensatory increase in CBF and a sixfold increase in cerebral glucose metabolism.

Pure hypoxemic injuries to the human brain rarely occur, partly because severe hypoxemia is required before neuronal death occurs, but also because one of the earliest effects of hypoxemia is cardiac dysfunction and resultant ischemia. Anesthesiologists have a great opportunity to cause hypoxemic brain injury if they render a patient hypoxemic and then artificially support the patient's blood pressure!

Ischemic injury is characterized by a decrease in oxygen delivery and also by a decrease in the supply of glucose and other metabolites. One of the earliest manifestations of cerebral ischemia is an abrupt reduction in the concentrations of

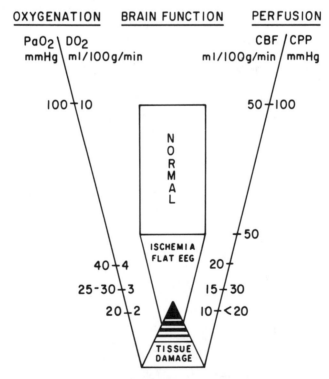

Figure 2-5 Graphic representation of brain function related to two measures of oxygenation and two measures of perfusion.

energy metabolites and eventually ATP. When tissue ATP is depleted, the $Na^+ - K^+$ ATPase-dependent ion pumps fail, leading to Na^+ influx, K^+ efflux, and membrane depolarization. Membrane depolarization results in an uncontrolled influx of Ca^{++}, which leads to disruption of mitochondrial and cell membranes and the release of free fatty acids including arachidonic acid. Ischemia leads to brain edema instantly. Edema can worsen ischemia and the cycle can quickly spiral into brain death.

Ischemia can be global or focal, complete or incomplete. With complete global ischemia the electroencephalogram becomes isoelectric in 15 to 25 seconds, the brain phosphocreatine concentration approaches 0 in approximately 1 minute, and the tissue high-energy phosphate concentration approaches 0 in 5 to 7 minutes.

Incomplete ischemia differs from complete ischemia in that there is a continuing supply of glucose despite tissue hypoxia. This supply of glucose sustains anaerobic metabolism with a resultant increase in brain lactic acid levels. Above a certain threshold lactic acid damages neurons. High brain glucose levels during periods of ischemia can produce toxic levels of lactic acid and increase tissue damage.

Brain protection addresses the preservation of neuronal integrity during periods of hypoxemia and ischemia. Brain protection and brain resuscitation are fundamentally different. Protection is instituted prior to an insult; resuscitation is administered following an insult. This section addresses only the issue of protection.

To prevent neuronal death from ischemia or hypoxemia, two basic strategies can be employed: either prevention of tissue hypoxia primarily, or modification of the events that lead to cell injury and death subsequent to energy failure. The prevention of tissue hypoxia can be divided into two general categories: decreasing tissue oxygen demand and increasing tissue oxygen supply. There are not many techniques to decrease true tissue oxygen demand, i.e., the level Po_2 required for neuronal survival. Hypothermia, however, is such a technique. Hypothermia decreases the oxygen requirements for both synaptic transmission and cellular maintenance. A temperature reduction from 38°C to 28°C decreases $CMRO_2$ to 45% of the normothermic value. A temperature of 18°C lowers the $CMRO_2$ to 20% of the normothermic value.

Short of hypothermia, the major way we affect tissue hypoxia is by increasing oxygen supply. Normal blood hemoglobin, arterial Po_2, cardiac output, and tissue blood flow all serve the function of maintaining oxygen delivery. However, we can also significantly affect tissue oxygen tension by the use of drugs, frequently anesthetics.

Some semantic confusion exists regarding the oxygen supply-demand balance effects of anesthetic agents. Both isoflurane and barbiturates decrease $CMRO_2$ by a maximum of 55%. This $CMRO_2$ suppression comes from abolishing neuronal synaptic transmission. However, the amount of oxygen required for the maintenance of cellular integrity is not decreased. Hence, the lower limit of acceptable local hypoxia is not altered as it is with hypothermia. This is where the semantic confusion exists. The reduced oxygen consumption by the brain with high doses of isoflurane or barbiturates essentially increases the supply of oxygen to the distal watershed areas of the capillary bed. The earliest sites of tissue hypoxia will be those areas farthest from the microcirculation at the venous end of the capillaries. By retarding synaptic transmission and hence oxygen consumption of the upstream (in the capillary sense) neurons, anesthetics decrease the amount of tissue at risk during ischemic periods by increasing the supply of oxygen to the most vulnerable areas of the capillary bed.

In addition to decreasing $CMRO_2$, the barbiturates may have several actions that provide brain protection. Barbiturates decrease intracranial pressure and cerebral edema and thereby improve cerebral blood flow. They may also increase the supply of oxygen to areas of regional ischemia by an inverse steal phenomenon.

Suggested Reading

Algotsson L, Messeter K, Nordstrom CH, Ryding E. Cerebral blood flow and oxygen consumption during isoflurane and halothane anesthesia in man. Acta Anaesthesiol Scand 1988; 32:15-20.

Archer DP, Labrecque P, Tyler JL, Meyer E, Trop D. Cerebral blood volume is increased in dogs during administration of nitrous oxide or isoflurane. Anesthesiology 1987; 67:642-648.

Artru AA. Relationship between cerebral blood volume and CSF pressure during anesthesia with isoflurane or fentanyl in dogs. Anesthesiology 1984; 60:575-579.

Barker J. Cerebral circulation, intracranial pressure, and the pharmacophysiology of anesthetic agents. Int Anesthesiol Clin 1982; 20:77-87.

Chin WP, Imai S, Nakano U, et al. Effects of drugs on the cerebral circulation of the dog in relation to the cerebral oxygen consumption. Br J Pharmacol 1983; 79:897-906.

Cucchiara RF, Theye RA, Michenfelder JD. The effects of isoflurane on cerebral metabolism and blood flow. Anesthesiology 1974; 40:571-574.

Drummond JC, Todd MM, Scheller MS, Shapiro HM. A comparison of the direct cerebral vasodilating potencies of halothane and isoflurane in the New Zealand white rabbit. Anesthesiology 1986; 65:462-467.

Ellinggen I, Hauge A, Nocolaysen G, Thoresen M, Walløe L. Changes in human cerebral blood flow due to step changes in PaO_2 and $PaCO_2$. Acta Physiol Scand 1987; 129:157-163.

Gisvold SE, Steen PA. Drug therapy in brain ischemia. Br J Anaesth 1985; 57:96-109.

Graham DI. The pathology of brain ischemia and possibilities for therapeutic intervention. Br J Anaesth 1985; 57:3-17.

Grubb RL, Raichle ME, Eichling JO, Ter-Pogossian MM. The effects of changes in $PaCO_2$ on cerebral blood volume, blood flow, and vascular mean transit time. Stroke 1974; 5:630-639.

Heiss WD. Flow thresholds of functional and morphological damage of brain tissue. Stroke 1983; 14:329-331.

Kety SS, Schmidt CF. The determination of cerebral blood flow in man by the use of nitrous oxide in low concentrations. Am J Physiol 1945; 143:53-65.

Lassen NA. Cerebral circulation and anaesthesia. Acta Anaesthesiol Scand (Suppl) 1978; 70:53-55.

Martin WRW, Powers WJ, Raichle ME. Cerebral blood volume measured with inhaled $C^{15}O$ and positron emission tomography. J Cereb Blood Flow Metab 1987; 7:421-426.

Messick JM, Milde LN. Brain protection. Advances in Anesthesia 1987; 4:47-88.

Newberg LA, Milde JH, Michenfelder JD. The cerebral metabolic effects of isoflurane at and above concentrations that suppress cortical electrical activity. Anesthesiology 1983; 59:23-28.

Plum F, Posner JB, Zee D. The relationship of cerebral blood flow to CO_2 tension in the blood and pH in the CSF, respectively. Scand J Clin Lab Invest (Suppl 102) 1968; 22:8F.

Risberg J, Ancri D, Ingvar DH. Correlation between cerebral blood volume and cerebral blood flow in the cat. Exp Brain Res 1969; 8:321-326.

Siesjo BK. Cerebral circulation and metabolism. J Neurosurg 1984; 60:883-908.

Steen PA, Newberg L, Milde JH, Michenfelder JD. Hypothermia and barbiturates: Individual and combined effects on canine cerebral oxygen consumption. Anesthesiology 1983; 58:527-532.

Symon L. Flow thresholds in brain ischaemia and the effects of drugs. Br J Anaesth 1985; 57:34-43.

Todd MM, Drummond JC. A comparison of the cerebrovascular and metabolic effects of halothane and isoflurane in the cat. Anesthesiology 1984; 60:276-282.

Donald L. Boos, M.D., and Joseph A. Stirt, M.D.

Pharmacology 3

Inhalation Agents

The inhalational anesthetics are usually chosen on the basis of cardiovascular actions, but it is their central nervous system (CNS) effects that assume somewhat greater importance in the neurosurgical patient. The profound impact that these agents have on cerebral physiology must be understood in order to exploit their beneficial properties and minimize those that are undesired. The issues involved are complex and sometimes controversial. The following is a discussion of the various inhalational agents, summarizing their respective CNS effects.

The inhalational agents produce dose-dependent depression of the CNS, which is reflected by progressive slowing of the electroencephalogram (EEG). The point at which the EEG becomes isoelectric or flat corresponds to a maximal suppression of neuronal function. Since metabolism is proportional to function, this is also the point of minimum cerebral metabolic rate ($CMRO_2$), approximately 40 to 50% of normal. Unless the brain is hypothermic, a further reduction in $CMRO_2$ represents a toxic effect, an incursion into the obligate metabolism required for CNS integrity. This is seen in decreased brain levels of ATP and phosphocreatine and an increase in lactate, evidence of anaerobic metabolism.

Normally, $CMRO_2$ is relatively constant and determines cerebral blood flow (CBF) such that the ratio of CBF to $CMRO_2$ is also constant, roughly 14 to 18:1 in the awake brain. This relationship, referred to as coupling, is disrupted by the inhalational anesthetics because they are all cerebral vasodilators and produce a dose-dependent impairment of autoregulation while simultaneously lowering $CMRO_2$ (Fig. 3–1). The ratio of CBF to $CMRO_2$ increases with increased inhalational agent concentration.

The net CBF observed for a particular inhalational anesthetic depends on two opposing effects. One is direct vasodilation, which increases CBF and is similar for all volatile agents. The other is the reduction in $CMRO_2$, which tends to decrease CBF and varies considerably between anesthetics. Thus, the more $CMRO_2$ is reduced, the lower the observed CBF will be. It should be mentioned that the CBF response to changes in $PaCO_2$ is enhanced by inhalational anesthetics.

Despite the common emphasis on CBF as a measure of cerebral vasodilation, cerebral blood volume (CBV) is actually a more important determinant of intracranial

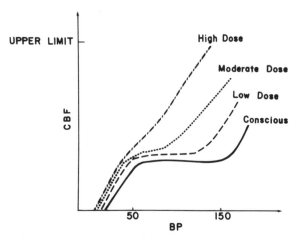

Figure 3-1 Schematic representation of the effect of a progressively increased dose of a typical volatile anesthetic agent on CBF autoregulation. Both upper and lower thresholds are shifted to the left. (From Shapiro HM. Anesthesia effects upon cerebral blood flow, cerebral metabolism, electroencephalogram, and evoked potentials. In: Miller RD, ed. Anesthesia. Vol 2. 2nd ed. New York: Churchill Livingstone, 1986:1263. Reproduced with permission.)

pressure (ICP). CBV is a measure of the total intracranial blood volume, including both arterial and venous systems. In contrast to increases in CBF that may minimally affect CBV, changes in venous capacitance as a result of altered venous tone, drugs, neck compression, or position changes are capable of markedly increasing CBV. All volatile anesthetics initially produce a similar increase in CBV (about 10%) that fails to normalize with time, unlike CBF, which drops to preanesthetic levels after 3 hours (Table 3-1). Furthermore, changes in CBV occur within minutes and are responsible for early increases in ICP.

Another determinant of ICP is cerebrospinal fluid (CSF) volume, but changes in this system are gradual and take longer to manifest. After 2 hours or more of inhalational anesthetic administration, CSF volume becomes a major contributor to increases in ICP. Total CSF volume depends on rate of formation (V_f), normally 20 to 25 ml/hr, rate of absorption (V_a), and resistance to absorption (R_a), each factor capable of being altered independently by anesthetic agents (Table 3-1).

Inhalational anesthetics affect evoked potentials by increasing latency (except for nitrous oxide) and decreasing amplitude. The concentrations compatible with clinically useful monitoring remain controversial. Some suggest that 0.5 maximum allowable concentration (MAC) of either enflurane or isoflurane or 1.0 MAC of halothane is the upper limit, while others place the figures at 1.0 and 0.75 MAC, respectively. Therefore, doses less than 1.0 MAC are probably acceptable for monitoring evoked potentials. This is certainly the case for brainstem auditory evoked potentials (BAEPs), which are the most resistant to anesthetic alteration.

Ventilatory effects of inhalational anesthetics are also significant. During spontaneous breathing, tidal volume decreases and respiratory rate increases, but not

Table 3-1 Effects of Anesthetics on Cerebral Physiology

Drug	CBF	CMRO$_2$	CBF/ CMRO$_2$	CBV	CSF Forma- tion (V$_f$)	CSF Resis- tance to Absorp- tion (R$_a$)	CPP*
Inhalational							
N$_2$O	↑	0†	↑	0	0	0	↓
Halothane	↑	↓	↑	↑	↓	↑	↓
Isoflurane	↑	↓	↑	↑	0	↓	↓
Enflurane	↑	↓	↑	↑	↑	↑	↓
Intravenous							
Barbiturates	↓	↓	0	↓	↓	↓	0
Etomidate	↓	↓	0	↓	↓	↓	0
Propofol	↓	↓	0	↓	?	?	↓
Ketamine	↑	0	↑	↑	0	↑	↓
Midazolam	↓	↓	0	?	↓‡	↓	0
Morphine	0	0	0	?	?	?	↓
Fentanyl	0	0	0	↓	0	↓	0
Alfentanil	0	0	0	?	?	?	↓
Sufentanil	↑(?)	0	0	?	?	?	↓

* Depends on ICP and blood pressure
† No effect
‡ At very high doses
Modified from Michenfelder JD. Anesthesia and the brain. New York: Churchill Livingstone, 1988:41, and Artru AA. New concepts concerning anesthetic effects on intracranial dynamics: CSF and CBV. ASA Annual Refresher Course Lectures, No. 133, 1987.

enough to maintain normal minute volume; hence, resting PaCO$_2$ rises. Inhalational agents produce a dose-dependent reduction in ventilatory response to CO$_2$, an effect that normalizes after approximately 5 hours. The normal increased ventilatory response to hypoxemia is almost abolished at clinical anesthetic doses.

These agents are all negative inotropes, particularly halothane and enflurane. They also alter cardiac conduction, which may be a factor when added to other drugs with similar properties that the patient may be receiving.

Nitrous Oxide

Long considered a relatively benign drug with few adverse CNS effects, N$_2$O continues to be used extensively in neuroanesthesia. This practice may evolve as a deeper appreciation develops of the effects of N$_2$O on the CNS.

Unlike the volatile anesthetics, N$_2$O has little impact on, or slightly increases, CMRO$_2$, implying a more complex action on the brain than previously thought. In addition, N$_2$O is a potent cerebral vasodilator, increasing CBF by 100% or more at approximately 0.5 MAC. Even when added to a background of 1.0 MAC halothane, a threefold increase in CBF is noted. Interestingly, N$_2$O appears to produce nonuniform changes in CBF with increases in anterior regions and decreases posteriorly. These changes in CBF are attenuated by barbiturates, narcotics, and hypocapnia. Nitrous oxide affects neither CBV or CSF dynamics (see Table 3-1).

Nitrous oxide 30% in oxygen results in loss of alpha waves on the EEG. At a 50% concentration or greater, a fast wave (30 to 40 Hz), primarily frontal pattern, emerges and the patient loses consciousness. EEG slowing never occurs. Nitrous oxide does not appear to cause seizures, although a few anecdotal reports do exist.

Halothane

Halothane lowers $CMRO_2$ less than the other volatile anesthetics. At a concentration of 1.5%, $CMRO_2$ is decreased by 25%; 4.5% is required to produce a 50% decrease and isoelectric EEG. However, halothane concentrations greater than 2% are associated with toxic metabolic effects, probably caused by disruption of mitochondrial respiration. Brain lactate levels increase while high-energy compounds decline as the dose of halothane is increased.

Halothane increases CBF twice as much as the other volatile anesthetics, with marked impairment of autoregulation. CBV increases by 12%. The rate of CSF formation slows but this is negated by a greater resistance to its absorption (see Table 3-1). The inevitable ICP increase is attenuated by hyperventilation if instituted well before the administration of halothane is begun. Contributing to intracranial hypertension is the disruption of the blood-CSF and blood-brain barriers that occurs with halothane.

Ischemia is less tolerated with halothane than with other inhalational anesthetics (except for N_2O) and develops at higher mean arterial pressures. Critical CBF values (onset of EEG changes) during carotid artery occlusion may be higher with halothane than with isoflurane.

Enflurane

Enflurane, although an isomer of isoflurane, has significantly different CNS effects. Chief among these is its propensity to cause seizures at moderate doses, especially during hypocapnia. This property makes it a poor anesthetic choice in the neurosurgical setting.

Enflurane lowers $CMRO_2$ more than halothane but less than isoflurane. Some have noted a 50% decrease at 2.0 MAC, while others have observed a maximum drop of 30% occurring at 1.0 MAC or greater. With the onset of seizures, however, $CMRO_2$ jumps 400% with a subsequent increase in CBF far above that normally seen with enflurane. In fact, CBF increases little during clinical use because of the concomitant decrease in blood pressure. At clinical concentrations of enflurane, CBV increases approximately 15%.

Another notable and undesirable effect of enflurane is its impact on CSF dynamics. It increases formation and resistance to absorption, producing the greatest net increase in CSF volume of any inhalational anesthetic agent. This becomes an important factor in prolonged use.

The EEG with enflurane shows dose-dependent slowing to 1.0 MAC, with spike waves appearing at 1.5 MAC. Seizures are common at 2.0 MAC, especially if $PaCO_2$ is less than 30. The EEG never becomes isoelectric.

Isoflurane

Isoflurane is the inhalational agent of choice for neuroanesthesia. It profoundly lowers $CMRO_2$ by as much as 50% at 2.0 MAC. This decrease in $CMRO_2$ corresponds to a flat EEG. Since $CMRO_2$ effects with isoflurane are caused by decreases in neuronal function and not metabolic toxicity, higher doses of isoflurane do not produce further changes similar to thiopental. Thus, it is not surprising that these agents are of no benefit during ischemia severe enough to produce a flat EEG. For incomplete global ischemia, such as occurs during deliberate hypotension, both isoflurane and thiopental improve outcome. For incomplete regional ischemia, however, isoflurane is considerably less effective than thiopental. Isoflurane, a cerebral vasodilator, may shunt blood from ischemic regions with vasomotor paralysis. In contrast, thiopental is a cerebral vasoconstrictor and can redistribute flow to those same regions (i.e., inverse steal).

With isoflurane, CBF typically increases less than with the other inhalational anesthetics. Autoregulation is impaired but remains functional up to 1.5 MAC. The response to hypocapnia is intact to 2.8 MAC, but at this dose increases in $PaCO_2$ fail to affect CBF, presumably because cerebral vessels are maximally dilated. With isoflurane, cerebral blood volume increases, and there is a decrease in resistance to CSF absorption (see Table 3-1). With hyperventilation, ICP changes are minimal. As expected, the EEG shows a dose-dependent slowing with burst suppression occurring at 1.5 MAC and isoelectricity at 2.0 MAC. Because of its vasodilating properties, isoflurane has been associated with coronary "steal," a potential problem in the neurosurgical patient with concomitant coronary artery disease.

Barbiturates

Barbiturates are useful neuroanesthetic drugs for a number of reasons. Most importantly, they decrease $CMRO_2$ by greatly reducing CNS neuronal activity. This results in coupled reductions in CBF and ICP. The elevated cerebrovascular resistance (CVR), however, only decreases CBF in normal regions. Because of vasomotor paralysis, vessels within injured or ischemic zones fail to react and remain maximally dilated. The result is the shunting of blood from normal to ischemic areas (i.e., inverse steal). There is no effect on CSF dynamics per se (see Table 3-1). Dose-dependent CNS depression is reflected by the EEG, which progressively slows. Cerebral metabolic rate is maximally lowered to approximately 50% of normal, at which point the EEG is flat. Higher doses of barbiturates have no further effect on $CMRO_2$.

Barbiturates work by enhancing inhibitory and blocking excitatory synaptic transmissions by their interaction with the gamma-aminobutyric acid (GABA) receptor complex, at a site different from that of benzodiazepines. By prolonging GABA occupancy, the duration of GABA inhibition is extended. They may also act presynaptically to decrease availability of excitatory neurotransmitters. In addition, nonselective depression of transmission occurs at higher doses.

Barbiturates have other CNS effects. They decrease free radical activity, possibly preventing further injury in ischemic zones. They ameliorate the cytotoxic cerebral edema often seen following ischemia. They are also potent anticonvulsants. Because of these salutary effects, barbiturates have been used for cerebral protection. They are moderately effective for incomplete or focal ischemia, much less so for global ischemia. However, favorable responses are observed when barbiturates are used during cardiac surgery for suspected air emboli and during carotid artery surgery. Their use in severe head injury has met with conflicting results. A recent study found them beneficial, but only when cardiovascular complications, particularly hypovolemia, were absent. Their main use in patients with head injury is to control ICP, usually as a last resort after other methods have failed.

Barbiturate-induced EEG changes are similar to those produced by other sedative hypnotics. Small doses increase beta activity, with increasing doses ultimately resulting in isoelectricity. Induction doses of barbiturates do produce a transient period of burst suppression, but not always a flat EEG. Evoked potentials are largely unaffected by those same doses, but higher doses will increase latency and decrease amplitude. Somatosensory evoked potentials (SSEPs) obtained from the spinal cord are altered slightly but not abolished even in the presence of a flat EEG.

A major disadvantage in using barbiturates is dose-dependent cardiovascular depression, a combination of both central and direct actions. Myocardial contractility is decreased owing to a lack of available calcium, but increases in heart rate help maintain cardiac output, even in mild congestive heart failure. The myocardial depression is less than that produced by volatile anesthetics. Peripheral vasodilatation occurs because of lowered sympathetic tone and depression of medullary pressor centers. The net result may be a reduction in blood pressure with an attendant decrease in cerebral perfusion pressure (CPP). Barbiturates should be used with great caution in patients who are hemodynamically compromised, especially those who are hypovolemic. Slow injection fails to alter these effects and only results in higher required total doses.

Barbiturates are also central respiratory depressants. The effect is usually transient, peaking 1 to 1.5 minutes after administration, but may be prolonged in patients with chronic obstructive pulmonary disease (COPD). Apnea occurs, but usually lasts less than 30 seconds. At doses employed clinically, the laryngeal and cough reflexes remain intact, as does the sympathetic response to intubation.

Tolerance, both acute and chronic, occurs with barbiturate use. In patients receiving barbiturates chronically, dose requirements may be up to six times normal. Because of the possibility of cross-tolerance, this may be of concern in the substance abuser with intracranial pathology.

Drug entry into the CNS is determined by lipid solubility, degree of ionization, protein binding, and plasma concentration. The highly lipid-soluble barbiturates easily penetrate the CNS. They are weak acids and largely un-ionized (50% for thiopental, 75% for methohexital) at physiologic pH, which facilitates CNS entry. Acidemia results in an even greater fraction of un-ionized drug and reduces dose requirements. Barbiturates are highly protein-bound and may be displaced by other agents, thereby increasing the amount of free drug having access to the brain. Similarly, low protein states (e.g., renal failure) also lower dose requirements. Plasma concentration depends on the dose and speed of administration; therefore, high doses and rapid injection increase the amount of barbiturate entering the CNS.

After an induction dose of barbiturate, brain uptake occurs in less than 30 seconds, with peak levels at 45 seconds. Termination of effect is caused by redistribution to lean tissues. Fat, with its poor vascularity, has a much slower uptake—peak levels occur at 2.5 hours—but will become a reservoir, whose size will depend primarily on dose.

For neuroanesthesia, thiopental is the barbiturate most frequently employed, but methohexital and thiamylal are also used. Despite much shared pharmacology discussed above, important differences exist. These will be discussed below. See Table 3-2 for a comparative summary and Table 3-3 for pharmacokinetic data.

Thiopental

Thiopental is metabolized in the liver at a rate of 10 to 25% per hour. Most is converted to inactive metabolites, but a small amount of long-acting pentobarbital is produced. It has a low hepatic extraction ratio—clearance divided by hepatic blood flow (HBF)—and its elimination depends on enzyme capacity rather than HBF. At low doses, elimination follows first-order kinetics with a $t_{1/2\beta}$ of 6 hours. However, at high doses zero-order kinetics are followed with a $t_{1/2\beta}$ of 60 hours. Saturation of hepatic enzymes begins at plasma levels of 30 to 50 μg/ml, and the shift to nonlinear kinetics occurs at 60 μg/ml.

Table 3-2 Pharmacology and Use of Barbiturates

	Thiopental	Thiamylal	Methohexital
Induction dose (mg/kg)	4-5	4-5	1-2 IV (25-30 PR)
Time to awakening (min)	5-10	5-10	3-8
Respiratory effects	Minimum depression with hypnotic dose progressing to apnea with high doses Laryngeal/cough reflexes intact	Similar to thiopental	Similar to thiopental with a shorter duration
Hemodynamic effects	Vasodilation, myocardial depression Blood pressure decreases markedly if hypovolemia present Reflex increase in heart rate Small amount of histamine release	Similar to thiopental	Similar to thiopental
CNS effects	↓ CBF, $CMRO_2$, ICP Flat EEG with induction dose	Similar to thiopental	Similar to thiopental Increased excitatory phenomena Seizures common after withdrawal of high dose infusion Increased seizure activity
Complications (%)			
Cough/hiccup	5	5	25
Pain/phlebitis	9/1	9/1	12/8
Movements	7	7	35

Adapted from Stoelting RK. Barbiturates. In: Pharmacology and physiology in anesthetic practice. Philadelphia: JB Lippincott, 1987:102-116, and Corssen G, et al. Barbiturates. In: Intravenous anesthesia and analgesia. Philadelphia: Lea & Febiger, 1988:85.

The slow elimination of thiopental allows it to accumulate when large doses are infused, making it necessary to monitor blood levels if zero-order kinetics are to be avoided. Once that point is reached, it may take 80 to 100 hours after thiopental is discontinued before neurologic evaluation is possible.

Dosing is listed in Table 3-2. Children require 5 to 6 mg/kg for induction if unpremedicated. In contrast, elderly patients require much less. This is due to the decline in volume of distribution (V_D) with age. When used for intraoperative control of ICP, 1 to 3 mg/kg every 20 to 30 minutes as needed usually suffices. The maximum

Table 3-3 Pharmocokinetic Values for Intravenous Anesthetics

Drug	$t_{1/2\alpha}$ (min)	$t_{1/2\beta}$ (hr)	VD_{ss} (L/kg)	Clearance (ml/kg/ min)	Protein bound (%)	pk_a	Un-ionized at pH 7.4 (%)
Barbiturates							
Thiopental	2–4	10–12	2–3	3–4	75	7.45	50
Methohexital	5–6	3–5	1.5–3	7–13	75	7.9	75
Benzodiaze-pines							
Diazepam	10–15	20–40	1.9	0.4	98	3.4	>90
Midazolam	7–15	2–4	1.7	7	95	6.2	90
Lorazepam	3–10	10–20	1.3	1.2	95	1.5 and 11.5	?
Ketamine	11–17	2–3	1–3	17	low	7.5	50
Etomidate	2–4	2–5	4.5	14	75	4.2	>90
Propofol	2–4	1–3	5–20	20–30	98	11	<10
Narcotics							
Morphine	10–20	2–4	3–5	15	30	8.0	25
Fentanyl	5–20	2–4	3–5	11.5	85	8.4	<10
Sufentanil	5–15	2–3	2.5	10	93	8.0	20
Alfentanil	5–20	1–2	0.5–1.0	6.4	93	6.5	90

Modified from Youngberg JA. Intravenous induction agents. In: Attia RR, et al, eds. Practical Anesthetic Pharmacology. Norwalk, CT: Appleton & Lang, 1986:42–43.

beneficial dose is approximately 15 mg/kg and corresponds to a flat EEG. A comparison with other induction agents is made in Table 3–4.

Thiamylal

Thiamylal is very similar to thiopental and is not discussed in detail. See Table 3–2.

Methohexital

Methohexital is metabolized considerably faster than thiopental. Its hepatic clearance is three times that of thiopental and its hepatic extraction ratio is 0.5 (vs. 0.15 for thiopental), making accumulation less likely.

Interestingly, methohexital enhances epileptogenic activity in patients with focal seizures. Seizures have also been reported in patients without a history of previous seizures at doses exceeding 24 mg/kg, especially after discontinuance of infusions. Excitatory phenomena are more common with methohexital than thiopental or thiamylal.

Dosing information is contained in Table 3–2. Age-related adjustments in doses should be considered. Faster recovery follows a methohexital induction; pain on injection is common. One advantage of methohexital is its effectiveness via administration per rectum, usually in children, at 25 to 30 mg/kg. Peak plasma values are achieved at 14 minutes. Sedation adequate for diagnostic radiology requires only 10 to 20 mg/kg per rectum or 10 mg/kg IM.

Table 3-4 Comparative Pharmacology of Intravenous Induction Agents

Agent	Induction	Cardio-vascular	Respiratory	Anal-gesia	Amnesia	Emergence
Thiopental	Smooth/rapid	Depression	Transient depression	None	Minimal	Smooth/rapid
Ketamine	Excitatory/rapid	Stimulation	Minimal	Yes	Minimal	Stormy/intermediate
Etomidate	Smooth/rapid	None	Transient depression	None	Minimal	Smooth/rapid
Propofol	Smooth/rapid/pain	Depression	Depression	None	Minimal	Smooth/rapid
Diazepam	Smooth/slow/pain	Minimal	Depression	None	Yes	Smooth/prolonged
Midazolam	Smooth/intermediate	Vasodilation	Depression	None	Yes	Smooth/intermediate
Alfentanil	Smooth/rapid/rigidity	Depression	Depression	Yes	Minimal	Smooth/rapid
Sufentanil	Smooth/rapid/rigidity	Minimal	Depression	Yes	Minimal	Smooth/intermediate

Adapted from White PF. Clinical use of newer intravenous induction drugs. Cleveland: IARS Review Course Lectures, 1988:102–112.

Propofol

Propofol is a newer intravenous anesthetic effective for maintenance of anesthesia as well as for induction. It lowers CBF by 30%, $CMRO_2$ by 30%, and ICP, but CPP also decreases because of the large decrease in blood pressure seen with induction doses (see Table 3–1). With continuous infusion, CPP appears to be maintained, making this route more suitable for neuroanesthesia. As with other sedative hypnotics, there is dose-dependent CNS depression. The EEG shifts from alpha to delta waves; burst suppression occurs with higher doses. Recovery is rapid, as is the return of the alpha EEG pattern. No epileptiform activity occurs despite the movements; twitches or tremors are observed in 15% of patients. Propofol decreases amplitude and increases latency of somatosensory evoked cortical potentials (SECPs) but does not alter SSEPs at the spinal cord. The latter therefore remain useful during propofol anesthesia. BAEPs are likewise unaffected.

Propofol causes greater cardiac depression than thiopental. Blood pressure typically drops by 15 to 30%, without any reflex increase in heart rate, and is used to gauge depth of anesthesia. Propofol is more effective than thiopental or etomidate in blunting the response to laryngoscopy and intubation.

With propofol there is marked respiratory depression, with a longer duration of apnea than that seen with other intravenous induction agents, lasting up to 2 minutes even in unpremedicated patients. Minute volume decreases despite increases in respiratory rate.

Propofol provides no analgesia, but is capable of substituting for a volatile agent for maintenance of anesthesia. Emergence is smooth with little nausea or vomiting. Pain on injection is common, though less than that observed with methohexital or etomidate. See Table 3–4 for comparative pharmacology and Table 3–5 for dosing information. Table 3–3 contains pharmacokinetic values.

Narcotics

Narcotics comprise a group of drugs that produce morphine-like effects and bind stereospecifically to any of several types of opioid receptors. With some overlap, each receptor type mediates different effects and demonstrates affinities for the various agonists. Opioid receptors are concentrated in the CNS, particularly those regions involved in nociception. Narcotic agonists trigger presynaptic events that result in decreased neurotransmitter release, specifically affecting acetylcholine, dopamine, substance P, and norepinephrine. Because of the receptor locations, it is not surprising that most narcotic effects are centrally mediated.

Narcotics produce dose-dependent EEG slowing, eventually replacing the original alpha pattern with high voltage, low-frequency delta waves. Unlike other CNS depressants, narcotics do not produce a continuum of depression progressing to burst suppression, but rather exhibit a ceiling effect, never producing an isoelectric EEG. Cerebral metabolic rate is submaximally reduced with preservation of coupling. Cerebral blood flow and potentially ICP are reduced accordingly (see Table 3–1). However, the magnitude of these changes is probably small and appears to depend on background anesthetics and technique (e.g., hyperventilation). Despite reports in animals, narcotic-induced seizures have never been documented in humans. Resistance to CSF absorption is decreased, which may contribute to any observed reductions in ICP.

Narcotics produce sedation, some possibly even anesthesia. It is speculated that this is caused by blocked afferents rather than generalized CNS depression. Conscious patients usually experience a euphoric tranquility, but dysphoria occasionally predominates. Amnesia is not reliably produced despite profound analgesia, and recall is possible if narcotics are used alone.

The principal effect of narcotics on the heart is bradycardia. This is caused by a central vagotonic action and direct depression of the sinoatrial (SA) and atrioventricular (AV) nodes. It is somewhat dependent on dose and speed of administration and is attenuated by slow injection or prior administration of a vagolytic agent. Heart rate is infrequently increased because of opiate-induced catecholamine or histamine release. When used alone, except for meperidine in high doses, narcotics preserve myocardial

Table 3-5 Propofol

Use	Dose (mg/kg)	Onset	Duration (min)
Induction	2–3	Rapid	5–10
Maintenance	50–150 μg/kg/ min	——	5–10 after stopped

contractility, but in combination with nitrous oxide they can cause cardiac depression. The net hemodynamic consequences depend on underlying heart disease, but most decreases in blood pressure are probably a result of lowered sympathetic tone.

Narcotics produce dose-dependent depression of respiratory centers, affecting ventilation rate, rhythm, CO_2 response, and minute and tidal volumes. Clinically, this is usually seen as a decreased respiratory rate, partially compensated for by an increased tidal volume. The diminished CO_2 response results in hypercapnia, which increases CBF and CBV. For the patient with reduced intracranial compliance, this results in potentially dangerous elevations of ICP with subsequent reductions in CPP. The elderly, infants, and patients with lung disease are particularly sensitive to drug-induced respiratory depression, necessitating even greater caution in the use of narcotics in these groups.

A potentially serious complication of opiate use in neurosurgical patients is muscle rigidity. Generally, its incidence and intensity increase with increasing potency, dose, and speed of administration. By making it difficult to ventilate the patient, especially during induction, rigidity contributes to hypoventilation from respiratory depression and further elevates PaCO$_2$. In addition, CVP increases, which reduces intracranial venous drainage, thereby increasing CBV and, potentially, ICP. The relationship between CVP and ICP in nonlinear, small elevations in CVP may produce disproportionately large increases in ICP. Attempts to attenuate opiate-induced rigidity with benzodiazepines and barbiturates have met with little success. Muscle relaxants given before opiates work best.

Narcotics have several effects on the gastrointestinal tract. Most common are postoperative nausea and vomiting caused by (1) direct stimulation of the chemoreceptor trigger zone, (2) vestibular-related position changes, (3) decreased gastrointestinal motility, and (4) increased gastric volume. In addition to increasing the risk of aspiration, retching may adversely affect blood pressure and ICP.

Opiates can cause urinary retention and urgency because of increases in bladder sphincter and detrusor tone. This is not a problem in the catheterized patient.

Narcotics are excellent antinociceptives; they serve to "smooth out" an anesthetic course by their action in controlling blood pressure as well as decreasing coughing and straining at extubation. Despite shared pharmacology, the various opiates have important differences. They are discussed individually in the following paragraphs. Table 3-3 contains phramocokinetic data, and Table 3-6 contains dosing recommendations.

Table 3-6 Clinical Doses of Narcotics

Drug	IV Dose	Onset (min)	Approximate Duration
Morphine	0.05-0.3 mg/kg	5-10	3-5 hours
Meperidine	0.5-1.0 mg/kg	5-10	2-3 hours
Fentanyl	1-5 μg/kg	2	45 min-2 hours
	5-10 μg/kg*		1-3 hours
Sufentanil	0.5-2 μg/kg	<1	2 hours
Alfentanil	10-40 μg/kg	<1	<30 min
	30-80 μg/kg*		<60 min
	0.5-3.0 μg/kg/min		Discontinue 10-15 min prior to end of case

*Larger doses will result in increase duration

Morphine

Morphine is lipid insoluble and poorly penetrates the CNS; it is slow to enter and exit. Only a fraction of the administered dose actually reaches the brain, determined more by CBF than by degree of ionization. After a single intravenous dose, it takes 15 to 30 minutes for the CSF level to peak, followed by a slow decay. Plasma levels change more rapidly. Consequently, onset and duration of central effects correlate poorly with blood levels, making morphine inferior to other narcotics for use during anesthesia, particularly for induction.

Of the cardiovascular effects produced by morphine, the decrease in blood pressure is most significant and may occur for several reasons. A decrease in heart rate may be a factor but is usually negligible with morphine. Diminished sympathetic tone produces venodilation with a subsequent decrease in venous return. The effect on blood pressure via this mechanism depends on existing volume status, the largest decrease occurring in the presence of hypovolemia. A third mechanism involves histamine release, which becomes substantial when morphine is given at a rate greater than 5 mg/min. The resulting drop in blood pressure, but not the amount of histamine released, can be attenuated by prior administration of H_1 and H_2 blockers. Histamine, a cerebrovasodilator, may contribute to any decrement of CPP if the increase in CBV is sufficient to raise ICP.

Morphine demonstrates first-order kinetics even at high doses. It is metabolized by the liver and to a lesser extent by the kidneys. The latter are responsible for the elimination of 80% of the metabolites; the remainder are excreted via the biliary tract. Morphine has a high hepatic extraction ratio, which means that most of what is presented to the liver is removed. This makes its metabolism dependent on hepatic blood flow. The decline in plasma levels is due primarily to elimination. Liver disease prolongs $t_{1/2,\beta}$ but clinical duration seems little affected.

Meperidine

Meperidine has one-tenth the potency of morphine and possesses some undesirable properties. CNS excitation and seizures can occur with the accumulation of the active metabolite, normeperidine. This is most common after infusion, large doses, or when used in the presence of renal failure, and may be heralded by tremulousness (awake patients) and tachycardia.

Because of its structural similarity to atropine, meperidine usually produces an increase in heart rate. It is also a direct negative inotrope, unlike the other narcotics, and may cause hypotension at high doses because of decreased cardiac output.

Meperidine is further distinguished from other narcotics because it lacks antitussive properties and produces mydriasis, another atropine-like effect. It is metabolized primarily in the liver with a small portion excreted unchanged by the kidneys. Overall, this opiate is not the best choice for neuroanesthesia.

Fentanyl

Fentanyl is considered by many to be the narcotic of choice for neuroanesthesia. It is 100 times more potent than morphine, with a faster onset and shorter duration. It lowers ICP slightly (at least in the presence of nitrous oxide) and maintains CPP better than sufentanil or alfentanil (Fig. 3-2). Fentanyl also decreases the resistance to CSF absorption and results in a 10% reduction in CBV (see Table 3-1). High doses ($>50\ \mu g/kg$)

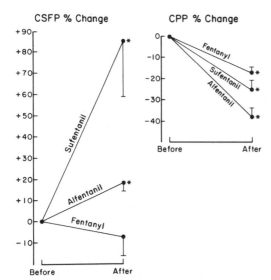

Figure 3-2 Peak changes in cerebrospinal fluid pressure (CSFP) and cerebral perfusion pressure (CPP) before and 10 minutes after administration of fentanyl, sufentanil, or alfentanil during N_2O-O_2- vecuronium anesthesia, expressed as percent change from control. (From Marx W, et al. Sufentanil, alfentanil, and fentanyl: impact on CSF pressure in patients with brain tumors. Anesthesiology 1988; 69:A627. Reproduced with permission of JB Lippincott.)

lower MAC by 65%. Much smaller doses, however, are more appropriate for neurosurgical patients and produce less dramatic MAC reductions.

Bradycardia, produced largely by fentanyl's enhancement of central vagal tone and depression of the SA and AV nodes, is more pronounced than with other narcotics. When used with vecuronium, fentanyl has been reported to cause unacceptably low heart rates and even asystole, presumably because vecuronium is devoid of vagolytic effects. Prophylactic administration of an anticholinergic is preventive.

No histamine is released, giving fentanyl an advantage over morphine in patients with bronchospastic disease. Respiratory depression may outlast analgesia and persist well into the postoperative period. Even after apparent recovery, respiratory depression has been shown to recur. This is thought to be due to fentanyl washout from the lungs as abnormal $\dot{V}/\dot{Q}$ regions normalize.

Fentanyl is extremely lipid-soluble and has a large volume of distribution, binding to many inactive sites. It is metabolized primarily in the liver to inactive metabolites. At lower doses its short duration is due to rapid redistribution similar to thiopental. Recovery from respiratory depression closely follows plasma decay. Following a single intravenous dose, the largest decline in plasma levels and respiratory depression is complete by approximately 45 to 60 minutes after administration. Elimination half-time is increased with advanced age and aortic cross-clamping, but not with cirrhosis; dosing should be adjusted accordingly.

Sufentanil

Sufentanil is five to 10 times more potent than fentanyl but has the highest therapeutic index of the clinically used opiates. It is capable of reducing MAC by 90%, being very close to a complete anesthetic. It affords good hemodynamic stability but has recently been shown to increase ICP substantially, probably by cerebral vasodilation, with a moderate decrease in CPP (see Fig. 3-2). Therefore, in patients with reduced intracranial compliance, sufentanil is best avoided.

As with fentanyl, sufentanil has been reported to produce significant bradycardia, particularly when used with vecuronium. Again, anticholinergics are preventive.

Sufentanil is extremely lipid soluble and enters the CNS rapidly, with a peak onset of approximately 5 minutes. It has a lower volume of distribution than fentanyl and a high percentage bound to protein. Metabolism occurs in the liver, with elimination evenly split between the biliary system and the kidneys. As always, duration increases with age.

Alfentanil

Alfentanil is stated to be five to 10 times less potent than fentanyl but may actually be 70 times less. It has a rapid onset (1 to 2 minutes) and a duration much shorter than the other narcotics, and it has a very small volume of distribution. After a 50 μg/kg dose of alfentanil, only 10 minutes is required for resumption of spontaneous ventilation. Termination of effect is due to redistribution. Alfentanil is extensively metabolized to inactive metabolites.

Although alfentanil causes a slight increase in ICP, it dramatically lowers blood pressure, resulting in often unacceptable decreases in CPP (see Fig. 3-2). However, alfentanil reliably prevents the responses to painful stimuli, such as skull pinning and incision, in patients in whom tight control of blood pressure is critical (e.g., those with intracranial aneurysms). Rigidity can be a problem when alfentanil is used for induction.

Narcotic Antagonists

Naloxone is the most common antagonist used perioperatively. It should be titrated (40 μg increments) to maintain analgesia while decreasing the level of respiratory depression. It has a duration of 30 to 45 minutes after an intravenous dose. A longer duration, with sustained blood levels, can be obtained by an intramuscular dose twice that given intravenously. Rapid injection of a large dose may result in nausea and vomiting. Care should be exercised when using this drug, particularly in patients with coronary artery disease, because of the increase in sympathetic activity it produces. In addition to hypertension and tachycardia, pulmonary edema has been reported. Despite its problems, naloxone may be necessary for early neurologic evaluation and continued perioperative assessment. When used postoperatively, the patient should continue to be observed for respiratory depression, which may outlast the duration of naloxone.

Lidocaine

Lidocaine can be a valuable adjunct in the care of neurosurgical patients. Its suppression of synaptic transmission produces a 20 to 30% reduction in $CMRO_2$. Unlike the barbiturates or etomidate, lidocaine is capable of reducing $CMRO_2$ beyond that associated with the absence of neuronal transmission (i.e., flat EEG). Once a barbiturate-induced isoelectric EEG is established, neither the administration of additional barbiturate nor etomidate has any effect on $CMRO_2$. Lidocaine given in high doses under the same conditions has been shown to decrease $CMRO_2$ an additional 15 to 20%. Because of lidocaine's ability to block Na^+ channels, it is speculated that the Na^+–K^+ leak is diminished, thus reducing the load on energy-dependent ion pumps. However, during deep isoflurane anesthesia, lidocaine is associated with lower ATP levels, possibly because of a toxic effect on oxidative phosphorylation. Therefore, lidocaine may have a combination of protective and toxic effects.

In addition to decreasing $CMRO_2$, lidocaine directly raises CVR; both contribute to reductions in CBF and ICP. Lidocaine is as effective as thiopental at rapidly lowering ICP, but produces less cardiovascular depression and helps maintain CPP. Intravenous lidocaine has also proven useful in preventing elevations of ICP that often occur with endotracheal suctioning or endotracheal tube manipulations, presumably because of its ability to blunt laryngotracheal reflexes. Topical application is considerably less effective and acts as an airway irritant. Less importantly, lidocaine potentiates inhalational anesthetics and is anticonvulsant at therapeutic plasma levels. At levels approaching 10 μg/mg, lidocaine can actually cause seizures.

Etomidate

Etomidate is a useful induction agent for neuroanesthesia, particularly in less hemodynamically stable patients. It is a potent, direct cerebrovasoconstrictor (i.e., CVR is increased independent of changes in CMR), reducing both CBF and ICP. Cerebral metabolic rate is reduced by 50%, a result of depressed neuronal activity. Unlike the barbiturates, etomidate lowers $CMRO_2$ nonuniformly, from large reductions in the cortex to little or no change in the brainstem, the probable reason for the lack of cardiovascular depression. Etomidate confers cerebral protection and improved outcomes following ischemia, as do thiopental and isoflurane. Considerably less benefit is obtained when etomidate is administered as an infusion because of lower plasma levels.

Etomidate produces an EEG pattern very similar to that of the barbiturates. One minute after an induction dose, delta waves predominate, followed in 30 to 40 seconds by burst suppression. The initial beta-wave EEG activation seen during thiopental induction does not occur. The delta-wave stage is associated with a high incidence of myoclonic movement, but no epileptiform activity is evident. Etomidate has been successfully used to treat status epilepticus despite the reports of its precipitating seizures in patients with seizure disorders. Until the issue is clarified, etomidate is best avoided in patients with a history of seizures.

Etomidate's effects on evoked potentials include a markedly increased amplitude in SECPs with a smaller increase in latency, but the SSEP at the spinal cord is unchanged and remains a useful monitor of function.

What makes etomidate sometimes preferable to thiopental is its capacity to maintain cardiovascular stability. Cardiac index, systemic and pulmonary pressure, afterload and preload show minimal changes. There may be up to a 10% increase in heart rate and a 20% decrease in pulmonary vascular resistance. Also, histamine is not released. The sympathetic response to intubation still occurs, though less than with thiopental alone. Etomidate produces no analgesia.

During induction, there is a 20% incidence of hiccups or coughing followed by a 10- to 70-second period of apnea. Overall, there is less respiratory depression than occurs with the thiopental and only a 15% increase in $PaCO_2$.

The major argument against the use of etomidate is its adrenocortical suppression via 11-β-hydroxylase. Increased mortality has been noted with continuous use for sedation in the intensive care unit. Even when used solely for induction, a measurable, acute decrease in cortisol occurs. Nevertheless, etomidate's combination of cardiovascular stability and beneficial cerebral effects make it a useful agent to have available for neuroanesthesia.

It is metabolized exclusively in the liver (98%) and excreted by the kidneys, so duration may be prolonged in liver failure. Unlike the barbiturates, etomidate appears safe for patients with porphyria. Dosing information is summarized in Table 3-7, and complications of its use in Table 3-8. A comparison with other induction agents is contained in Table 3-4, and pharmacokinetic values can be found in Table 3-3.

Benzodiazepines

Benzodiazepines are sedative hypnotics, but they have a wider range of effects than other agents so classified. They are also anxiolytics, anticonvulsants, and amnesics. While qualitatively similar, there are individual differences in selectivity of actions which help determine use (Table 3-9). Their principal mechanism involves the facilitation of GABA inhibition in the CNS, but they also antagonize central serotonin and decrease the availability of acetylcholine in the brain.

Benzodiazepines produce a dose-dependent CNS depression with subsequent decreases in $CMRO_2$ and, ultimately, reductions in CBF and ICP (see Table 3-1). They afford some degree of cerebral protection, though less than that of the barbiturates.

Table 3-7 Etomidate

Use	Dose (mg/kg)	Onset	Duration (min)
Induction	0.2–0.4	Immediate	5–10
Infusion	100 μg/kg/min $\times$ 10 min then 10 μg/kg/min	2 min	10 after discontinued

Table 3-8 Complications of Etomidate Use

Adrenocortical suppression
  Via 11-β hydroxylase
  Decreases cortisol—persists for several hours after an induction dose
Myoclonic movements
  Occur in up to 80% of patients
  Not associated with seizure activity on EEG
  Use of muscle relaxants often required
Nausea and vomiting
  Occurs in 30–40% of patients
  Largest source of complaints
Pain on injection
  Due to high osmolarity of formulation
  High incidence of thrombophlebitis
  Decreased with use of larger veins

Table 3-9 Benzodiazepines

Drug	Induction	Preoperative Medication	Intra-operative Sedation	Amnesia	Night Hypnotic
Midazolam	++	+++	+++	−	+++
Diazepam	+	+++	+	++	++
Lorazepam	−	+++	−	++	+++
Triazolam	−	+++	−	++	++
Chlordiazepoxide	−	+	−	+	−
Flurazepam	−	−	−	++	−
Oxazepam	−	+	−	+	−
Prazepam	−	−	−	−	−
Temazepam	−	−	−	++	−
Alprazolam	−	+	−	−	−

Modified from Reves JG. Benzodiazepines. In: Prys-Roberts C, Hue CC, eds. Pharmacokinetics of anesthesia. Oxford: Blackwell, 1984.

Like other sedative-hypnotics they cause a shift in the EEG from a predominant alpha pattern to one of rapid, low-voltage beta waves followed by theta waves. This shift occurs primarily in the frontal and rolandic regions without the rostral spread seen with barbiturates. The benzodiazepines are also incapable of providing general anesthesia, unlike the barbiturates in high doses. Benzodiazepines do, however, decrease the MAC of volatile anesthetics.

Their effect on evoked potentials varies. SECPs exhibit a decrease in both amplitude and early potential latency with a prolongation of the late potential latency. SSEPs obtained at the spinal cord are not affected.

Of the many benzodiazepines, only those commonly used perioperatively are discussed individually. See Table 3-3 for pharmacokinetic values.

Diazepam

Diazepam is the standard to which the other benzodiazepines are compared. Its primary use is as an oral premedicant; peak blood levels are achieved at 1 hour in adults, 15 to 30 minutes in children. It is an excellent anticonvulsant and is the first-line treatment for status epilepticus. It is occasionally used for anesthesia induction because of its minimal cardiovascular depression, but its onset is delayed and recovery protracted (see Table 3-4). Hepatic metabolism produces long-acting metabolites responsible for much of diazepam's duration. Its elimination half-time of 24 to 48 hours is prolonged by age, cimetidine use, and liver disease ($t_{1/2\beta}$ may be 10 days in cirrhotic patients). Diazepam is largely protein-bound but is easily displaced by heparin, markedly increasing the amount of free drug. There is minimal respiratory depression when diazepam is used alone, but long periods of apnea are possible when it is combined with other CNS depressants, particularly the narcotics. Skeletal muscle relaxation occurs by inhibition of spinal afferents but does not affect neuromuscular blockade. Only slight anterograde amnesia results from premedicant doses.

For dosing information, see Table 3-10. Intramuscular diazepam is not recommended because of unpredictable absorption. Its use for intraoperative sedation

Table 3-10 Clinical Use of the Benzodiazepines

Drug	Dose	Comments
Midazolam	0.5-0.1 mg/kg IM premed 0.5-2.5 mg to 0.1 mg/kg IV sedation 0.2-0.4 mg/kg IV induction 4-6 mg/hr IV infusion	Shortest duration* 20 minutes of hypnosis after induction
Diazepam	0.1-0.2 mg/kg PO premed 0.3-0.6 mg/kg IV induction	Postoperative sedation may last for several hours
Triazolam	0.25-0.5 mg PO premed	Shorter duration than diazepam with less postoperative sedation and greater amnesia
Lorazepam	0.5-4 mg (max 0.05 mg/kg) PO premed 2-4 mg IM	Prolonged postoperative sedation Amnesia at higher doses for 6-8 hours

*Duration of benzodiazepines variable—sedation lasts much longer than hypnosis

has been superseded by midazolam because of the latter's shorter half-life and lack of pain on injection.

Midazolam

Midazolam has 3 to 4 times the potency of diazepam with both a faster onset and recovery ($t_{1/2\beta} = 1$–4 hours), making it a more suitable induction agent. However, there is less hemodynamic stability. Blood pressure decreases—precipitously in the presence of hypovolemia—as peripheral resistance and cardiac output are lowered. Midazolam produces 40% reductions of CBF and CMRO$_2$ and is more protective than diazepam, but less so than thiopental. Midazolam may also be a better anticonvulsant than diazepam because of its higher CNS penetration and potency. There is no analgesia and no blunting of the response to laryngoscopy and intubation. Respiratory depression is slightly greater than with diazepam, especially in large doses or when narcotics are used concurrently. Anterograde amnesia is prominent, lasting 1 hour after an intramuscular premedication dose (absorption is reliable for intramuscular midazolam) and 2 hours after an intravenous induction dose. Patients may be responsive but demonstrate no recall shortly after its administration.

Metabolism occurs in the liver without production of active metabolites; it is not affected by H$_2$ blockers. Midazolam is supplied as an ionized, water-soluble drug at pH 3.5, but once injected the higher physiologic pH ensures that most of the drug is un-ionized and highly lipid-soluble. If used for intraoperative sedation, it is best titrated to produce a calm but not sleeping patient. Otherwise, confusion or a "startle" reaction is possible with sudden awakening.

Lorazepam

Lorazepam is not often used for neuroanesthesia because of prolonged postoperative sedation despite the lack of active metabolites. Recovery can be hastened if lorazepam is given the night before rather than the morning of surgery. Oral doses of 1 to 2 mg are used for sedation, 2 to 4 mg if amnesia (approximately 6 hours) is desired.

Triazolam

Triazolam is a shorter-duration oral benzodiazepine that has been used as a premedicant on the day of surgery. Recall is slightly lower than with diazepam.

Because of the possibility of prolonged sedation, benzodiazepines, including midazolam, should be used judiciously for neurosurgical patients in whom early postoperative evaluation is important. Increasing a dose may greatly prolong sedation while affecting hypnosis only slightly. Soon, this may be less of a problem with the release of flumazenil (RO 15-1788), a specific benzodiazepine antagonist capable of reversing both sedation and amnesia. It has been effectively used to treat benzodiazepine overdose. Flumazenil is given in increments of 0.1 to 0.2 mg IV every 60 seconds until adequate reversal is achieved. Rarely have doses greater than 0.5 mg been necessary. If flumazenil is given too rapidly or in too great a dose, CNS excitation can occur. Partial return of CNS depression may occur 45 to 60 minutes after the initial and second doses are employed.

Ketamine

Ketamine is a unique anesthetic with limited applicability in neuroanesthesia. A cerebrovasodilator, it increases CBF by 60 to 80%, producing a subsequent elevation of ICP that may be attenuated by hyperventilation or barbiturates. Ketamine also increases the resistance to CSF reabsorption, which over time may increase ICP beyond that produced by CBF increases alone. Cerebral metabolic rate is unchanged, though regional differences may exist.

Ketamine is known to activate limbic structures (increasing the cerebral metabolic rate for glucose) while depressing other regions (decreasing the cerebral metabolic rate for glucose), especially the cortex and associative fibers. However, this only occurs at anesthetic plasma levels. At subanesthetic levels, ketamine produces generalized CNS excitation with global increases in $CMRO_2$. Thus, a hypermetabolic brain is to be expected during recovery from ketamine anesthesia. The brain also becomes disorganized and incapable of properly interpreting sensory information. For this reason ketamine is an exceptional somatic analgesic. A summary of CNS effects is contained in Table 3-1.

Despite enhanced muscle tone, purposeless movements, and signs of CNS excitation with ketamine, no epileptiform activity is observed on the EEG. In fact, ketamine is able to suppress such activity and has even been used to treat refractory seizures. However, in epileptic patients both cortical and subcortical seizures have been reported. The typical EEG demonstrates a shift to theta waves (4 to 6 Hz) coincident with unresponsiveness, followed by high-amplitude delta waves (less than 4 Hz). There is no burst suppression as seen with barbiturates.

An interesting property of ketamine is its antagonism of glutamate, an excitatory amino acid released after injury that mediates neuronal cell death. The noncompetitive antagonism of glutamate receptors, most numerous in the limbic structures, may be responsible for ketamine's actions and hypothetically provide some protection to a region particularly vulnerable to ischemia. This is not a justification for using ketamine in elective neurosurgical cases where ICP is a potential problem. For the multiple-injured patient requiring emergency surgery, however, ketamine may not be as harmful as once thought.

Ketamine is a vasodilator but its sympathetic stimulation dominates, resulting in increases in heart rate, cardiac output, and blood pressure. This increases myocardial

O_2 consumption and may precipitate ischemia. It is also a direct-acting myocardial depressant and can lower blood pressure, especially in patients with high preexisting sympathetic tone. Slow injection minimizes this effect.

Airway obstruction is minimal with ketamine, making it a desirable anesthetic when access to the patient is limited. Respiratory depression occurs less frequently than with other agents, but apnea can occur with large doses or if ketamine is used with sedative hypnotics. Increased secretions can be minimized with anticholinergics. Airway resistance will be decreased only if initially elevated.

Emergence from ketamine anesthesia can be marked by hallucinations and agitation. Benzodiazepines greatly lower the incidence of these phenomena. Such occurrences may well be a manifestation of the CNS excitation produced by subanesthetic levels of ketamine and will impair neurologic evaluation. Blurred vision is common and persists for hours.

Ketamine is a lipid-soluble drug with excellent CNS penetration. It has a short duration but is cumulative with repetitive dosing. Metabolism occurs in the liver with elimination by the kidney. Clinical use is outlined in Table 3-11. See Table 3-4 for comparison with other intravenous induction agents and Table 3-3 for pharmacokinetic values.

Droperidol

Droperidol is primarily used as an antiemetic or in combination with a narcotic for neurolept techniques. Alone, it is a vasoconstrictor that decreases CBF and potentially ICP without altering $CMRO_2$. Theoretically, this could worsen ischemia, since CBF may fail to meet demand. Some have reported a synergistic decrease in $CMRO_2$ when droperidol and fentanyl are used in combination, but this is likely due to the effect of the background anesthetic. A useful adjunct for neuroleptic awake intubations or neurodiagnostic procedures, droperidol may result in unwanted postoperative sedation lasting up to 12 hours and provides neither analgesia nor amnesia.

Droperidol enhances the ventilatory response to hypoxemia when used alone but in no way overcomes the respiratory depressant effects of simultaneously used agents. Side effects—dyskinesia, akathisia, hallucinations, agitation—may confuse a postoperative neurologic evaluation. As an alpha-adrenergic blocker, droperidol may produce mild decreases in blood pressure.

Droperidol has a rapid distribution with a slow half-life. Onset is approxi-

Table 3-11 Ketamine—Clinical Use

Use	Dose (mg/kg)	Onset	Duration (min)†
Induction			
IV	1–2	Immediate	6–10
IM	5–10	2–3 min	10–25
Repeat doses (IV)	½ of initial*	Immediate	8–15
Infusion	1–2 mg/kg/hr*		

* Much lower if used with N_2O or narcotic
† May be markedly prolonged if used with volatile anesthetics

mately 3 to 10 minutes. As an antiemetic, a dose of 0.5 to 2.5 mg is used. It is usually not given alone because of the possibility of profound anxiety, at times resulting in patients' refusing subsequent surgery.

Muscle Relaxants

Muscle relaxants are used to facilitate tracheal intubation, provide surgical relaxation, and to ensure an immobile patient. They are chosen on the basis of (1) side effects, (2) duration, and (3) route of elimination. Side effects may include changes in ICP and blood pressure, the determinants of CPP, and are of obvious importance to the neurosurgical patient. The duration of muscle relaxation should correspond to that of the procedure to permit early neurologic evaluation, and requires the consideration of routes of elimination and how they may be affected by any coexistent disease. Below is a review of both depolarizing and nondepolarizing muscle relaxants with special emphasis on their use in the neurosurgical setting.

Depolarizing Relaxants

Succinylcholine is the only depolarizing muscle relaxant in common use. It is essentially a dimer of acetylcholine and acts as an agonist at the same receptor sites. At the neuromuscular junction it produces a rapid depolarization at the endplate but is degraded much more slowly than acetylcholine. Its continued presence at receptor sites rendors the motor endplate unexcitable to any incoming neuronal action potentials. Clinically, this sequence of events appears as fasciculation followed by profound relaxation.

Succinylcholine acts postsynaptically, producing a block that is monitored by a decrease in twitch height without tetanic fade, train-of-four fade, or post-tetanic facilitation, all of which are thought to represent presynaptic events. It should be noted, however, that succinylcholine can produce a so-called phase II block. This type of block is heralded by tachyphylaxis, followed by the development of characteristics of nondepolarizing blockage (e.g., train-of-four fade). Phase II block may occur after as little as 30 minutes of succinylcholine infusion at total doses of 2 to 6 mg/kg in the presence of volatile agents and 7 to 13 mg/kg with narcotic techniques. Pharmacologic antagonism is not uniformly successful and may complicate and prolong the inevitable spontaneous recovery, and is thus discouraged.

Succinylcholine does not act solely at the neuromuscular junction. It is an agonist at ganglionic nicotinic receptors and at cardiac muscarinic receptors. The chief clinical effect is a sinus bradycardia (prevented by prior administration of atropine) that is most often observed in children less than 1 year of age and in patients receiving a second dose of succinylcholine shortly after the first. Minor effects are catecholamine release and a lowered threshold for cardiac dysrhythmias. This may explain the nodal rhythms and ectopy, especially in the presence of hypercapnia and hypoxia, which often follow the use of succinylcholine.

The duration of action of succinylcholine is normally limited to 5 to 10 minutes because of rapid hydrolysis by plasma cholinesterase (PChE). When PChE activity is low, however, the duration may be substantially prolonged. This is evident in patients with atypical cholinesterase and those taking certain medications. Increased PChE activity has little clinical significance.

Succinylcholine has no effect on CSF dynamics but increases ICP independent of fasciculations, probably by cerebral vasodilatation. Despite the use of hyperventilation and thiopental during induction, larger increases in ICP have been noted with succinylcholine than with pancuronium. This increase is prevented by a complete nondepolarizing blockade and, more important, by "defasciculating" doses of metocurine (Fig. 3–3). Therefore, if ICP is a concern and succinylcholine is deemed necessary, its use should be preceded by a small dose of nondepolarizer (i.e., pretreatment), allowing 3 to 4 minutes for it to be effective.

Succinylcholine should be used cautiously in patients with neurologic or muscular diseases because of the potential for life-threatening hyperkalemia. The same warning applies to trauma and burn victims. Instead of the expected 0.5 mEq/L increase, potassium levels high enough to cause cardiac arrest may occur. Pretreatment with nondepolarizing relaxants is not protective. The mechanism of this complication is a proliferation of extrajunctional receptors that are very sensitive to agonists and are responsible for large fluxes of potassium (Fig. 3–4). The hyperkalemic response becomes evident within hours of trauma, days of burns, and 1 to 2 weeks of stroke. Rather than being comforted by a presumed grace period, however, it seems prudent to avoid succinylcholine whenever possible in patients at risk. For a list of various neuromuscular disorders and their responses to succinylcholine, see Table 3–12.

Other complications attributed to succinylcholine have been witnessed,

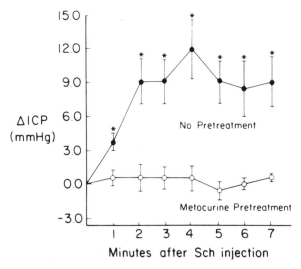

Figure 3-3 Changes (mean ± SEM) in intracranial pressure (ICP) after administration of succinylcholine (Sch) 1 mg/kg to anesthetized patients with malignant brain tumors. Open circles indicate values after administration of metocurine 0.03 mg/kg and Sch (group I); solid circles indicate values after administration of saline and Sch (group II). Baseline values prior to Sch were similar; after Sch, ICP increased significantly in group II and remained elevated. *P ≤ 0.5 compared to baseline value prior to Sch injection. (From Stirt JA, et al. "Defasiculation" with metocurine prevents succinylcholine-induced increases in intracranial pressure. Anesthesiology 1987; 67:50–53. Reproduced with permission of JB Lippincott.)

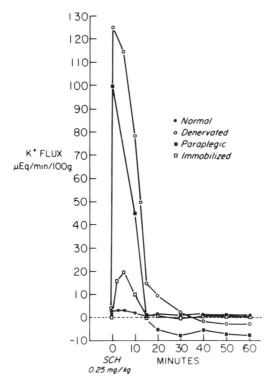

Figure 3-4 Potassium ion fluxes of normal, immobilized, paraplegic, and denervated canine skeletal muscle after injection of succinylcholine (Sch). (From Thiagarajah S. Anesthetic management of spinal surgery. In: Frost, EM, ed. Practical Neuroanesthesia. Anesthesiol Clin North Am 1987; 5:593. Reproduced with permission of WB Saunders.)

primarily in the pediatric population. These include the connection with malignant hyperthermia, masseter spasm and its possible link to malignant hyperthermia, pulmonary edema, and myoglobinemia. This has led some to abandon the routine use of succinylcholine in children. Despite its numerous shortcomings, succinylcholine remains a useful drug for emergency airway management. It produces a profound, rapid-onset block of short duration and can be given intramuscularly in a dose of 5 to 10 mg/kg (onset several minutes with this route). Contraindications are summarized in Table 3-13.

Nondepolarizing Relaxants

The nondepolarizing muscle relaxants (NDMRs) act as competitive antagonists primarily at postsynaptic, but also at presynaptic, cholinergic receptors at the neuromuscular junction. Blockade of the latter interferes with a positive feedback loop that modulates the availability of acetylcholine for neuronal release and is presumably responsible for the fade and post-tetanic facilitation that characterize a nondepolarizing block. The pharmacology of these agents varies considerably. Their selection must be based predominantly on cerebral physiology and the maintenance of CPP. This necessitates avoiding hypotension and elevations in ICP.

Atracurium

Atracurium has no effect on ICP despite mild histamine release. Blood pressure may drop somewhat with the rapid administration of large doses. Employing smaller divided

Table 3-12 Responses to Muscle Relaxants in Neuromuscular Disorders

Disorder	Response to Nondepolarizers	Response to Succinylcholine
Intracranial lesions		
Hemiplegia	Decreased	Hyperkalemia
Parkinsonism	Normal	Normal
Multiple sclerosis	Normal	Hyperkalemia
Diffuse head injury	?	Hyperkalemia
Encephalitis	?	Hyperkalemia
Ruptured cerebral aneurysm	?	Hyperkalemia
Tetanus	Normal	Hyperkalemia
Spinal cord lesions		
Paraplegia/quadriplegia	Increased	Hyperkalemia
Amyotrophic lateral sclerosis	Increased	Contracture
Poliomyelitis	Increased	?
Acute anterior horn disease	?	Hyperkalemia
Peripheral nerve lesions		
Neurofibromatosis	Increased	Resistance
Peripheral neuropathies	Decreased	?
Muscular denervation	Normal	Contracture/hyperkalemia
Neuromuscular junction lesions		
Myasthenia gravis		
Active	Increased	Resistance (early phase II block)
Remission	Normal	?
Muscular lesions		
Myasthenic syndrome	Increased	Increased
Myotonia	Normal/increased	Unpredictable Malignant hyperthermia association
Muscular dystrophy	Normal/increased	Hyperkalemia Malignant hyperthermia (Duchenne)
Ocular muscular dystrophy	Increased	?

Modified from Azar I. The response of patients with neuromuscular disorders to muscle relaxants: a review. Anesthesiology 1984; 61:173-187.

Table 3-13 Contraindications to Succinylcholine

Absolute Contraindications	Relative Contraindications
History of malignant hyperthermia	Increased ICP*
Severe burns ≤ 6 mo of age	Open eye injury
Severe trauma	Severe glaucoma
Upper motor neuron lesions	Hyperkalemia
Denervation	History of masseter
Neuromuscular disorders	spasm

* Attenuated or prevented by pretreatment

doses eliminates this problem. Otherwise, cardiovascular stability is well maintained (Tables 3–14 and 3–15).

Metabolism occurs in both tissue and plasma—two-thirds by ester hydrolysis, one-third by Hofmann degradation. The latter route yields the metabolite laudanosine which is capable of CNS excitation but not at concentrations observed clinically. This unique metabolism gives atracurium an unusual plasma decay curve that is unaffected by liver or renal failure. Its duration is 30 to 40 minutes following an intubating dose. It may be the relaxant of choice for myotonic dystrophy. It crosses the placenta to a moderate extent, potentially affecting the newborn.

Because of its relatively short duration despite large doses, atracurium is useful

Table 3-14 Muscle Relaxant Effects on Hemodynamics and ICP

Drug	Mean Arterial Pressure	Heart Rate	Intracranial Pressure
Succinylcholine	—	↓	↑
Atracurium	↓	↑	—
Vecuronium	—	—	—
Pancuronium	↑	↑↑	—
Metocurine	↓	↑	—
d-Tubocurarine	↓↓	↓ or ↑*	↑†
Gallamine	↑	↑↑↑	— to ↑
Pipecuronium	—	—	?
Doxacurium	—	—	?
Mivacurium	↓	↑	?

* Initially increased because of histamine release; as this dissipates the ganglionic blockade predominates
† Caused by histamine release

Table 3-15 Muscle Relaxants: Autonomic and Histamine Effects

Drug	Effect on Cardiac Muscarine Receptor	Effect on Autonomic Ganglia	Histamine Release
Succinylcholine	Stimulates	Stimulates	Slight
Atracurium	—	—	Slight
Vecuronium	—	—	—
Pancuronium	Moderate block	—	—
Metocurine	—	Weak block	Slight
d-Tubocurarine	—	Moderate block	Moderate
Gallamine	Strong block	—	—
Pipecuronium	—	—	—
Doxacurium	—	—	—
Mivacurium	—	—	Slight

Modified from Miller RD. The rational approach to the choice of a muscle relaxant. ASA Refresher Course No. 52, 1986.

for rapid-sequence induction. Its short duration makes infusion appropriate. Infusion rate should begin at 0.3 to 0.5 mg/kg/min after intubation, and then be titrated to effect. There is no cumulation, and duration is not increased with prolonged infusion. Atracurium should be diluted with normal saline because of its more rapid degradation in lactated Ringer's solution.

Vecuronium

Vecuronium does not affect CSF dynamics or ICP. Because of the large separation of neuromuscular and autonomic effects, cardiovascular stability is well maintained even at doses eight times the ED95 (i.e., 0.4 mg/kg; see Table 3–14). However, marked bradycardia may occur when used with narcotics, presumably because of the latter's unopposed vagotonic activity. Prior treatment with atropine is preventive.

Metabolism occurs in the liver, but failure of this organ only results in slight prolongation of duration because recovery occurs in its distribution rather than its elimination phase. Metabolites, one of which is moderately active, are excreted in bile. There is a small degree of cumulation. Vecuronium is safe in obstetric use.

Like atracurium, vecuronium is useful for rapid-sequence induction because of its duration. However, at higher doses used for rapid-sequence induction, its duration may be considerably prolonged. A maximum decrease in onset time is achieved with a dose of 0.3 mg/kg. Vecuronium may be used as an infusion; starting dose after an initial bolus is 0.05 to 0.1 mg/kg/hr, with titration to effect.

Pancuronium

Pancuronium has no direct effects on ICP but does have prominent autonomic effects. It is vagolytic, an indirect sympathomimetic, and alters conduction in the SA and AV nodes. The result is tachycardia, frequently nodal, with occasional ectopy and modest increases in cardiac output and blood pressure (see Table 3–14). These effects may be desirable in children or to maintain CPP in some patients, but may also unnecessarily increase CBF and ICP in those with impaired autoregulation and reduced intracranial compliance.

Pancuronium is metabolized in the liver and excreted by the kidneys. It is long-acting and cumulative. It is safe for use in obstetric and malignant hyperthermia patients. It is not as useful as other agents for rapid-sequence induction.

Metocurine

Metocurine does not directly affect ICP but does liberate a significant amount of histamine when administered rapidly. Given slowly, it has relatively few cardiovascular effects and its ganglionic blockade is of little consequence (see Table 3–14 and 3–15). It is sometimes used in combination with pancuronium because of the balanced side effects of the mixture. Metocurine is excreted largely unchanged by the kidneys. It is long-acting, cumulative, and seldom used for rapid-sequence induction.

d-Tubocurarine

Curare has no direct effects on CBF, CVR, or $CMRO_2$, yet it raises ICP in patients at risk. Presumably, this is due to the large histamine release that follows it administration. Histamine causes vasodilatation, hypotension, reflex tachycardia, and mild positive inotropy and increases vascular permeability, which in the brain results in cerebral edema. Although attenuation is possible by prior H_1 and H_2 receptor blockade and slow administration, this relaxant should not be used when ICP is a concern. Following the histamine response, heart rates tend to be low-normal. Curare exhibits stronger ganglionic and presynaptic blockade than the other NDMRs (see Tables 3–14 and 3–15).

Without significant metabolism, most is excreted unchanged by the kidney and to a lesser extent by the biliary system. It is long-acting and cumulative.

Gallamine

This seldom-used relaxant is similar to pancuronium but has even greater autonomic effects. It produces large increases in heart rate and cardiac output (see Table 3–14). It releases norepinephrine and predisposes to dysrhythmias. Gallamine is long-acting, cumulative, and excreted unchanged by the kidneys.

Pipecuronium

This is a new steroidal relaxant without cardiovascular effects. Cerebral effects are not likely to occur but have yet to be examined in detail. It is very similar to pancuronium in duration. It may afford few advantages over vecuronium.

Doxacurium (BW 938U)

This is a potent long-acting relaxant without side effects (see Table 3–14). It has unknown effects on ICP and appears to be similar to the other long-acting agents. It is excreted unchanged by the kidneys.

Mivacurium (BW 1090U)

The effects of mivacurium on ICP are not known. This drug does release histamine and may therefore lower blood pressure and increase ICP (see Table 3–14). It is a short-acting relaxant, is noncumulative, and was designed for infusion. Mivacurium is hydrolyzed by PChE at 90% of the rate of succinylcholine, giving it a duration 1.5 to 2.0 times that of single-dose succinylcholine. Infusion dose is 5 to 10 μg/kg/min.

Dosing guidelines for induction for all the relaxants discussed above are provided in Tables 3–16 and 3–17. Maintenance doses are one-quarter to one-half those required for intubation. If volatile agents are used, lower doses are needed because of potentiation, particularly with isoflurane and enflurane. Neuromuscular blockade is titratable using small, intermittent doses; pharmacokinetically, nothing is gained by using large initial doses.

In children, dosing is similar to that in adults despite the increased sensitivity of the myoneural junction in infants less than 2 months of age. The onset of actions of all NDMRs is faster in children, and the duration of atracurium and vecuronium is shorter. In the elderly, there is slower onset and prolonged recovery because of the decline in kidney function with age.

For rapid-sequence induction, succinylcholine is currently unparalleled, but its many contraindications often preclude its use. The onset of action of NDMRs can be hastened by increasing the doses, but only at the expense of increased side effects and duration. This makes the short-acting relaxants must suitable for this purpose. Its lack of side effects at high doses makes vecuronium a good choice for neurosurgical patients. Some believe that onset time can be further shortened with "priming," in which

Table 3-16 Guidelines for Clinical Use of Muscle Relaxants

Drug	Normal Intubating Dose (mg/kg)	Onset to 100% block (min)	Duration (min)
Succinylcholine	1.0	0.5–1.0	5–10
Atracurium	0.5	2.5	30–45
Vecuronium	0.1	2.5	45–60
Pancuronium	0.1	3	120
Metocurine	0.4	4	150
d-Tubocurarine	0.5	4	150
Pipecuronium	0.1	4	120–150
Doxacurium	0.05	4	100–120
Mivacurium	0.2	1.5–2	≤30

Adapted from Savarese JJ. The newer muscle relaxants. ASA Annual Refresher Course Lectures. No. 321, 1987.

Table 3-17 Rapid Sequence Induction (Intubation within 90 sec.)

Drug	Priming Dose (mg/kg)	Intubation Dose (mg/kg)	Duration* (min)
Succinylcholine	—	1 (1.5 mg/kg with pretreatment)	5–10
Atracurium	0.07	0.6–1.0	45–60
Vecuronium	0.01	0.2–0.3	60–90
Mivacurium	0.03	0.25	15

* Minimum to 25% twitch recovery
Reprinted with permission from Savarese JJ. The newer muscle relaxants. American Society of Anesthesiologists, Inc., No. 142, 1986.

approximately 10% of the total dose is given 4 to 6 minutes before the remainder. Timing of the split doses is critical, and 7% of the population may experience an undesired degree of blockade. It must be remembered that good intubating conditions depend not only on muscle relaxation but adequate anesthesia. When both are achieved, intubation can be accomplished in 90 seconds.

Anticholinesterases

Anticholinesterases are used to antagonize nondepolarizing neuromuscular blockade. Edrophonium, neostigmine, and pyridostigmine all temporarily disable acetylcholinesterase with subtle mechanistic differences and increase the amount of acetylcholine able to compete with NDMR at the neuromuscular junction.

The doses, onsets, and durations of the anticholinesterases are provided in Table 3-18. The larger doses are necessary for reversal of profound blockade, but supranormal doses have not proven helpful. It may take 30 to 40 minutes, even with edrophonium, to reverse profound paralysis. If reversal is inadequate 30 minutes after the anticholinesterase is given, consider electrolyte and acid-base problems or drug interactions. If muscle relaxation cannot be reversed, the patient should be ventilated mechanically until recovery is adequate (1 to 2 twitches) before a second dose of

Table 3-18 Anticholinesterases

Anti-AchE	Dose (mg/kg)	Onset (min)	Duration (min)
Edrophonium	0.5–1.0	1–2	60
Neostigmine	0.04–0.07	7–10	70
Pyridostigmine	0.2–0.35	12–16	120

anticholinesterase is given. If edrophonium is used to antagonize a profound block, the full 1.0 mg/kg should be used. Edrophonium and neostigmine have equal durations of antagonism, but many prefer the latter in cases of profound blockade. Despite differences in onset and duration, no advantage is obtained by combining these agents.

When used in patients with renal failure, there may be a slight delay in reversal, but "recurarization" is unlikely to occur because the anticholinesterases outlast the NDMR. In patients with neuromuscular disease, anticholinesterases may elicit abnormal responses such as increased paralysis or tonic contractions. Using a short-acting NDMR and attempting to forgo reversal may be preferable for such patients.

Although mentioned as a possible adjunct to antagonism of neuromuscular blockade, calcium cannot be recommended in the presence of brain injury because its role in cell death makes it potentially detrimental. It is better to ventilate the patient mechanically until adequate reversal is possible.

The anticholinesterases result in generalized muscarinic receptor stimulation because of the resulting increase in acetylcholine. Clinically, the bradycardia is of most concern; it is prevented by coadministration of an anticholinergic, either glycopyrrolate or atropine. For doses and effects, see Table 3-19. Glycopyrrolate's slower onset makes its use more suitable when given with neostigmine or pyridostigmine. It should be given several minutes earlier if used with edrophonium.

When used with the anticholinesterase agents, atropine may cause a temporary but undesirable elevation in heart rate. Atropine also causes CNS effects and may not be

Table 3-19 Pharmacology of Anticholinergics

	Atropine	Glycopyrrolate
Dose		
With edrophonium	7 μg/kg–10 μg/kg	0.01†
With neostigmine	15 μg/kg	0.01
With pyridostigmine	15 μg/kg*	0.01
Duration	15–30 min	2–4 hr
Effect on CNS	Mild sedation	None
Secretions	↓↓	↓↓↓
Smooth muscle tone	↓↓	↓↓↓
Heart rate	↑↑↑	↑↑

* Not recommended because of differences in onsets
† Give several minutes before edrophonium because of differences in onsets

desirable for the neurosurgical patient. The anticholinesterases, by increasing bronchial smooth muscle tone and secretions, can precipitate bronchospasm in patients with reactive airways. For such patients a larger than usual dose of glycopyrrolate given well in advance of the anticholinergic is helpful.

Suggested Reading

Bevan DR, et al. Muscle relaxants in clinical anesthesia. Chicago: Year Book, 1988.

Michenfelder JD. Anesthesia and the brain. New York: Churchill Livingstone, 1988.

Miller RD, ed. Anesthesia. 2nd ed. New York: Churchill Livingstone, 1986.

Stoelting RK. Pharmacology and physiology in anesthetic practice. Philadelphia: JB Lippincott, 1987.

C. Morgan Cooper, M.D., and Joseph A. Stirt, M.D.

Monitoring 4

Basic Monitoring

The primary goal in monitoring any patient undergoing a neurosurgical procedure is to have timely information about relevant physiologic variables in order to protect neuronal function. Monitoring of blood pressure, heart rate and rhythm, adequacy of ventilation, and temperature should be considered routine in all patients. Additional monitoring may be needed, depending on the patient's preoperative physiologic status.

Monitoring blood pressure using noninvasive Doppler/oscillotonometry (Dinamap) is mandatory in all patients undergoing a neurosurgical procedure. This is especially important in patients who are positioned prone or in those who have sustained multiple trauma. If indicated, direct arterial pressure monitoring is also used, but the noninvasive blood pressure cuff remains applied and ready for use if needed.

A continuous tracing of the electrocardiogram is also required for all neurosurgical operations. Manipulation of the brain stem is associated with changes in the rate and rhythm of the heart. Patients with head injuries may have associated changes in wave morphology and patterns including inverted T waves, large U waves, widened P-R, Q-T, and QRS intervals, plus wandering atrial or ventricular pacemakers.

Insertion of a pulmonary artery catheter should be completed preoperatively if the patient has significant underlying cardiovascular disease. If fluid balance is in doubt, a central venous pressure (CVP) catheter may be used.

Precordial or esophageal stethoscopes are employed to monitor heart and lung sounds. Often the patient's head, airway, and upper thorax are not accessible to the anesthesiologist, so continuous monitoring of heart and breath sounds is most important. This is especially critical when the patient is in other than the supine position.

Temperature monitoring is extremely important, since a large amount of body heat can be lost from a craniectomy or laminectomy incision. Hypothermia may delay wake-up time at the end of the procedure. Signs of increased body temperature should be addressed, since for every degree above 37°C, there is an exponential increase in $CMRO_2$ while cerebral blood flow (CBF) increases linearly. Above 42°C, direct thermal damage occurs. Deliberate hypothermia and circulatory arrest, once a popular technique for repair of complex intracranial vascular lesions, is rarely used today in neurosurgery.

Monitoring oxygen saturation with pulse oximetry has become the standard of care for almost all surgical procedures and should be employed in all patients requiring general anesthesia.

Depending on the type of surgery, the length of the procedure, and the preoperative physiologic assessment of the patient, additional monitors should be added to those discussed above. Justification for using a specific monitor depends on its utility in determining a patient's course and outcome and its ability to identify events that have a reasonable chance of occurring. Noninvasive techniques are preferred to invasive monitors if the information gained is of equal value.

Brain Monitoring

The purpose of monitoring the brain is to prevent changes that result in cerebral ischemia. The cerebral metabolic and neurodynamic effects of different therapies are discussed in Chapter 3. Usually no single parameter can define the degree to which ischemia is present, because the brain is a markedly nonhomogeneous organ. CBF may range from 20 ml per 100 g/min to 80 ml per 100 g/min in white and gray matter, respectively. Autoregulation maintains a constant CBF in normal adults by arteriolar adjustment to mean arterial blood pressure, $PaCO_2$, and PaO_2. CO_2 may alter flow by as much as 1.75 ml per 100 g/min for each 1 mm Hg change in $PaCO_2$. PaO_2 below 50 mm Hg will increase CBF (Fig. 4–1).

Monitoring devices must help to define the adequacy of cerebral perfusion pressure (CPP):

CPP = mean arterial blood pressure (MAP) − intracranial pressure (ICP)

CPP is the driving force behind CBF, and the control of CBF is maintained by autoregulation. Sustained ICP greater than 20 mm Hg may be significant in the face of

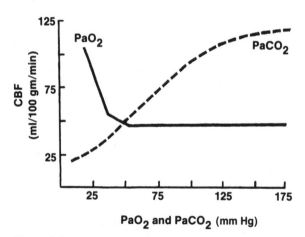

Figure 4-1 Changes in cerebral blood flow due to alterations in PaO_2 and $PaCO_2$. (From Shapiro HM, et al. Intracranial hypertension. Anesthesiology 1975;43:447. Reproduced with permission of JB Lippincott.)

hypotension, resulting in marginal CBF and CPP. Normal CPP in a normotensive adult is approximately 100 mm Hg. The lower limit of acceptable CPP in a healthy, normotensive patient with intact autoregulation is 50 mm Hg.

For all craniotomy patients, an indwelling arterial line should be routine for blood pressure monitoring. Mean arterial pressure is measured with the transducer at the level of the external auditory canal. Use of an arterial line allows for close monitoring so that wide swings in MAP may be avoided. It also allows for adjustment in $PaCO_2$ by intermittent measuring of arterial blood gas tensions. Because MAP and $PaCO_2$ greatly affect ICP, an arterial line should be placed prior to induction in any patient with symptoms of elevated ICP.

Intracranial hypertension is defined as sustained elevation of ICP greater than 15 mm Hg in the supine position. Invasive ICP monitoring of the high-risk neurosurgical patient may be required preoperatively if extreme signs of elevated ICP are present, such as a midline shift greater than 5 mm on computed tomography of the head, papilledema, vomiting, severe headache, or transient blindness. ICP monitoring during induction of anesthesia allows for appropriate adjustments in technique with titration of various anesthetic agents. Acute increases in pressure may occur during patient positioning (which has the potential for limiting venous return), at the conclusion of surgery (ICP may rise with application of head dressing), and postoperatively (rebleeding). Thus, ongoing monitoring of ICP would appear desirable and useful, but controversy persists about whether ICP monitoring affects outcome in any significant way.

There are four basic methods of monitoring ICP (Fig. 4-2): (1) epidural, (2) subdural (bolt or catheter), (3) intraventricular, and (4) intraparenchymal.

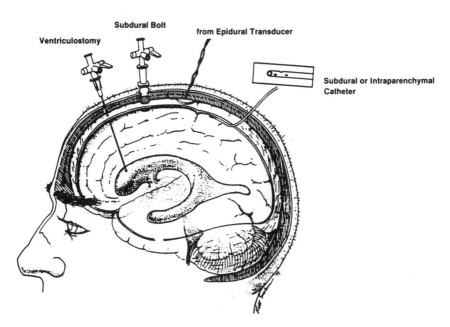

Figure 4-2 Commonly employed techniques and sites for ICP measurement. (From Shapiro HM. Neurosurgical anesthesia and intracranial hypertension. In: Miller RD, ed. Anesthesia. Vol 2. 2nd ed. New York: Churchill Livingstone, 1986:1577. Reproduced with permission.)

Epidural ICP Monitoring

Epidural pressure can be monitored by placement of a pressure sensor or transducer directly in contact with the surface of the dura. The advantage of this technique is that the parenchyma of the brain and dura are not disturbed, and problems with localization of a compressed ventricle are not present. When the transducer is located on the dura, recalibration of the system is impossible, and a variance of approximately 5 mm Hg in 24 hours remains a problem. This technique is accurate enough to distinguish relative changes in pressure and to give the physician an indication of rising ICP, although absolute values may not be accurate. Errors usually occur on the high side, and there have been no reports of patients with falsely negative readings who in fact had elevated ICP.

Extradural pressure readings may be 5 to 30 mm Hg higher than pressure measured by intraventricular methods. This may be due to the angle of placement against the dura or excessive pressure on the dura. The incidence of infection is low with this technique.

Subdural ICP Monitoring

Subdural pressure monitoring involves placement of a threaded bolt into the subdural space over the cerebral hemisphere. The hollow bolt is threaded into the subdural space through a 5-mm twist drill hole. The advantage of this technique is that it does not require brain penetration and location of ventricular position. What is important is that during placement the venous sinuses and proposed surgical site be avoided. Plugging of the subarachnoid bolt with cortical tissue and the inability to drain cerebrospinal fluid (CSF) therapeutically are major problems with this technique. Measurements are not as reliable as those obtained through a ventricular catheter, and infection remains a problem.

A second form of subdural monitoring employs a soft catheter placed through a burr hole into the subdural space. In children, a 22-g intravenous catheter may be used to obtain CSF from the anterior fontanelle and, if successful, left in place for monitoring purposes.

Intraventricular ICP Monitoring

Ventricular pressure monitoring requires placement of a catheter through the brain into the ventricular system, the catheter then being connected to an external electrical transducer. This is accomplished through a single-twist drill or burr hole placed through the skull, usually along the coronal suture line. Usually the ventricle contralateral to the side of the lesion is chosen for cannulation. The transducer is then zeroed at either the heart or the external auditory canal, thereafter keeping the reference point constant. An advantage of this type of monitoring is that CSF can be removed as a therapeutic measure to treat elevated ICP, or saline can be injected into the ventricle to calculate an intracranial compliance curve. Disadvantages include passage of the catheter through viable brain tissue, accidental release of CSF, difficulty placing the catheter in a compressed or distorted ventricle, and significant risk of infection.

Ten percent of catheterized patients have positive CSF cultures, although only 1% are clinically significant. Duration of monitoring, line breaks, and types of monitors affect infection rates. Other risk factors for infection are intraventricular bleeding, ICP greater than 20 mm Hg, or a neurosurgical operation. Prophylactic antibiotics have little or no effect on reducing the incidence of infection. Rates of infection increase significantly after 3 days, and essentially all patients become infected within 10 days.

Intraparenchymal ICP Monitoring

A small (4 French) fiberoptic transducer-tipped pressure-monitoring catheter system has been used intraparenchymally to measure ICP. This system measures pressures by optically detecting the movement of a light-reflecting membrane placed at the tip of the catheter. Any change in pressure causes a change in reflected light that is received and analyzed by a microcomputer, then converted into digital or analog signals. Calibration of the system occurs prior to insertion and is not affected by hydrostatic forces. The major disadvantages of this system are that the catheter enters neural tissue, the fiberoptic cables are relatively expensive and may fracture, and calibration can only be performed prior to insertion. The ease of use and resistance to artifact interference, however, make this type of monitor attractive.

Intracranial Pressure Waveforms

Three types of spontaneous pressure waves have been described by Lundberg based on their shape, duration and magnitude:

A waves: Sustained pressure waves (50 to 100 mm Hg) recurring relatively infrequently (5 to 20/min). A waves are life threatening.

B waves: Smaller, sharper waves (0 to 50 mm Hg) recurring rhythmically at a frequency of about 1/min, ranging from ½ to 2/min. These may be seen concomitantly with Cheyne-Stokes respirations and may be precursors of A waves.

C waves: Small, rhythmic oscillations (0 to 20 mm Hg) with a frequency between 4 and 8/min. These are usually related to changes in systemic arterial pressure.

If a disruption in the cranium exists, compliance of the system is increased, and thereafter even small elevations in ICP may represent a significant compromise in CBF. Perfusion may be decreased as a result of intracranial contents shifting toward the area, allowing for release of pressure (e.g., suture diastasis, bony defects).

Infratentorial–Posterior Fossa Surgery

Operations in the posterior fossa present many of the same concerns as procedures performed above the tentorium. Surgery here has special importance in that cardiovascular and respiratory control centers can be directly affected by manipulation of the brain stem or by a mass effect causing increasing pressure in the posterior fossa. Positioning the patient may pose additional concerns since the prone, sitting, or lateral "park bench" positions, while offering the surgeon optimal working conditions, may also compromise cardiovascular and ventilatory mechanisms and increase the risk of venous air embolism. In addition, severe flexion of the neck may kink the endotracheal tube or increase brain edema by limiting venous drainage of the head.

Manipulation of the brain stem or the cranial nerves, especially nerves V, IX, and X, may cause cardiac arrhythmias. Asystole, bradycardia, premature ventricular contractions, and ventricular tachycardia or other arrhythmias may occur in up to 50% of adults and 15% of children undergoing brainstem manipulation. For these reasons, close electrocardiographic (ECG) monitoring is critical. Good communication between the neurosurgeon and anesthesiologist will help correct these events, since most resolve when brain retraction eases.

Venous Air Embolism

Often the neurosurgeon, in order to maximize gravitational drainage of blood and CSF and to enhance surgical exposure when operating in the posterior fossa, will place the patient in the sitting position. By elevating the operative site above the level of the heart, the potential exists for the entrainment of air into the venous system (venous air embolism, or VAE). This occurs when veins encased in bone or held open by fibrous tissue (dural sinuses) fail to collapse. Air enters the venous system and flows down a pressure gradient into the right side of the heart, where it may eventually obstruct the pulmonary outflow tract, leading to cardiac failure and death.

Air may cross over into the arterial system, causing a paradoxical air embolism. Approximately 30% of the population has a potentially patent foramen ovale which predisposes them to such paradoxical air emboli. If air is entrained under certain conditions, such as during positive pressure ventilation or after prolonged time in the sitting position, the normal pressure differential between the right and left atria may become reversed, allowing air to enter the left atrium. From here its distribution to the brain or coronary arteries can have devastating consequences. Paradoxical air emboli have also been known to occur via the pulmonary vascular bed. During intracranial surgery, the first 60 minutes is the most common period for occurrence of VAE.

Monitoring for Venous Air Embolism

Routine Monitors

Blood Pressure.   Routine placement of a blood pressure cuff is mandatory. Postural hypotension occurs in approximately 30% of patients placed in the sitting position. A fall in MAP of 20 to 30 mm Hg is not unusual. This may be treated in the usual fashion with pressors and fluids. In the detection of VAE, a fall in blood pressure secondary to impaired cardiac output is a late finding.

Electrocardiography.   As with the monitoring of blood pressure, use of ECG, while mandatory as a first-line modality, is an insensitive method of detecting VAE. When changes occur on the ECG, physiologic deterioration has already begun. Signs of VAE on ECG include an increase in heart rate, peaking of the P wave, S-T segment suppression, and finally premature ventricular beats.

Esophageal Stethoscope.   The esophageal stethoscope is useful for listening to both heart tones and breath sounds. Auscultatory findings in VAE do not occur until air at a rate of 1.7 cc/kg/min is entrained into the venous system and cardiopulmonary compromise has occurred. The classic "mill-wheel" murmur is a continuous murmur heard during both systole and diastole. It has been described as the sound produced by shaking a plastic bag full of water and air. When the murmur is heard, it is a late finding and an ominous sign of impending cardiovascular collapse.

The esophageal stethoscope is the only way of detecting the "gasp" reflex, which occurs as a result of alveolar stimulation, this event being the first physiologic change seen with VAE.

Airway Pressure.   VAE results in decreased pulmonary compliance and increased peak airway pressures of 25% or greater. This is thought to be due to bronchoconstriction secondary to the release of various mediators.

Invasive Monitors

Arterial Line.   Any patient who is at significant risk for VAE should receive invasive arterial monitoring. Invasive monitoring provides not only the ability to quantify accurately beat-by-beat variability in blood pressure, but also allows for easy sampling of arterial blood for blood gas tension determinations and offers a more accurate measurement for calculating cerebral perfusion pressure. If the patient is placed in the three-quarters prone or "park bench" position, placement of the arterial line in the down-sided radial artery is preferred, because it allows the anesthesiologist to monitor axillary compression as well.

The transducer should be positioned at the level of the external auditory canal so cerebral perfusion pressure can be easily assessed.

Central Venous Catheter.   Placement of a CVP catheter is best accomplished by insertion via the median basilic vein of the arm, with the external or internal jugular approach as second choices. The arm is preferred in order to avoid any risk of pneumothorax or hemothorax, and to avoid confusing neck hematoma with postoperative signs of posterior fossa hemorrhaging. The CVP catheter allows the anesthesiologist to measure right atrial filling pressures and to aspirate air in case of VAE.

Air tends to collect high in the right atrium, and this is where the CVP catheter should be positioned. Accurate positioning may be accomplished by fluoroscopy or chest radiography. When chest radiography is used, if the film shows positioning of the tip of the catheter over the body of T7, the tip should be located properly near the right atrium. This approach can be time consuming, and even after a spot film is taken, warming of the catheter or changes in patient position may cause the tip to migrate out of ideal position.

A second method of CVP catheter positioning employs intravascular electrocardiography for catheter tip placement. Care must be taken to avoid cardiac microshock, and monitors should be properly isolated. A current leak of less than 10 microamperes is recommended. A metal stopcock can be inserted onto the catheter hub and this, in turn, wired to an isolation amplifier. The right shoulder ECG lead is then attached to the amplifier. As the tip is advanced, the morphology of the P wave on lead II changes as follows:

Superior vena cava: inverted P wave

Superior vena cava–right atrial junction: W-shaped wave

Midatrial: biphasic P wave

Conducting solutions of 8.4% $NaHCO_3$ or 4% saline are flushed through the catheter. Using a multiorificed catheter, electrical interference may occur with current flowing through the more proximal catheter openings. A multiorifice catheter is best placed over the superior vena cava–right atrial junction with the patient at 80 degrees in the sitting position. A single-orifice catheter is optimal when placed 3.0 cm above the cavoatrial junction. Some investigators have used a balloon-tipped CVP catheter which, with inflation, would "float" to the air-blood surface and allow for removal of entrained air. Aspiration flow rates of 240 cc/min are necessary to remove significant amounts of air from the central venous circulation. Therefore, a large-bore, multiorifice catheter should be used whenever possible.

Noninvasive Monitors

End-Tidal CO₂. Continuous end-tidal CO_2 monitoring ($P_{ET}CO_2$) is an intermediately sensitive way to monitor for venous air embolism. Normally, venous blood flows through the pulmonary artery to the lungs where delivered CO_2 is eliminated. When an airlock is formed in the pulmonary outflow tract, CO_2 cannot be delivered to the lungs, and end-tidal CO_2 falls. The decrease in $P_{ET}CO_2$ is roughly proportional to the size of the venous air embolism. Any event causing an increase in physiologic dead space may cause a fall in $P_{ET}CO_2$.

Present methods to monitor CO_2 include infrared in-line analysis, aspiration, and mass spectrometry. Argon laser analysis is a more recent variation.

End-Tidal O₂. The airlock described above also blocks the delivery of oxygen to arterial blood through the pulmonary capillaries. This will cause the end-expired O_2 tension to rise, and a change may also be seen thereafter on pulse oximetry as hemoglobin saturation subsequently decreases.

End-Tidal N₂. Venous air embolism will cause a rise in the end-expired N_2 concentration. Air is approximately 79% nitrogen and the appearance of end-tidal nitrogen in a patient breathing an O_2 and non-nitrogen mixture implies either a leak in the anesthetic circuit that is allowing entry of room air or VAE.

The combination of a fall in $P_{ET}CO_2$ and rise in $P_{ET}N_2$ should make the anesthesiologist highly suspicious of the occurrence of VAE.

Doppler Ultrasonography. Precordial Doppler monitoring is the most sensitive monitor of those typically used in the operating room for the detection of intracardiac gas. It is approximately 40 times more sensitive than the end-tidal CO_2 monitor in this regard. A bolus of air as small as 0.25 cc or air infusion as small as 0.015 cc/kg/min can be detected using this technique, making the Doppler an excellent prophylactic tool in the detection of early subclinical air entrapment. The anesthesiologist and surgeon can then be forewarned of significant VAE, and possible cardiovascular collapse can be avoided.

The correct placement of a 2.0 to 2.5 MHz ultrasonic probe is over the right atrium, usually between the third and fifth rib interspaces on the right side of the sternum.

Rapid injection of 3 to 5 cc of agitated saline into a central line will help verify proper positioning of the Doppler probe. The noise produced by the reflection of sound waves bounced off moving air bubbles in blood has been described as a high-pitched scratching noise similar to moving a phonograph needle over a record.

One of the major problems with the use of the Doppler is interference from electrocautery devices. A switch to turn off the Doppler may be incorporated into the electrocautery foot pedal control.

Transesophageal Echocardiography. Transesophageal echocardiography (TEE) is a recent modality being used by some centers in the monitoring of VAE. It appears to be just as sensitive as precordial Doppler, but offers enhanced specificity, since air can be seen. Another advantage of TEE is that paradoxical air emboli can also be detected. The theoretical advantages of TEE must be weighed against the cost, technical difficulties, and added impact on the anesthesiologist's attention to other patient-related functions. Some argue that if TEE is used, a trained technician should assist the anesthesiologist in order to prevent distraction from his or her primary tasks. Figure 4–3 depicts the various methods of monitoring VAE and shows when they are effective.

Neurophysiologic Monitoring

Electroencephalographic Monitoring

Ideally, electroencephalography (EEG) appears to be a superb, noninvasive monitor of cerebral function in the unconscious or anesthetized patient. Anything interfering with cerebral metabolic function such as hypoxia, ischemia, hypercapnia, or anesthesia should be reflected by changes on the EEG.

In its infancy EEG monitoring equipment was bulky, time consuming, and extremely difficult to use. As with any advanced electronic monitoring equipment, the use of EEG in the operating room places it in an electrically hostile environment. Interference from external sources, such as other monitors or electrocautery, will introduce artifact, decreasing the utility of the device. In order to minimize these effects, more advanced equipment incorporates electronic amplifiers and filters to improve the signal-to-noise ratio. In recent years many manufacturers of EEG equipment have modified the original design and have added computer capabilities to help make it more user friendly. Still, with all the simplifications there are concerns that (1) this monitoring modality requires the attention of a trained technician to assist the anesthesiologist in the care of the patient, and (2) simplifying the data might result in the loss of its integrity.

Why should the anesthesiologist bother monitoring the EEG? Obviously, one answer is that the EEG can provide information useful in determining if the patient is "asleep." This means that the EEG can help guide delivery of optimal anesthetic management. At this point in time, the technical considerations, expense, and time involved in set-up and operations outweigh the benefits. There are other, time-honored methods for determining the depth of anesthesia.

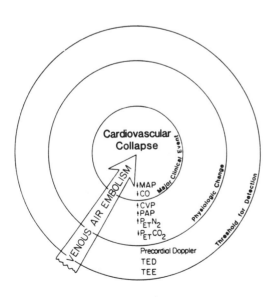

Figure 4–3 Clinical continuum of venous air embolism. Continuous venous air embolism produces a progression of clinical manifestations ranging from detectable air without physiologic change to eventual cardiovascular collapse. Symbols: TED = transesophageal Doppler; PCD = precordial Doppler; TEE = transesophageal echocardiography; $P_{ET}CO_2$ = end-tidal CO_2; $P_{ET}N_2$ = end-tidal nitrogen; CVP = central venous pressure; PAP = pulmonary artery pressure; MAP = mean systemic arterial pressure. (From Lucas WJ. How to manage air embolism. Problems in Anesthesia 1987;1:299. Reproduced with permission of JB Lippincott.)

The second reason is that the EEG provides a tool for the diagnosis of impending neurologic injury. It is presumed that if early warning of ischemia to the nervous system is known to the anesthesiologist, proper action to correct the insult can be undertaken in a timely fashion, and permanent injury will be avoided. Early intraoperative therapeutic measures might include elevating cerebral perfusion pressure, deepening anesthesia, or administering steroids or anticonvulsants.

The EEG may also serve as a predictor of outcome. The Mayo Clinic reported a large series in which no patient awakened with a new neurologic deficit that could not have been predicted from the intraoperative EEG.

EEG monitoring is currently used most often for cerebrovascular surgery, cardiopulmonary bypass, and deliberate hypotension. During these procedures, hypoxia or ischemia resulting from inadequate cerebral perfusion will adversely affect neuronal function, and it has been clearly established that cerebral metabolic and electrical activity correlates well with the mean frequency of the EEG.

Basic Principles of Electroencephalography

EEG waves are the summation of excitatory and inhibitory synaptic potentials generated by the pyramidal cells of the cerebral cortex, generally influenced by rhythmic discharges from the thalamus. Electrical activity is linked to metabolic activity, and the EEG, being a measure of electrical activity, is therefore affected by anything influencing metabolic activity, such as oxygen uptake or cortical blood flow.

Within any individual's EEG, variations are very small. This makes the EEG a useful parameter for monitoring, since any change from a stable baseline indicates a significant change in the brain's metabolic activity. During surgery, any transient EEG abnormality that is immediately recognized and corrected usually results in a normal recovery. In contrast, when a major EEG abnormality persists from the time of the insult to the end of the surgery, there is a significantly higher chance of permanent neurologic injury.

Technical Aspects of Electroencephalographic Recording

Figure 4–4 shows the standard reference point for electrode placements using the International 10–20 Electrode System. Placement of electrodes is calculated using a percentage of the patient's head circumference, interaural and nasion-inion distance. By convention, the left side of the skull is given odd numbers, the right side even. The code used is as follows:

F_p—frontal pole
F—frontal
C—central
P—parietal
O—occipital
z—midline

In the operating room, all available channels usually are not used. Much has been written about proper lead placement and the number of leads required for any given procedure. This remains the subject of much debate.

All channels of the EEG use two active electrodes and a reference electrode (monopolar montage, Fig. 4–5). A reference point G is chosen and measurements are made between F–G and C–G. The difference between these measurements results in a

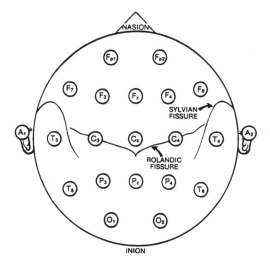

Figure 4-4 Position for EEG electrodes according to the International 10-20 Electrode System.

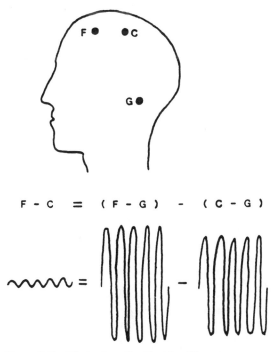

Figure 4-5 Elimination of artifact by difference amplification. To obtain the signal between F and C, a reference point G is selected. Since electrical artifact appears to be of equal amplitude for F-G and C-G, subtracting these two electronically produces F-C, the desired signal, free from electrical interference.

measurement of F–C. Electrical artifact common to each is processed out, and amplification of the difference between F and C is performed. This technique is called common mode rejection.

In Figure 4–6, the difference between bipolar and common reference montage is shown. With a common reference montage you have five channels available, with differences between adjacent electrodes being measured using the reference electrode at A_1. The advantage of this set-up is that the amplitude of the tracings is high, and this is significant in the electrically hostile operating room. The main disadvantage is that if there is any technical difficulty with A_1, all five channels become inoperable. The bipolar montage on the right side of the diagram records four channels. Even if one electrode fails in this configuration, some information remains.

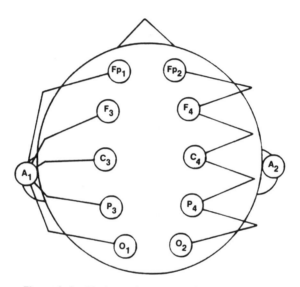

Figure 4-6 Bipolar and common reference montages. The left parasagittal electrodes are connected in a common reference montage using the left earlobe (A_1) as the common reference electrode. Five channels would be recorded, each of them between the parasagittal electrode and the ear electrode. Differences among these channels would represent the differences in cerebral activity among the various parasagittal electrodes, because each channel is recorded as the difference between the activity at the parasagittal electrode and the activity at the ear electrode. For comparison, the right parasagittal electrodes have been connected in a bipolar chain. In this configuration, only four channels of EEG data are recorded. Each channel of data represents the electrical difference between the two adjacent electrodes. (From Levy WJ. Monitoring. In: Kaplan, ed. Cardiac Anesthesia. 2nd ed. Orlando, FL: Grune & Stratton, 1987:323. Reproduced with permission of WB Saunders.)

Electrode Positions (Montage)

Since the EEG signal is normally symmetrical, lead placement is also symmetrical. Asymmetry in the face of a previously symmetrical pattern is suggestive of a catastrophic occurrence.

Electrode placement is somewhat dependent upon what information is sought. The gold-standard remains the classic 16-channel EEG. For detection of global ischemia, for the patient with therapeutically induced barbiturate coma, or for monitoring of anesthetic depth, a simple 2-channel lead placement as shown in Figure 4–7 can be used, since clinical studies indicate that most changes that may result from the typical responses to surgery and anesthesia in the operating room can be monitored without a complex montage.

A basic principle is that the EEG recorded at an electrode represents the electrical activity immediately adjacent to that electrode. The closer an electrode is to an area that becomes ischemic, the better are the chances of seeing a change. However, widely spaced scalp electrodes are also sensitive to cortical events in areas far greater than the area of cortex directly beneath the electrode. This is primarily due to the impedance of the skull. Therefore, some have advocated the simple montage shown in Figure 4–7 (A).

Placement of electrodes in a frontomastoid configuration alone might be adequate for accessing global ischemia, but is probably inadequate for monitoring middle cerebral artery ischemia. Thus, when using less than a 16-channel montage, electrodes ideally should be located so that the middle cerebral artery watershed area is being monitored. Figure 4–7 (B) shows a montage that accomplishes this goal.

To make the measurements required for adequate placement of the EEG electrodes, the following procedure is recommended:

1. Measure the distance from nasion to inion along the midline through the vertex and make a preliminary mark at the midpoint C_z. This point should be placed at an intersection with a line measured in the coronal plane from the root of the zygoma just anterior to the tragus bilaterally.
2. Placing the tape along the midline through C_z, points are marked at 10%, 20%, 20%, 20%, 20%, and 10% of the total nasion-inion distance. These will locate the positions of F_{pz}, F_z, C_z, P_z, O_z.

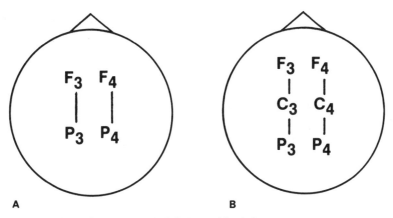

A   **B**

Figure 4–7   (A) 2-channel and (B) 4-channel lead placement

3. Reapply the tape transversely through C_z and mark points at 10%, 20%, 20%, 20%, 20%, and 10% of the total distance between the preauricular anchors. These mark the positions of T_3, C_3, C_z, C_4, and T_4. Remember, by convention the odd-numbered positions are on the left and the even numbers on the right.

4. Measure the distance between F_{pz} and O_z by applying the tape along the great circle passing through T_3 and again marking points at 10%, 20%, 20%, 20%, 20%, and 10% of this length. These note the positions of F_{p1}, F_7, T_3, T_5, O_1.

5. This is then repeated on the right side and using the same percentages, and the positions of F_{p2}, F_8, T_4, T_6, and O_2 are determined.

6. The distance between F_{p1} and O_1 is then measured by applying the tape along the great circle passing through C_3 and marking 25% intervals. These then give the positions of F_3, C_3, and P_3.

7. This procedure is again repeated on the right side and the positions of F_4, C_4, and P_4 are determined. All the F leads in the anterior coronal section should be equidistant as should the P leads, T5, and T6 in the posterior coronal plane.

Many types of electrodes have been developed to make the application easier and more efficient. The basic principles that apply are as follows:

1. The location should be clear of hair, oil, dirt, and dead skin. To improve contact and to reduce impedance, a degreaser and abrasive gel may be used.

2. The type of electrode will depend on the montage required. For those areas over the scalp beyond the normal hairline, or in less hirsute individuals, simple pregelled adhesive patches can be applied. When electrodes are to be placed over areas of normal hair growth, a silver disk electrode filled with conductive paste and cemented in place with collodion works well. It should be remembered that some cleansers and adhesives are flammable and are best used away from and prior to the application of any other electrical devices.

3. Stainless steel needle electrodes can be rapidly applied into the skin and in the properly premedicated patient produce only minimal discomfort. Hematomas, edema, and a nidus for infection can form around needle electrodes, thus increasing their impedance, which is further increased by their small surface area. The use of needle electrodes for cardiopulmonary bypass is contraindicated because of the degree of anticoagulation required.

Interpretation and Normal Findings

The EEG signal generated in the cerebral cortex is of low energy, around 2 to 200 mv as compared with the 500 to 1,000 mv for the ECG. Interpretation of the EEG involves measuring frequency and amplitude as well as evaluating the morphology of the waveform.

Frequency. The electrical waveform of the EEG is subdivided into sine waves of specific frequencies (cycles/sec, or Hertz [Hz]) as follows (see also Fig. 4–8):

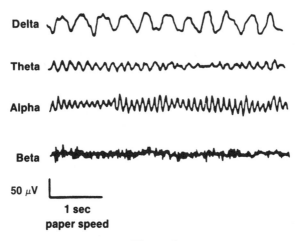

Figure 4-8   Four basic EEG waveforms

Delta (δ) 0 Hz to 3 Hz. These are high voltage, low-frequency waves consistent with stage 4 "deep sleep," deep anesthesia, or neuropathologic states.

Theta (Θ) 4 Hz to 7 Hz. Theta waves are seen predominantly in premature infants, healthy children during sleep, and during hyperventilation. They are also prominent during general anesthesia.

Alpha (α) 8 Hz to 13 Hz. Alpha waves are typically seen in a person who is relaxed, alert, and with eyes closed. Alpha waves originate primarily from the parieto-occipital regions. The typical alpha range averages approximately 10 to 11 Hz, with this baseline slowing with advancing age. In children, the mean frequency is within the low 8 Hz range, advancing to higher frequencies of 10 to 11 Hz during adulthood. Light anesthesia is characterized by a dominance of 10 to 14 Hz frequencies.

Beta (β) 14 Hz to 30 Hz. Beta waves are low voltage, fast activity rhythms typically seen in the awake, alert individual.

An isoelectric (flat line) EEG signifies electrical inactivity and is consistent with ischemia, hypothermia, barbiturate coma, greater than 2 MAC isoflurane anesthesia, or brain death.

Amplitude.   Amplitude refers to the peak-to-peak measurement of the wave form and is expressed in microvolts:

> Low amplitude: less than 20 μV
>
> Medium amplitude: 20 to 50 μV
>
> High amplitude: greater than 50 μV

Symmetry.   Normal brain activity demonstrates symmetry. Acute asymmetry signifies a potentially devastating event. However, an asymmetrical pattern during a neurovascular procedure such as a carotid endarterectomy, where the watershed area of the middle cerebral artery is affected, is commonly seen with slowing of the EEG relative to the contralateral side, without change in outcome.

Anesthetic Effects

Under general anesthesia, interindividual variability of the EEG decreases, and regional differences in frequency and amplitude become minimal. Patterns become similar throughout, and this is another reason some neuroanesthesiologists feel application of a simple bilateral fronto-occipital or frontoparietal montage can be justified. The EEG will vary according to the type of anesthetic agent being given, but since most anesthesiologists employ a combination of drugs, this is of little practical importance. The changes typically seen with increasing depth of anesthesia are primarily dose-dependent rather than agent-specific.

Induction. Induction with usual doses of thiopental characteristically produces a change in the beta pattern, with increases in amplitude, dispersion, and then a slowing in frequency toward the alpha range.

Sub-MAC Anesthetic Concentrations. As the alpha rhythm gives way to increased beta activity, a widespread anteriorly rhythmic pattern is seen in the low beta and alpha frequencies. As anesthesia deepens, the excitement phase disappears, and there is a progressive slowing in frequency.

Supra-MAC Anesthetic Concentrations. Large doses of anesthetics shift the EEG from theta to delta with increased slowing and finally a decrease in amplitude with burst suppression and ultimately an isoelectric EEG. Table 4–1 shows the effects on the EEG of various physiologic and anesthetic conditions.

Processing

The raw EEG records the changes of voltage over time. Computerized analysis converts this complex data through the use of fast Fourier transformation into power (amplitude squared) versus frequency. Fourier analysis uses a complex mathematical manipulation to reduce the complex EEG waveform into its component harmonically related sine waves. Displays of the unprocessed EEG signal are still very important and give the

Table 4–1 Factors Affecting the EEG

Increasing Frequency	Low Frequency, High Amplitude
Hyperoxia	Hypoxia
Hypercarbia	Hypocarbia
Hypoxia	Hypothermia
Seizures	Barbiturates
Low-dose barbiturates	Etomidate
Low-dose benzodiazepines	Narcotics
Nitrous oxide 30–70%	Inhalational agents >1 MAC
Inhalational agents <1 MAC	
Ketamine	
Low Frequency, Low Amplitude	Isoelectric
Hypoxia	Brain death
Hypercarbia	Hypoxia (Pa_{O_2} <25 mm Hg)
Barbiturates	Hypothermia (<17°C)
Hypoglycemia	Barbiturate coma
	Isoflurane-2 MAC

observer the chance to assess the validity of the processed data. Thus, the 16-channel EEG monitored by an experienced electroencephalographer remains the gold standard.

Cerebral Function Monitor.   The cerebral function monitor is a simplified version of the EEG in which the amplitude of the sine waves are measured and displayed as the average peak voltage on a strip chart recorder. This modality traces the product of power and frequency. The trace of the upper border represents peak-to-peak amplitude at its highest point, while the lower border represents the lowest point of the peak-to-peak amplitude. The monitor was originally designed to follow EEG activity in the intensive care setting. It remains a fairly good monitor for global ischemia, but is poor at detecting focal ischemia and is a poor choice for the measurement of depth of anesthesia.

Cerebral Function Analyzing Monitor.   This is an advanced version of the cerebral function monitor and offers the user a component breakdown of frequency and amplitude.

Power-Spectrum Analysis.   Power-spectrum analysis breaks the EEG down, analyzes it, and digitizes it using fast Fourier transformation. To simplify the data, a one-dimensional (univariate) descriptor of the power spectra may be determined. As the waveform is simplified into these univariate descriptors, much of the information inherent in the waveform is deleted. At times the information obtained can be somewhat misleading. The advantages of this technique are simplicity, and its ability as an indicator of global ischemia. However, it is quite sensitive to artifact and baseline drift.

Compressed Spectral Array.   Compressed spectral array is a three-dimensional display of frequency and power over time. Frequency is described on the X-axis, power on the Z-axis, and time on the Y-axis. Time and amplitude are then rotated onto the same axes. This graphic display of information is presented with clarity on a two-dimensional screen (Figs. 4–9 and 4–10). One of the concerns with this type of display is that high-

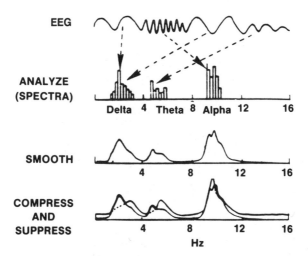

Figure 4-9   Steps in the generation of a compressed spectral array from segments of raw EEG data.

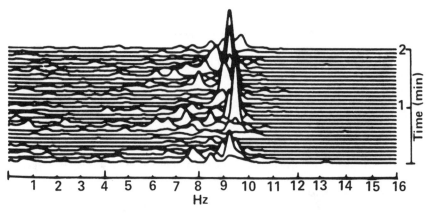

Figure 4-10 Compressed spectral array of a normal adult, showing a large peak corresponding to the alpha rhythm. (From Klass DW, Daly DD, eds. Current practice of clinical electroencephalography. New York: Raven Press, 1979:461. Reproduced with permission.)

amplitude activity tends to obscure concurrent low-amplitude activity at the same frequency. This results in the loss of some data and becomes significant when one looks at trends. This type of display may also include the spectral edge frequency, which is the frequency below which 97% of the power is found. Spectral edge frequency may be of greater benefit in measuring depth of anesthesia, but it does not accurately reflect a bimodal EEG and therefore might miss areas of focal ischemia.

Density-Modulated Spectral Array.   In order to avoid the loss of data behind the peaks within the compressed spectral array display, density-modulated spectral array (DMSA) uses light intensity or density of a dot matrix to represent the power at any frequency. This type of display currently appears to be enjoying the most popularity among clinical neuroanesthesiologists.

Monitoring in Carotid Endarterectomy

The role of EEG monitoring and the need for surgical shunting is the subject of serious debate. Nevertheless, 10% of patients undergoing carotid endarterectomy have EEG changes when the carotid artery is clamped, and just under 4% have a significant change requiring therapeutic intervention. Some clinicians recommend the use of a 16-channel EEG in monitoring for this procedure, but monitoring fewer channels appears simpler and almost as effective, as long as there are recordings that allow a comparison of symmetry. Ipsilateral slowing is significant for cerebral ischemia (Fig. 4-11).

Some centers use only frontopolar, central, parietal, occipital, or midtemporal placements. An example of both 2-channel and 4-channel montage is seen in Figure 4-7. A typical 2-channel montage might include F-P bilaterally, while a 4-channel lead placement might include F-C-P bilaterally. Frequencies are monitored between 1 and 30 Hz with a sensitivity of 5 μv/mm. A 10-minute baseline is usually obtained prior to clamping, and the EEG monitoring is continued for at least 10 minutes after release of the cross-clamp. Some centers go so far as to monitor the EEG continuously from the preinduction awake state to the awake state postoperatively. Even a normal EEG does not exclude the possibility of postoperative sequelae, since catastrophic events may occur once monitoring has been completed.

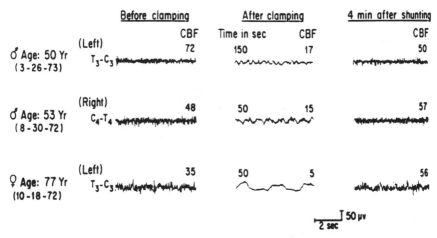

Figure 4–11 Carotid EEG. (From Sundt TM Jr, et al. Correlation of cerebral blood flow and encephalographic changes during carotid endarterectomy. Mayo Clin Proc 1981; 56:533. Reproduced with permission of the publisher.)

Cardiopulmonary Bypass

Identification of cerebral hypoxia is the primary reason for monitoring the EEG during cardiopulmonary bypass. Under controlled hypothermia, the EEG may be indistinguishable from that seen in hypoxia. This makes interpretation difficult. Seizure activity may also be seen secondary to either hypotension or an embolic event on cardiopulmonary bypass. Cerebral function monitoring has been used in the past for the detection of these acute events. It appears, however, that this is not adequate for monitoring focal ischemia. Four-channel monitoring may be preferable for detection of embolic phenomena, although this has yet to be determined by prospective study.

Monitoring for Depth of Anesthesia

Depth of anesthesia, arousal, and response to painful stimuli may be monitored using the EEG. At the present time, power-spectrum analysis appears the method of choice for assessing depth of anesthesia.

Anesthetic agents produce quite variable EEG patterns, from burst suppression to an isolectric EEG with increasing dosage of barbiturates and 2.0 MAC isoflurane, seizure activity with enflurane, and EEG slowing with large doses of narcotics. The EEG must therefore be interpreted in light of the known anesthetic (and surgical) conditions under which it is recorded.

Deliberate Hypotension

When blood pressure is lowered to an MAP of 50 mm Hg, there is always some risk of ischemic brain damage. EEG monitoring of brain function in this situation offers additional safety to the patient. The use of power-spectrum analysis has been shown to be effective in the detection of both focal and global cerebral ischemia.

Evoked Potentials

Principles of Evoked Potentials

While the EEG measures the surface summation of random spontaneous electrical cortical activity, an evoked potential is the response of the nervous system to an externally applied stimulus. As such, normal somatosensory evoked potentials (SSEPs) reflect the integrity of the pathway being studied. These pathways are ascending sensory tracts usually involving a peripheral or cranial nerve. If the study of evoked potentials is to be useful during anesthesia, four criteria must be met:

1. Neural pathways at risk must be accessible to monitoring.
2. Appropriate sites must be available for stimulating and recording data.
3. Skilled technicians must be available for data interpretation and equipment assessment.
4. If abnormal evoked potentials appear, the possibility for therapeutic intervention must exist.

Typically, evoked potentials tend to get buried in the EEG signal because of their low amplitude (1 to 5 μV). Signal averaging helps to amplify the evoked potential, while extraneous random EEG activity and other "noise" is filtered out electronically. However, when a large portion (25%) of any evoked potential waveform is eliminated, the waveform generated may be misleading.

Various factors such as electrical noise, hypothermia, ischemia, changes in $PaCO_2$, anesthesia, age, gender, stimulus characteristics, and electrode placement can affect evoked potentials. Figure 4–12 is a typical example of an SSEP.

Classification and Terminology

Latency. Latency is the elapsed time between application of the stimulus and its recording. It is measured in milliseconds and increases with hypothermia, anesthesia, and ischemia.

Amplitude. The amplitude of the evoked potential is approximately an order of magnitude less than the EEG (evoked potentials are approximately 1 to 5 μV in amplitude as compared to the EEG, which runs approximately 10 to 200 μV in amplitude). The amplitude may also be affected by anesthesia, ischemia, hypothermia, and the strength and site of the application of the neural stimulus.

Near-Field Potentials. Near-field potentials are stimuli that are recorded by electrodes close to the neurogenerative source (e.g., the sensory cortex) (Table 4–2). Because the source of the stimulus is in the cortex of the brain, it is anatomically close to the surface scalp recording electrode. Although close, the latency period is relatively long (<100 msec) because the stimulus must travel across multiple synapses before reaching the scalp electrode. The voltage of a near-field potential is preserved with normal synaptic function.

Far-Field Potentials. Far-field potentials arise from subcortical neurogenerative sources that are relatively "far away" anatomically from the scalp electrode (e.g., the brain stem) (Table 4–2). Any stimulus applied peripherally will, as it travels up the spinal cord, reach the brain stem first. From there it is conducted rapidly through neural tissues

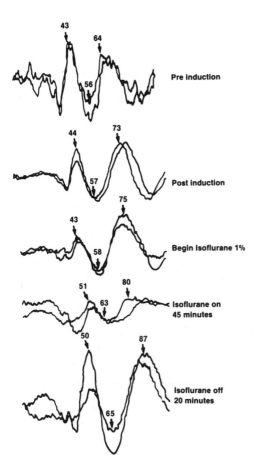

43
64
56
Pre induction

44
73
57
Post induction
75

43
58
Begin Isoflurane 1%

51
80
63
Isoflurane on
45 minutes

50
87
Isoflurane off
20 minutes
65

Figure 4-12 Cortical somatosensory evoked potentials for an awake and an anesthetized patient. The posterior tibial nerve of a patient was stimulated 1,024 times with 5.1 stimuli/sec. All cortical responses were averaged. In order to suppress extraneous signals a filter was used to eliminate all frequencies below 30 Hz and above 250 Hz. The numbers attached to the positive and negative potentials represent the time (in milliseconds) that elapsed after the stimulation, also called the latency. Thus all recorded potentials arose with a latency of less than 100 msec. Such potentials are called near-field potentials. These are assumed to arise in nervous tissue near the scalp electrode, in other words, in the cortex of the patient's brain. The figure shows how isoflurane increases the latency and decreases the amplitude of the near-field evoked somatosensory evoked potential. (From Gravenstein JS, Paulus DA, eds. Clinical monitoring practice. Philadelphia: JB Lippincott, 1987:265. Reproduced with permission.)

Table 4-2 Characteristics of Near-Field and Far-Field Evoked Potentials

Near-Field Potentials	Far-Field Potentials
Cortical neurogenerator	Brainstem neurogenerator
Longer latency (<100 msec)	Short latency (<45 msec)
Shorter distances	Longer distances
Larger amplitude (higher voltage)	Lower amplitude (lower voltage)
Less amplication required	Requires more amplification
Fewer individual responses required (50–200)	Requires more rapid rates of stimulation (1,000s)
More sensitive to anesthetic/ physiologic effects	Less sensitive to anesthetic/ physiologic effects

to the surface scalp electrode. Although the distance traveled is significantly longer anatomically, the speed of conductance is quite fast. This results in a short latency (<45 msec).

Another feature of far-field potentials is that, because of the longer distance they travel, signal strength fades, resulting in relatively low voltage and therefore lower amplitude. In order to enhance the reception of these potentials, increased amplification of multiple, repeated stimuli is required.

Types of Evoked Potentials

Somatosensory Evoked Potentials.   The technique used by most electrophysiologists is to monitor two channels, with electrodes placed over the anatomic pathways to be studied. Sites are chosen so that pathways below and above the proposed surgical site are monitored. For scoliosis or aortic surgery, typically the median nerve above and the posterior tibial nerve below are stimulated respectively along with corresponding cortical sites (Fig. 4–13). If there is a thoracic or lumbar-level insult, a change may be seen on the posterior tibial trace. Interruption of the conduction pathway at any point between site of stimulation and the cerebral cortex can alter the cortical SSEPs. This may occur secondary to ischemia, retraction, or direct surgical disruption. Surgical treatment of scoliosis is associated with a 1 to 3% risk of spinal cord damage, depending on the technique used in the application of Harrington or Luque fixation.

Traditionally a "wake-up" test is performed to see if, after instrumentation and prior to closure, the patient can voluntarily move his or her legs. Depending on the results, the patient is either reanesthetized and possible corrections instituted, or closure of the incision is completed. While SSEP monitoring is a valuable tool for the diagnosis of spinal cord ischemia, false-negative results have been reported. The wake-up test provides proof of intact function; however, it does so only at a single point in time. SSEP enhance surveillance by offering an acceptably reliable continuum in the measurement of sensory pathway integrity. Depending on the institution, a wake-up test may be performed prior to closure in all patients undergoing scoliosis repair, or immediately intraoperatively only in those with changes in the SSEP. It remains prudent to monitor SSEP continuously for changes intraoperatively while still undertaking the wake-up test just before closure, even in the presence of normal waveform morphology.

Brainstem Auditory Evoked Potentials.   Brainstem auditory evoked potentials (BAEPs) are generated by an audible click delivered to each ear in sequential fashion in order to stimulate the eighth cranial nerve and associated brainstem pathways. The signal is then recorded by scalp electrodes positioned over the vertex. BAEP monitoring is used at present during surgery involving the eighth cranial nerve, such as for acoustic neuromas or with surgery in the posterior fossa, such as microvascular decompression for trigeminal neuralgia, where the brain stem may be at risk.

BAEPs are short-latency potentials that may be affected by surgical retraction of the eighth cranial nerve or by any of the other variables previously described. Loss or alteration of waveform may be reversible if intervention occurs in a timely fashion. No patient with preserved BAEPs has been reported to incur permanent hearing loss; therefore, loss of the BAEP waveform may be a highly specific prognostic indicator of unilateral deafness.

Visual Evoked Potentials.   Visual evoked potentials (VEPs) are generated by flashes of light presented monocularly through the closed eyelid. The eyes are protected in the

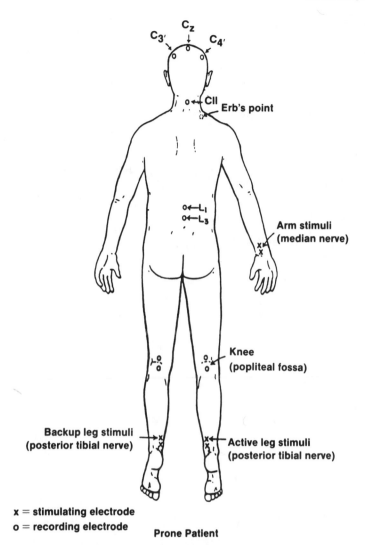

x = stimulating electrode
o = recording electrode

Prone Patient

Figure 4-13 The median nerve and posterior tibial nerve of a patient are stimulated. Electrode locations for both stimulating and sensing are shown (patient is prone). $C_{3'}$ is located centralateral to the site of stimulation, 3 cm posterior to C_3. $C_{4'}$ is ipsilateral to the stimulation; it is 3 cm posterior to C_4. (From Gravenstein JS, Paulus DA, eds. Clinical monitoring practice. Philadelphia: JB Lippincott, 1987:270. Reproduced with permission.)

usual fashion with ointment and clear plastic tape. Intraoperative monitoring using VEP has been performed during surgery for pituitary lesions and resection of lesions in the anterior cranial fossa. VEPs are quite variable and are very sensitive to metabolic changes and anesthetics. At this time, VEP is considered unreliable and of little value in the operating room.

Suggested Reading

Friedman WA, et al. Monitoring of sensory evoked potentials is highly reliable and helpful in the OR. J Clin Monit 1987; 3:38.

Ginzburg HH, et al. Postoperative paraplegia with preserved intraoperative somatosensory evoked potentials. J Neurosurg 1985; 63:296.

Levy WJ. Intraoperative EEG patterns: implications for EEG monitoring. Anesthesiology 1984; 60:430.

Levy WJ, et al. Automated EEG processing for intraoperative monitoring: a comparison of techniques. Anesthesiology 1980; 53:223.

Michenfelder JD. Intraoperative monitoring of sensory evoked potentials may be neither a proven nor an indicated technique. J Clin Monit 1987; 3:45.

Rampil IJ, et al. Prognostic value of computerized EEG analysis during carotid endarterectomy. Anesth Analg 1983; 62:186.

Sundt TM, et al. Correlation of cerebral blood flow and electroencephalographic changes during carotid endarterectomy. With results of surgery and hemodynamics of cerebral ischemia. Mayo Clin Proc 1981; 56:533.

Richard J. Sperry, M.D.

Positioning in Neurosurgery 5

Proper patient positioning and the physiologic consequences of positioning are not given active attention in most anesthesiology training programs. These subjects are usually left for residents to discover on their own. However, many preventable injuries occur when an anesthesiologist does not pay scrupulous attention to details during patient positioning. Also, the consequences of positioning need to be anticipated so that adequate preparations may be made. Hence the irony in our lack of formal training.

This chapter discusses proper ways to place a patient in the supine, prone, and sitting positions. The physiology, common injuries, and complications of these positions are also covered. No suggestion is made that these are the only ways to safely position a patient. Rather, one or two safe and proven methods are presented.

The Supine Position

Although the supine position is not unique to neurosurgery, many neurosurgical procedures are performed in this position. This chapter reviews this common position and serves as a springboard to compare the effects of other positions.

The physiologic alterations seen with positioning the healthy, awake patient may be different from those seen in a patient under anesthesia. The compensatory actions of the central nervous system and the cardiovascular system will be depressed in direct proportion to the anesthetic concentration. The picture of depression will vary, depending on anesthetic techniques and the patient's disease, age, and medication regimen. Therefore, it is vital that the patient be closely monitored during any major position change, especially if there is significant cardiovascular or pulmonary disease.

The major physiologic changes seen in the supine patient are in the cardiovascular and respiratory systems.

Cardiovascular Effects

In the supine position, venous return increases, producing an increase in stroke volume and cardiac output. Sympathetic tone decreases, yielding a decrease in mean arterial blood pressure, heart rate, and peripheral vascular resistance. The systolic blood pressure remains at about the same level; however, the diastolic blood pressure is decreased and the pulse pressure is therefore increased.

Respiratory Effects

There is a reduction of the functional residual capacity (FRC) upon assuming the supine position and a further reduction with the induction of general anesthesia. The supine, anesthetized patient has an FRC decrement of approximately 1 liter. This may have significant implications for oxygen exchange in the lung for some patients.

Closing capacity is important as it relates to FRC. Closing capacity is the lung volume when distal airways begin to close, excluding distal lung units from ventilatory gas exchange. Units that remain closed during tidal ventilation become atelectatic and contribute to intrapulmonary shunt. Units that close early are poorly ventilated and contribute to ventilation-perfusion mismatch. Small airway closure normally occurs at a significantly smaller lung volume than FRC, and all lung units remain functionally patent. However, if FRC is reduced, as in the supine, anesthetized patient, or closing capacity is increased by age or disease, airways may begin to close, producing relative hypoxia.

Anesthesia administered in the supine position may also alter normal ventilation-perfusion relationships. In the upright position, gravitational influences provide a gradient of blood flow in the lung (least in the apex and greatest in the base). Because of an intrapleural pressure gradient from apex to base and the shape of the pulmonary compliance curve, ventilation is also greatest in the bases. Thus, ventilation and perfusion are normally well matched.

In the supine position, gravity causes perfusion to be greatest in the dorsal aspect of the lung. The abdominal contents force the dorsal portion of the diaphragm more cephalad, placing it on a more advantageous part of its length-tension curve. Thus, a spontaneously breathing patient ventilates the dorsal lung best and ventilation-perfusion relationships remain intact.

However, during controlled ventilation the abdominal contents decrease the compliance of the dorsal lung. The ventral lung thus receives more ventilation but the same amount of perfusion. Thus, ventilation and perfusion are not well matched, and hypoxemia may result.

Central Nervous System Effects

Since many neurosurgical patients undergo surgery in the supine position and nearly all patients are nursed in this position, it is important to discuss the effects of the supine position on cerebral blood volume and intracranial pressure.

In any position, adequate venous drainage must be assured. Cerebral venous congestion will lead to an increase in cerebral blood volume and thereby intracranial pressure if intracranial compliance is reduced. The head must be maintained in an unobstructing posture, allowing the internal jugular veins to drain properly. Extremes of neck flexion and rotation must be avoided in patients with an intracranial mass. Elevation of the head 15 to 30 degrees will encourage venous drainage.

Complications

All positions are associated with potential positioning trauma or other complications. This section covers the complications associated with the supine position. However, many of these complications apply equally to other positions.

It is important to determine the points of weight bearing imposed by a given position. These points must be appropriately padded and protected. The weight of the supine patient is borne by the occiput, scapulae, elbows, sacrum, calves, and heels. These points should be padded and should rest on soft material that is not wrinkled. Wrinkled material can produce secondary skin and subcutaneous tissue pressure that may lead to an ischemic insult. Several case reports exist that describe tissue necrosis at these weight-bearing points following prolonged procedures.

After the induction of general anesthesia and the onset of muscle relaxation, the musculoskeletal system is susceptible to abnormal stress. Joints are normally protected from hyperextension by muscle tone, pain sensation, and proprioceptive reflexes. With all these protections lost under anesthesia, the patients' joints may be placed in abnormal flexion or extension, resulting in injury. This is particularly true when a patient is turned, placed prone, or moved to the sitting position.

The cervical spine is of particular concern during positioning because it is very susceptible to injury and such injury can have grave consequences. The head forms a pendulum on the end of the neck and can produce great torque and other disruptive forces. The head must be stabilized and held midline during positioning.

Stress and stretch can be placed on the elements of the thoracic and lumbar spine with the onset of muscle relaxation and, with a flat operating table, the normal lumbar lordosis is lost and ligaments can be stretched. Backache is a common postoperative complication. This can be minimized by some lumbar support or with pillows placed under the legs.

The peripheral nerves are also vulnerable in an anesthetized patient and are frequent sites of injury. The brachial plexus and its branches are the nerves most commonly injured. The ulnar nerve passes along the medial side of the humerus and becomes very superficial at the medial epicondyle. Compression of the ulnar nerve at the elbow is likely if the elbow is not protected. The ulnar nerve is most vulnerable with the hand and the forearm in pronation. Supination places the ulnar nerve in a more protected position.

The brachial plexus is also subject to stretch injury with extreme abduction of the arm. The radial and axillary nerves may be compressed by the ether screen poles or other attachments to the operating table. The median nerve is adjacent to major blood vessels at the elbow and can be injured during attempts at vascular cannulation.

The brachial plexus and its branches can be protected by following these guidelines:

1. Pad the elbow
2. Never abduct the arm more than 90 degrees
3. Supinate the hand and forearm
4. Protect the arm from compression by the operating table attachments

Function of the various upper extremity peripheral nerves can be tested rapidly, as shown in Figure 5-1.

The Prone Position

Most procedures on the thoracic and lumbar spine, many procedures on the cervical spine, and some intracranial procedures are performed in the prone position.

Patients may be pronated either before or after the induction of anesthesia. Awake pronation can be useful in patients with a compromised spinal canal and a neurologic deficit that may be worsened with handling. The patient can indicate pain

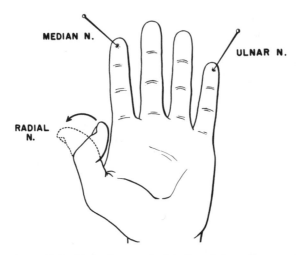

Figure 5-1 Method to test the function of the major upper extremity nerves. Injury to the musculocutaneous nerve causes loss of biceps function and inability to flex the forearm. Injury to the axillary nerve causes loss of deltoid function and inability to abduct the arm. (From Martin JT. Positioning in anesthesia and surgery. 2nd ed. Philadelphia: WB Saunders, 1987. Used with permission.)

upon assuming a certain position. Also, a quick neurologic examination can be performed to document the absence or presence of progression of neurologic deficits. If progression of a deficit is found, the faulty positioning can be corrected.

Awake pronation requires adequate sedation and topical anesthesia to permit awake intubation. After adequate positioning, general anesthesia is produced by the intravenous or inhalational method.

Pronation of the patient following the induction of anesthesia requires planning and the coordination of many members of the operating team. Injuries can occur to both patient and team members alike.

Optimal pronation of an anesthetized patient requires a level of anesthesia that blunts autonomic reflexes, but that is not so deep as to risk hypotension. If narcotics are to be used as a part of the anesthetic, it is useful to administer a loading dose to the patient prior to pronation. A fluid bolus of about 500 ml can stabilize the patient's hemodynamics. Neuromuscular blockade should also be achieved prior to pronation.

To pronate the patient, first move the bed parallel and directly adjacent to the operating table. Two assistants stand on the free side of the table to receive the patient, and two stand on the free side of the stretcher. One assistant manages the feet. If the cervical spine is stable, the anesthesiologist manages the head and coordinates the turn. If the cervical spine is unstable, the neurosurgeon handles the head during pronation and coordinates the turn. Place and keep the arms of the patient alongside the body. At the signal from the person managing the head, disconnect the patient from the anesthesia machine and turn him gradually onto the outstretched arms of the receiving assistants. Hold the arms alongside the body and the head in the sagittal plane during the turn.

After the turn is complete, reconnect the patient to the anesthesia machine and auscultate the lung fields for appropriate endotracheal tube position. The assistants then move their arms from under the patient, who remains supported by appropriate chest rolls. The chest rolls should support the lateral edge of the torso from clavicle to pelvis.

Next, gently rotate the head toward the anesthesia machine and place it on a headrest. Special attention must be given to the downside eye and ear. No pressure should be placed on either of these two structures.

Secure the arms either alongside or in front of the patient.

Cardiovascular Effects

The cardiovascular system usually adapts well to the prone position. Depending upon the level of the legs in relation to the heart, venous pooling may reduce cardiac filling pressures and cardiac output. Improper positioning may obstruct the femoral veins or inferior vena cava, causing a decrease in venous return and blood pressure. Wrapping the legs in elastic or pneumatic stockings helps prevent venous pooling. This assists in maintaining cardiac filling pressures and thereby cardiac output and blood pressure.

Respiratory Effects

The respiratory system can be significantly compromised by incorrect prone positioning. A prone patient who is allowed to breathe spontaneously must raise the entire thoracic mass off the sternum to expand the pleural cavity. This can significantly increase the work of breathing. The work of breathing is increased further by the force exerted on the diaphragm by the abdominal contents, which are forced cephalad because of compression from the weight of the dorsal trunk.

If the patient is appropriately supported by chest rolls, the chest and abdomen will hang free. Ventilation would thus be accomplished with normal pressures. The FRC decrement seen in the supine position is not found in a properly positioned prone patient.

Central Nervous System Effects

The vertebral venous plexus forms an important anastomotic channel with the femoral veins and the inferior vena cava. When these venous channels are obstructed, blood will return from the lower extremity to the heart through the vertebral veins. Distention of the vertebral veins will lead to increased intraoperative bleeding and potentially decreased surgical visibility.

Proper positioning of a prone patient on chest rolls has many benefits. Ventilation is accomplished at lower airway pressures, decreasing the chance of barotrauma. As ventilation proceeds with a free abdomen and thorax, there is less motion of the back, motion which is exaggerated under the microscope, and cerebrospinal fluid flux in the wound is less. A properly supported patient also decreases vertebral venous engorgement and bleeding.

Complications

The prone position has much potential for patient injury. The endotracheal tube may become displaced, and vascular access lines and monitors are more precarious. These must be adequately secured prior to pronation and must be guarded during the turn.

Attention must be afforded various soft tissues such as breasts and genitalia. The breasts should be placed medially between the chest rolls. The delicate skin of the nipple and areola should not be stretched.

Both male and female genitalia should be in the midline. These tissues should have no stretch or pressure placed on them.

The eyes should be lubricated and taped shut so as to avoid drying and injury to the cornea. The padded head support must not place pressure on the eye or ischemia may result. Multiple case reports document the potential for blindness following eye compression. This is of particular concern when a horseshoe headrest is used. The head supports must be spaced widely enough to allow both eyes to be free. A pin-based head holder may be a better alternative for head fixation than a horseshoe headrest.

The downside ear should be flat and not folded upon itself. Ischemic injury to the ear may result if this remains unnoticed. Plastic reconstruction of an external ear is difficult, and results are often poor.

Additionally, pressure must not be placed in the preauricular area. The facial nerve is superficial in this area and can be injured.

Care must be taken during chest roll placement and arm positioning to protect the brachial plexus and its branches. The head of the humerus can be forced into and may compress the neurovascular bundle if the arms and axillae are not relaxed. The ulnar nerve and radial nerve are also susceptible to compression at the elbow and should be protected as described on page 93.

Undue neck rotation cannot only cause postoperative neck pain but may also add to brachial plexus stretch.

Pathologic joints, found in the rheumatoid arthritis patient, must not have force applied to them during positioning. All such patients should be considered to have pathologic cervical vertebrae.

The Sitting Position

Perhaps no position has created more controversy and comment than the sitting position. Although some institutions utilize the sitting position only rarely, others perform procedures in this position almost daily.

The usual surgical argument in favor of this position centers on better anatomic orientation, better visualization for the surgical assistant, and a drier surgical field (blood and cerebrospinal fluid drain away from the operative field). Some claim these factors yield better operative results. The antecedents have basis in fact and consensus. The conclusion, however, has neither support nor refutation in the literature.

Arguments against the sitting position revolve around the added risk and the physiologic consequences produced by this position. The risks associated with the sitting position do not disappear with acceptable alternative positions for a given procedure. Hence, the situation is not one of risk versus no risk, but rather one of degree. The ultimate decision to use the sitting position should be one of judgment: Do the perceived benefits outweigh the perceived risks for a given procedure in a given patient? Since abilities and skills of both neurosurgeons and anesthesiologists vary, it is likely that the risk-benefit ratio will be unique in a given situation.

The patient's physiologic status and anatomy enter into this decision. For patients who have poor cardiac reserve, an alternative to the sitting position may be preferred. The presence of a ventriculoatrial shunt is also a contraindication to the sitting position. It would thus be unwise to make an all-encompassing statement about the use of the sitting position.

This chapter presents the technical aspects of the sitting position, the physiologic sequelae, and the injuries associated with the sitting position. The major issues of venous air embolism and paradoxical air embolism along with special monitoring requirements are discussed in Chapter 8.

Following the application of the usual intraoperative monitors, general anesthesia is induced. Intra-arterial monitoring, a urinary catheter, and a central catheter (if used) can be placed before or after the induction of anesthesia. Endotracheal intubation is perhaps optimal and safest if a reinforced nonkinkable tube is used.

The patient's legs are then wrapped to promote venous return and prevent venous stasis. Compression boots may also be applied. The patient is then ready for gradual adjustment of the table to achieve the sitting position.

Although there is controversy concerning the best way to put a patient in the sitting position, a common method is described here.

First, place a three-point skull clamp on the patient while he is still supine. While constantly monitoring the blood pressure, adjust the operating table (Fig. 5-2). Flex the table fully and lower the foot section 45 degrees. Next, slowly elevate the back section while placing the chassis in the Trendelenburg position. Then, raise the back further until the desired sitting position is achieved. Finally adjust the foot section of the table to the horizontal position. Optimally, the legs will rest at the level of the heart. (Fig. 5-3).

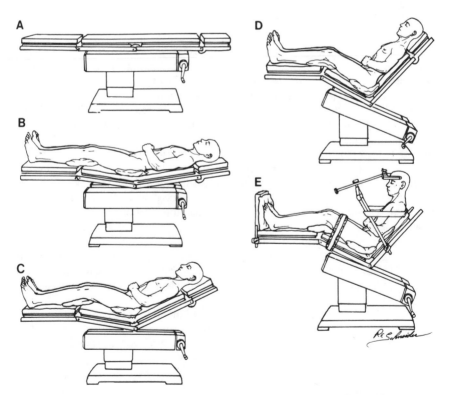

Figure 5-2 The procedure for establishing the sitting position. (From Martin JT. Positioning in anesthesia and surgery. Philadelphia: WB Saunders, 1987. Used with permission.)

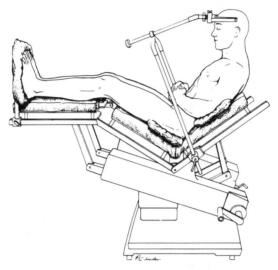

Figure 5-3 Close-up view of the correct final sitting position. (From Martin JT. Positioning in anesthesia and surgery. Philadelphia: WB Saunders, 1987. Used with permission.)

Remove the headrest and attach the skull clamp to a U-shaped frame which has been attached to the operating table. Then adjust the U-frame and skull clamp attachment to produce the desired neck flexion and head position.

The U-frame can be attached to the back section of the operating table, which would allow the head to be rapidly lowered by depressing the back section. Alternatively, if lateral access to the middle cranial fossa is required, the frame can be attached to the side of the thigh section. However, the latter placement may make it difficult to lower the head should it become necessary to do so.

Continuous monitoring of the blood pressure is essential while achieving the sitting position. Hemodynamic instability is usually not a problem if positioning is accomplished soon after the induction of anesthesia and if the level of anesthesia is not too deep. If hemodynamic instability is a problem, the level of anesthesia should be reduced and fluid administered. A fluid bolus of 500 ml of crystalloid or 250 ml of hetastarch or other iso-osmotic colloid is usually sufficient.

Once successful positioning is achieved a precordial Doppler is applied (see Chapter 8), and the patient is appropriately padded. Special care should be afforded such points as the heels, elbows, and portions of the legs or torso that may come into contact with the U-frame.

Pillows can be placed under the knees to minimize sciatic stretch. The arms can be conveniently folded across the lap to give appropriate arm support, to allow access to venous and arterial lines, and to lift the shoulders to minimize branchial plexus stretch.

Cardiovascular Effects

The effects of the sitting position on the cardiovascular system can be profound. Intrathoracic blood volume may decrease by 500 ml or more, resulting in a decreased (right greater than left) atrial pressure. Cardiac output falls 12 to 20%, and systemic vascular resistance increases 50 to 80%, yielding decreased renal blood flow but a variable change in blood pressure. The heart rate is generally unchanged or slightly increased. Cerebral blood flow may be decreased by up to 15%.

These changes may produce a great strain on an individual with significant cardiovascular disease. The ability to tolerate these hemodynamic alterations must be considered in the preoperative decision to use the sitting position.

Anesthetics used during the sitting position may depress the myocardium, enhance venous pooling, and decrease systemic vascular resistance. If the blood pressure is not closely monitored, these anesthetic agents may produce rapid cardiovascular deterioration. Neuromuscular relaxation should be provided to prevent potentially dangerous movement and the anesthetic titrated to optimal hemodynamic response. Hypotension should be treated promptly by using vasopressors, adjusting depth of anesthesia, and cautiously administering fluids.

Respiratory Effects

The respiratory system is not significantly stressed in the sitting position. In fact, the FRC decrement that occurs in the supine position is not found in the sitting position. However, one author has reported a decrease in the diffusing capacity for oxygen. This is thought to be secondary to an increased zone 1 of the lung resulting from decreased pulmonary perfusion. The clinical significance of this finding is uncertain.

Complications

The sitting position is associated with some interesting potential complications. The problems of venous air embolism, paradoxical air embolism, and arrhythmias are discussed in Chapter 8.

The head-elevated position can be associated with decreased cerebral perfusion pressure. The arterial line transducer is placed at head level. The cerebral mean arterial pressure (MAP) will differ from that measured at another, lower reference point in a predictable manner:

$$\text{Cerebral MAP} = \text{measured MAP} - (\text{cm height difference})/1.3$$

As cerebrospinal fluid drains from the cranial compartment, the brain tends to sag, placing traction on veins bridging between the brain and the venous sinuses. These bridging veins can tear, resulting in bleeding and in a site for air to enter the venous circulation.

Air enters the cranial cavity as cerebrospinal fluid drains, creating a pneumocephalus. This pneumocephalus is generally not an immediate threat to the patient. Rarely, delayed emergence from anesthesia is caused by a pneumocephalus. The chief concern about a pneumocephalus is the ability of nitrous oxide to expand the mass of air and create a tension pneumocephalus.

Edema of the face and tongue have been reported following surgery in the sitting position. Presumably flexion and rotation of the head and neck can obstruct veins and impede lymphatic drainage.

Brachial plexus and sciatic nerve injury can result from improper positioning. The weight of the arms pulling down upon the brachial plexus, combined with a fixed and occasionally rotated head, can stretch the neck and brachial plexus. To prevent this complication, avoid extremes of head rotation and gently support the arms in the patient's lap. The sciatic nerve can be injured if the thighs and knees are not gently bent and supported.

Rare but potentially devastating injuries to the cervical spine and spinal cord can occur in the sitting position. Pathologic cervical vertebrae can easily be injured with neck flexion and rotation. Flexion and rotation of the neck can also stretch the spinal cord and compromise spinal blood flow, resulting in quadriplegia. It is customary to limit neck flexion so that two fingers can be placed between the chin and the sternum.

Suggested Reading

Bagshaw RJ, Smith DS, Young MS, Bloom MJ. Anesthetic management of surgery in the vertebral canal. Anesth Rev 1985; 12:13–32.

Black S, Ockert DB, Oliver WC, Cucchiara RF. Outcome following posterior fossa craniectomy in patients in the sitting or horizontal positions. Anesthesiology 1988; 69:49–56.

Marshall WK, Bedford RF, Miller ED. Cardiovascular responses in the seated position—impact of four anesthetic techniques. Anesth Analg 1983; 62:648–652.

Martin JT. The head elevated positions. In: Martin JT, ed. Positioning in anesthesia and surgery. Philadelphia: WB Saunders, 1987:79.

Martin JT. The prone position. In: Martin JT, ed. Positioning in anesthesia and surgery. Philadelphia: WB Saunders, 1987:191.

Matjasko J, Petrozza P, Cohen M, Steinberg P. Anesthesia and surgery in the seated position: Analysis of 554 cases. Neurosurgery 1985; 17:645–702.

Standefer M, Bay JW, Trusso R. The sitting position in neurosurgery: A retrospective analysis of 488 cases. Neurosurgery 1984; 14:649–658.

Scott L. Mears, M.D., and Richard J. Sperry, M.D.

Fluid Management 6

The administration of fluid therapy is an essential component of any anesthetic technique. In addition to the general principles of fluid and electrolyte management, there are extra considerations for neurosurgical patients. The blood-brain barrier is a key element of fluid balance in the brain and is discussed first in this chapter. Osmotic therapy and the dangers of glucose as a component of fluid therapy are then covered. Finally the issues of whether to use crystalloid or colloid and how much fluid to administer are addressed.

Blood-Brain Barrier

The blood-brain barrier (BBB) is a term that designates the endothelial cells that line the inside of the cerebral capillary system. These capillaries are different from those found outside the central nervous system. The cerebral capillaries have a single-thickness inner lining of endothelial cells that are stuck to each other by tight junctions. These tight junctions "glue" the cells together so firmly that there are no leaks along the seam between the cells. In this way a complete seal is formed along the length of the capillary that will not allow substances to pass between the individual cells. Thus, the only way for molecules to pass from the blood stream into the brain is to pass through the endothelial cell itself. This is in contrast to capillaries outside the central nervous system where gaps between the endothelial cells allow passage of molecules from the blood into the interstitial space.

Different kinds of molecules pass through the cell in different fashions. Lipid-soluble substances cross the cell by simple diffusion, while non-lipid-soluble molecules are transported across the cell from the blood to the brain by carrier proteins. General anesthetics are a good example of lipid-soluble molecules that cross the BBB by simple diffusion. On the other hand, glucose and amino acids are insoluble in lipid and so cannot penetrate the cell membrane. Molecules like glucose and amino acids are bound to a carrier protein on the cell surface, which is then internalized, carried across the cell to the opposite surface, and released. This transport is not active and so uses no cellular energy, but it does require a concentration gradient to drive the molecule across the cell.

Hence the terms "carrier mediated transport" and "facilitated diffusion." The proteins that do the actual carrying are quite specific for the molecule carried.

Alterations in the BBB result in abnormal passage of large molecules and liquid from the blood stream to the interstitium of the brain. The common mechanism for a disrupted BBB is seam leakage, which results from a mechanical separation of the capillary endothelial cells by stretching or breaking of the tight junctions. For example, when hypertension exceeds cerebrovascular autoregulation, the cerebral capillaries are forcefully dilated and the endothelial cells are stretched. This causes gaps in the seams through which molecules can freely pass when driven by the increased hydrostatic pressure. Seam leaks also occur with endothelial cell death as is seen in trauma or with toxins.

The endothelial cells of the BBB are very resistant to hypoxic damage and can withstand significant periods of severe hypoxia (15 minutes) without impairment of function. This is of obvious benefit to an injured brain. Prolonged hypoxia will, of course, lead to endothelial cell death and blood-brain barrier disruption, but this process takes time and is most often seen 6 to 12 hours after the insult.

A leaky BBB is also found with intracranial tumors. As a tumor grows it releases tumor angiogenesis factor, which stimulates the growth of new blood vessels. The newly grown capillaries have an endothelial lining similar to that found in capillaries outside the brain. These vessels show fenestrations, wide intercellular junctions, and many pinocytotic vesicles. These "holes" inhibit the formation of a mechanical dam that is the primary element of the BBB. Consequently, the capillaries in and around the tumor will leak fluid and blood proteins, resulting in cerebral edema. The degree of edema can be documented by radiographic studies and correlates well with a greater risk for an intraoperative increase in intracranial pressure.

The treatment of a disrupted BBB is controversial. Dexamethasone is thought to stabilize or even partially reverse BBB damage from an intracranial tumor and from pseudotumor cerebri. Its use to treat other causes of BBB disruption (trauma, hypoxia) has not been associated with improved outcome. There is even some suggestion that the use of steroids in these cases may be harmful because of the associated hyperglycemia. Other therapy for a disrupted BBB is directed at minimizing the harmful effects of a leaking BBB and is the same as treating increased intracranial pressure. This includes elevation of the head, hyperventilation, oxygenation, blood pressure control, and seizure prophylaxis.

In summary, the BBB consists of a single layer of endothelial cells in the cerebral capillary. The cells are so tightly adherent to each other that they prevent leakage of molecules from the blood into brain tissue. Molecules enter the brain through the endothelial cells by lipid diffusion or by a specific transport system. Disease states such as tumors, hypoxemia, and trauma lead to a mechanical separation of the endothelial cells and result in "seam leaks" and the loss of BBB function.

Osmolarity

Typically the osmolarity of brain tissue is slightly greater than that of blood. The normal serum osmolarity is about 290 mOsm/L, and the normal blood-brain osmotic gradient is 3 mOsm/L. This gradient is maintained by the BBB. However, under pathologic conditions the integrity of the BBB is lost and fluid shifts from the blood into the brain, causing edema.

Mannitol and other osmotic agents given intravenously reverse the blood-brain osmotic gradient by markedly increasing the osmolarity of the blood. If the BBB is sufficiently intact, water shifts from the brain into the blood, decompressing the cerebral edema. An increase in the blood osmolarity of 10 mOsm/L removes 100 to 150 ml of water from the brain (see Chapter 7). The serum osmolarity should be maintained between 300 and 315 mOsm/L. Below 300 mOsm/L the blood-brain gradient is too low to be effective; above 315 mOsm/L both renal and neurologic dysfunction occur. If the serum osmolarity rises above 315 mOsm/L, all hypertonic fluids should be stopped and, if necessary, a 2.5% dextrose–0.45% saline solution carefully infused to reduce the serum osmolarity and to decrease the potential for hyperosmotic complications.

The peak change in serum osmolarity dictates the amount of brain water removed from the brain and consequently the degree of intracranial pressure reduction. In the case of mannitol administration, the peak osmolarity change is related to the total mannitol dose and to the rate of mannitol infusion. The peak osmolarity changes resulting from different doses of mannitol given by rapid infusion (2 ml/kg/min) in dogs is shown below:

1 g/kg	40 mOsm/L increase
0.75 g/kg	32 mOsm/L increase
0.5 g/kg	21 mOsm/L increase

If furosemide (0.7 mg/kg) is administered intravenously 15 minutes after mannitol, it potentiates the effects of mannitol by producing a large volume of hypotonic urine and thereby maintains a favorable osmotic gradient for a longer period of time.

Potential complications from mannitol therapy do, however, exist. Mannitol is a weak vasodilator and when administered can initially decrease the blood pressure. When vasodilation is coupled with intravascular volume expansion, an increase in cerebral blood flow and intracranial pressure can occur. The increase in intracranial pressure is usually short (1 to 2 minutes) but can be significant (10% increase). Intravascular volume expansion also leads to an acute increase in cardiac filling pressures. This may induce congestive heart failure in a patient with poor cardiac reserve. Intravascular volume expansion by extracellular water also decreases the serum sodium and potassium levels. This may induce cardiac arrhythmias, especially in digitalized patients.

Hyperosmolar states are usually not produced in patients with normal kidney function unless excessive mannitol is administered. However, the anephric patient does not excrete mannitol; thus, hyperosmolality and hypervolemia can easily occur. Mannitol administration to anephric patients should be avoided if possible. Mannitol remains in the patient's blood stream until removed by hemodialysis. The increased intravascular volume can be effectively treated with peritoneal dialysis; however, the intravascular volume will reaccumulate. Only hemodialysis corrects the osmotic derangement by removing mannitol.

Patients with renal failure who are not anuric will eventually excrete mannitol, but excretion will be quite delayed. The use of furosemide alone is recommended in these patients.

In addition to decreasing intracranial pressure, mannitol may also improve blood flow to ischemic areas of the brain. It does this in two ways. First, mannitol reduces red cell rigidity, which allows the blood to pass more freely through a narrowed microcirculation. Second, mannitol leads to hypervolemic hemodilution. When the hematocrit is reduced (30 to 35%) the blood viscosity is decreased, thereby improving cerebral blood flow to ischemic areas.

Glucose

For years it has been known that intravenous fluids containing glucose can cause cerebral edema. The mechanism for this cerebral edema stems from the passage of both sugar and water into the brain cell with the subsequent metabolism of the sugar leaving only the free water behind.

Recently, many studies have associated a high serum glucose level with poor neurologic outcome after regional and global brain ischemia. The proposed mechanism for this poor outcome is an increase in lactic acid formation from anaerobic cellular metabolism that is driven by an excess of glucose. Even when a dextrose infusion does not increase the serum glucose level outside the normal range, it appears to worsen outcome. It has also been shown that insulin-induced hypoglycemia does not improve postischemic outcome.

We still need more information pieces to complete the glucose puzzle. The optimal serum glucose level for patients with cerebral ischemia has not been determined. However, we do know that at least 4 hours of surgery for intracranial tumors can be performed without hypoglycemia or ketosis in nondiabetic patients given only normal saline. It is also apparent that glucose administration potentiates postischemic injury—even when that infusion does not result in hyperglycemia. When we consider the fact that nearly all neurosurgical procedures have a potential for ischemia, it is prudent to avoid intraoperative glucose infusions.

Crystalloid vs. Colloid

The controversy over crystalloid and colloid fluids for the neurosurgical patient has a long history. Here we examine this issue for three patient groups: patients with an intact BBB, trauma patients in shock, and patients with a dysfunctional BBB.

In patients with a normal BBB, colloids remain inside the blood vessel and do not lead to brain edema. For this reason colloid administration has historically been the mainstay of fluid therapy for neurosurgery. Crystalloid administration was thought to increase brain water content, and initial studies in animals with noninjured brains showed this to be true. Early thinking centered on the idea that the plasma colloid oncotic pressure was the major factor determining fluid flux across the BBB. However, it now appears that this may not be true. Recent studies have examined the effects of plasma oncotic pressure and serum osmolarity on the amount of water entering noninjured animal brains. In these studies when the serum osmolarity was maintained, the plasma oncotic pressure could be lowered by 12.5 mm Hg (nearly a 50% change) without producing brain edema. However, when the plasma oncotic pressure was maintained and the serum osmolarity reduced by 13 mOsm/kg (only about a 5% change), brain water content increased. Osmolarity thus seems to be the key factor in producing or preventing brain edema in noninjured brains (intact BBB). From the point of view of physiology, it doesn't seem to matter much whether crystalloid or colloid solutions are given to a patient with a normal blood-brain barrier if the serum osmolarity is not allowed to fall. The cost and complications associated with colloid solutions may, however, tip the scale in favor of crystalloids for these patients.

While crystalloid may be the "best choice" for patients with a normal BBB, it may not be the best choice for those patients who need rapid fluid volume resuscitation. If a patient needs volume replacement for hypotensive shock, the primary goal is to restore perfusion to the vital organs. If the hypotension is secondary to hemorrhage, blood is of course the best resuscitation fluid. Colloid and crystalloid solutions are alternatives to blood; however, colloid administration replenishes intravascular volume more efficiently than crystalloid. One liter of normal saline results in a 200-ml increase in the intravascular volume, 1 L of 5% albumin in a 500-ml increase, and 1 L of hetastarch in a 750-ml increase or more. But colloid is not without problems. Hetastarch has been incriminated in causing a coagulopathy if more than 1 to 1.5 L are administered. If crystalloid is used, normal saline administration should be combined with administration of lactated Ringer's solution. The osmolarity of lactated Ringer's solution is 273 mOsm/L; if used alone for massive fluid resuscitation it may lead to a fall in serum osmolarity with subsequent brain edema. Normal saline is also not benign. A large volume of normal saline may lead to hyperchloridemia and metabolic acidosis.

In patients with a disrupted BBB the answers remain unclear. If colloid is administered it may leak out of the vascular space and increase the tissue oncotic pressure, causing edema. If crystalloid is given it may pass into the interstitium and worsen edema. But which is the lesser evil? Which fluid has the longest effect? Which is worse acutely? We don't know. We do, however, know that both fluids are used with success. At present any specific recommendation of one fluid or the other is an extrapolation of experimental data and is based on theory. The animal models and the laboratory techniques used to address this issue have come of age, and more specific data should be available in the near future. In patients with a disrupted BBB there will always be an area of the brain with an intact BBB. It will vary in size and location, but it will be present. It makes intuitive sense to take advantage of what we know and to direct therapy at the normal area of the brain, especially if the normal area is much larger than the area that is damaged. We therefore recommend crystalloid therapy over colloid therapy. Some may argue that this approach is tantamount to the ostrich that hides its head in the sand and hopes the danger will pass if it is ignored. It is not that at all. Anesthesiologists are frequently required to make a decision without all the facts. We make *this* decision knowing that we might be proved wrong in the long run, but feeling that it is our best decision at the present time.

Our current recommendation for fluid therapy is to use crystalloid in all situations except volume resuscitation for shock, and to maintain the serum osmolarity near normal unless osmotic therapy is selected.

The question of how much crystalloid or colloid solution to administer must also be addressed. It is never desirable to withhold fluid to the point that cardiovascular stability is threatened. However, a "wet" patient is also usually not desirable. The terms "dry" and "wet" refer to ends of the spectrum of euvolemia. A euvolemic patient with cardiovascular stability is *always* the goal. Euvolemia requires that fluid deficits be replaced, that maintenance fluid be administered, and that third-space fluid and blood loss be replaced.

Patients who present for tumor surgery should be kept on the dry side of normal. Excess fluid administered to these patients may cause brain edema at the sites of blood-brain barrier disruption. Thus a dry but stable patient is optimum for tumor surgery.

Fluid resuscitation for shock and head trauma should produce a stable, euvolemic patient. As for tumor patients, an excess of fluid may encourage cerebral edema in the head trauma patient. However, a dry trauma patient may be at risk for hypoperfusion of vital organs—especially if the blood pressure is maintained by sympathetic activation. Thus, a euvolemic patient is optimum for head trauma.

A full vascular system and an elevated cardiac output may improve the symptoms of vasospasm. Thus, patients at risk for vasospasm (subarachnoid hemorrhage, intracranial aneurysm) may benefit from vigorous fluid therapy. However, the cardiovascular system should never be "stuffed" so full with fluid that pulmonary edema or cardiac dysfunction develops.

General Suggestions

1. Use no dextrose-containing solutions.
2. Use insulin to maintain serum glucose below 200 mg/dl.
3. Limit the volume of lactated Ringer's solution and use colloid and normal saline–lactated Ringer's solution for volume resuscitation.
4. Limit hetastarch to 1 to 1.5 L to avoid coagulopathy.
5. Maintain hematocrit at 30 to 35%.
6. Mild volume expansion for aneurysm clipping may help reduce vasospasm.
7. Keep patients with tumors dry, patients with trauma normal, and patients with aneurysms wet.

Suggested Reading

Albright AL, Latchaw RE. Intracranial and system effects of osmotic and oncotic therapy in experimental cerebral edema. J Neurosurg 1984; 60:481–489.

Cottrell JE, Robustelli A, Post K, Turndorf H. Furosemide and mannitol induced changes in intracranial pressure and serum osmolality and electrolytes. Anesthesiology 1977; 47:28–30.

deCourten-Myers G, Myers RE, Schoolfield L. Hyperglycemia enlarges infarct size in cerebrovascular occlusion in cats. Stroke 1988; 19:623–630.

Haupt MT, Rackow EC. Colloid osmotic pressure and fluid resuscitation with hetastarch, albumin, and saline solutions. Crit Care Med 1982; 10:159–162.

Joo F. The blood-brain barrier. Nature 1986; 321:197–198.

Kassell NF, Peerless SJ, Durward QJ, et al. Treatment of ischemic deficits from vasospasm with intravascular volume expansion and induced arterial hypertension. Neurosurgery 1982; 11: 337–343.

Lanier WL, Stangland KJ, Scheithauer BW, Milde JH, Michenfelder JD. The effects of dextrose infusion and head position on neurologic outcome after complete cerebral ischemia in primates: Examination of a model. Anesthesiology 1987. 66:39–48.

Levin AB, Duff TA, Javid MJ. Treatment of increased intracranial pressure: A comparison of different hyperosmotic agents and the use of thiopental. Neurosurgery 1979; 5:570–575.

Pollay M, Roberts PA. Blood-brain barrier: A definition of normal and altered function. Neurosurgery 1980; 6:675–685.

Poole GV Jr, Johnson JC, Prough DS, Stump DA, Stullken EH. Cerebral hemodynamics after hemorrhagic shock: Effects of the type of resuscitation fluid. Crit Care Med 1986; 14:629–633.

Wood JH, Kee DB. Hemorheology of the cerebral circulation in stroke. Stroke 1985; 16:765–772.

Zornow MH, Scheller MS, Todd MM, Moore SS. Acute cerebral effects of isotonic crystalloid and colloid solutions following cryogenic brain injury in the rabbit. Anesthesiology 1988; 69:180–184.

Zornow MH, Todd MM, Moore SS. The acute cerebral effects of changes in plasma osmolality and oncotic pressure. Anesthesiology 1987; 67:936–941.

Scott L. Mears, M.D., and Richard J. Sperry, M.D.

Supratentorial Surgery 7

The majority of intracranial neurosurgical procedures are performed for a supratentorial mass lesion. Supratentorial procedures include those for tumor, hematoma, or trauma. This chapter presents the principles of anesthetic management for these common procedures. Although the underlying pathology may be different for different lesions, the anesthetic considerations are the same.

Preoperative Evaluation

The preoperative visit begins with a complete medical history that probes deeply into the function of the heart and the lungs. Most perioperative morbidity and mortality result from poor cardiac or pulmonary function. Disease of either of these organ systems needs to be defined and then addressed in both the preoperative preparation of the patient and the anesthetic plan.

Patients for neurosurgery are also questioned specifically about central nervous system disease. Seizure disorders need to be assessed for type and for adequacy of therapy. Cerebral hemorrhages or prior strokes are noted, and any residual speech, sensory, or motor dysfunctions are recorded. Obtain the results of any recent intracranial surgery or diagnostic procedures, and consider the possibility of residual pneumocephalus or other possible anesthetic interactions.

Review the patient's list of medications, paying particular attention to those drugs that may have perioperative effects. Steroids increase serum glucose levels by stimulating gluconeogenesis and cause direct adrenal suppression that may lead to hypotension with surgical stress. Mannitol and other diuretics used to reduce cerebral edema can lead to hypovolemia and electrolyte imbalances. These can cause profound hypotension upon anesthetic induction and cardiac arrhythmias. Antihypertensive agents may alter the patient's intravascular volume status. Clonidine has been shown to predispose some patients to severe hypertension after naloxone administration. Tricyclic antidepressants and L-dopa have been incriminated for inducing intraoperative hypertension and cardiac arrhythmias. Benzodiazepines, phenothiazines, and butyrophenones can contribute to perioperative hypotension and cloud the sensorium.

The preoperative physical examination is directed toward the airway, the lungs, and the cardiovascular system. In addition to the patient's underlying medical conditions, look for specific signs of hypovolemia. Hypovolemia is a common finding in neurosurgical patients because they are often somnolent and have inadequate oral intake. They may also have increased urinary water loss resulting from x-ray dye or diuretics. Mild to moderate hypovolemia is usually well tolerated and desirable in this patient population. However, significant hypovolemia should be corrected before the induction of anesthesia.

Also, perform a brief neurologic examination, including an assessment of the level of consciousness. Document any focal motor or sensory deficits. The neurologic examination can be briefly repeated in the operating suite just before the induction of anesthesia to identify a rapidly progressing lesion.

The patient should also be examined for the signs and questioned about the symptoms of increased intracranial pressure (ICP). These include headache, nausea, vomiting, papilledema, and unilateral pupil dilation. As ICP increases, the patient's mental status deteriorates, followed by respiratory and cardiac dysfunction. A Cheyne-Stokes breathing pattern and bradycardia with hypertension are ominous signs of brainstem compression.

Routine preoperative laboratory work includes a complete blood count, blood chemistry, and coagulation studies. Other tests are ordered as indicated. Hyperventilation and diuresis will decrease the serum potassium level. Potassium supplementation should thus be considered early. A serum glucose level above 200 mg/dl is not acceptable, and insulin therapy should be begun to lower serum glucose to the normal range.

The preoperative radiographic studies provide essential information about tumor size and location, cerebral edema, and midline shift. Although the anesthesiologist is generally not expert at interpreting computed tomographic (CT) or magnetic resonance imaging (MRI) scans, he or she can get a good feel for potential problems and for the extent of surgery to be performed.

Preoperative sedative medication is contraindicated in patients with a decreased mental status. If preoperative medication is desired, diazepam (Valium), 0.1 to 0.2 mg/kg PO 1 to 2 hours before surgery, is recommended. Avoid narcotics because of the risk of raising ICP from vomiting or hypoventilation. Perhaps the best alternative is to withhold all preoperative sedatives until the patient is in the operating suite and then to administer an intravenous sedative agent while preparing the patient for surgery. In this way, the anesthesiologist can readily deal with any adverse drug effects that may arise.

Monitors

Routine monitors for supratentorial procedures include continuous electrocardiography (ECG), blood pressure cuff, esophageal stethoscope, FiO_2 monitor, pulse oximeter, temperature probe, peripheral nerve stimulator, and an indwelling urinary catheter. For patients with ischemic heart disease, use a modified V_5 ECG lead. Additionally, an arterial line is placed for continuous blood pressure display and for easy access to blood for laboratory analysis. End-tidal CO_2 measurement helps to monitor hyperventilation and endotracheal tube disconnections or kinks. All these monitors should be employed routinely.

The use of ICP monitoring for trauma and intracranial surgery has been controversial. Some clinicians advocate routine use; others point to the fact that no outcome studies have shown it to be effective. With ICP monitoring, the anesthesiologist can be more selective and administer decompressive therapy only to those patients who require it and thereby avoid exposing other patients to the risks of diuretic administration. In addition, occult increases in ICP can occur; these would go unnoticed without ICP monitoring. For example, positioning of the head can lead to obstruction of venous outflow through the jugular veins and cause increased ICP. Also, rapid tumor expansion secondary to hemorrhage leads to increased ICP that may be relieved only by rapid surgical decompression. The risk of infection (about 4%) negates the use of an ICP monitor in all patients undergoing craniotomy for tumor resection. However, in the subgroup of patients at risk for a large increase in ICP (tumor size > 3 cm with a midline shift or significant edema), there are potential advantages to ICP monitoring.

Anesthetic Management

Although induction of anesthesia for patients undergoing craniotomy can be performed with various agents, the best single class appears to be the barbiturates. Thiopental administration provides a profound reduction in cerebral metabolic rate ($CMRO_2$), cerebral blood flow (CBF), and ICP. Narcotics also reduce $CMRO_2$, but to a lesser extent than CBF. In theory, this could lead to ischemia; however, this has not been shown to be clinically relevant. Narcotics do provide excellent control of blood pressure and heart rate, which makes them very useful anesthetic adjuncts. Etomidate does not cause an increase in ICP when used for induction, but it may depress the pituitary adrenal axis. Ketamine causes an indirect increase in heart rate, blood pressure, and ICP and produces a seizure pattern on the EEG. For these reasons ketamine is a poor anesthetic agent for neuroanesthesia. The effect of anesthetic agents and other drugs on CBF and ICP is shown in Figure 7-1.

A smooth and gentle induction of general anesthesia is more important than the drug combination utilized. An acceptable induction sequence combines four steps:

1. Preoxygenation and self-hyperventilation.
2. Administration of thiopental, 3 to 4 mg/kg IV, followed by mask ventilation to assure airway patency.
3. Administration of vecuronium, 0.1 mg/kg IV, and mask hyperventilation with O_2:N_2O (50 : 50) until neuromuscular blockade is achieved. If there is a contraindication to the use of N_2O, add a small concentration of isoflurane to the O_2.
4. Administration of lidocaine, 1.5 mg/kg IV, and additional thiopental, 2 mg/kg IV, just before endotracheal intubation.

Naturally the dose of these induction agents may need to be adjusted for patients with cardiovascular instability. A combination of narcotics (fentanyl, 5μg/kg, or sufentanil, 0.5 to 1 μg/kg) and a small sleep dose of etomidate (6 to 8 mg) allows for ICP control and remarkable cardiovascular stability. As always, the key to the appropriate use of anesthetic agents is close patient monitoring with titration to effect.

A rapid-sequence induction can be performed with the same combination of drugs as a routine induction. However, cricoid pressure is applied, mask ventilation is

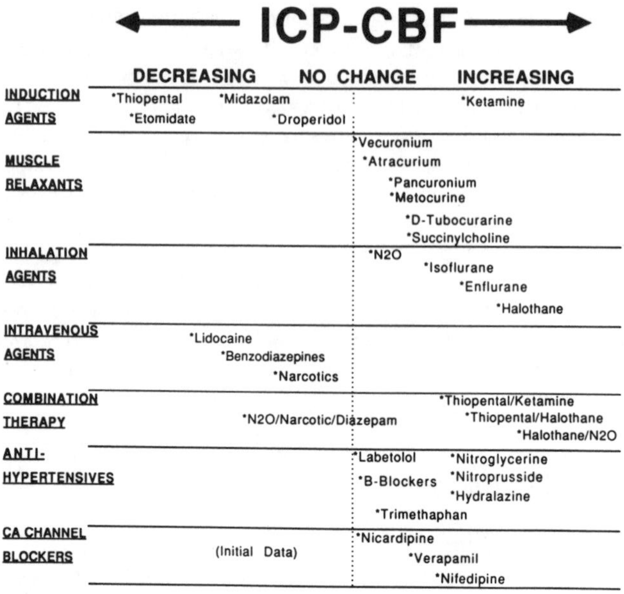

← ICP-CBF →

	DECREASING	NO CHANGE	INCREASING
INDUCTION AGENTS	*Thiopental *Etomidate	*Midazolam *Droperidol	*Ketamine
MUSCLE RELAXANTS		*Vecuronium *Atracurium *Pancuronium *Metocurine *D-Tubocurarine *Succinylcholine	
INHALATION AGENTS		*N2O *Isoflurane *Enflurane *Halothane	
INTRAVENOUS AGENTS	*Lidocaine *Benzodiazepines *Narcotics		
COMBINATION THERAPY	*N2O/Narcotic/Diazepam		*Thiopental/Ketamine *Thiopental/Halothane *Halothane/N2O
ANTI-HYPERTENSIVES		*Labetolol *B-Blockers *Trimethaphan	*Nitroglycerine *Nitroprusside *Hydralazine
CA CHANNEL BLOCKERS	(Initial Data)	*Nicardipine *Verapamil *Nifedipine	

Figure 7-1 The effects of various drugs and drug combinations on intracranial pressure and cerebral blood flow.

not delivered, and vecuronium, 0.15 mg/kg is used to facilitate endotracheal intubation. In a patient with a full stomach and a difficult airway, awake intubation should be performed. Heavy topical anesthesia and minimal intravenous sedation with subsequent oral endotracheal intubation using a lighted stylet is extremely effective in these patients.

If narcotics are to be used as a part of the anesthetic, it would be reasonable, even desirable, to administer these agents slowly during induction. Fentanyl or sufentanil can make induction and endotracheal intubation very smooth.

Three caveats must be given regarding the use of narcotics:

1. Neurosurgical patients may have a rapid clouding of their sensorium with any sedative agent. Hence, their protective airway reflexes may be blunted quickly.
2. Narcotics induce hypoventilation, which can be very dangerous in these patients.
3. The combination of thiopental and narcotics (particularly sufentanil) can produce a dramatic decrease in blood pressure. Hence, the dose of thiopental must be reduced for induction of anesthesia when a significant narcotic load has been administered.

Esmolol or labetalol may also be given prior to intubation. These drugs blunt the hypertensive response to intubation. As with narcotics, the dose of sodium pentothal must be adjusted if these drugs are administered or hypotension will result.

Maintenance of anesthesia can be accomplished in a number of ways. These techniques generally fall into two categories: primarily volatile agents and primarily narcotics. Either technique can be used. The most important feature of administering a given anesthetic is not which technique is used but rather how appropriately that technique is applied. This cannot be overemphasized.

Many authorities on neuroanesthesia feel that a narcotic-based anesthetic technique with either N_2O or low-dose (<1%) isoflurane in oxygen is optimum. If a narcotic-based anesthetic is chosen, either fentanyl or sufentanil may be used. The place of alfentanil and other new narcotics during neurosurgery has not yet been defined. However, sufentanil and alfentanil may affect intracranial pressure and cerebral perfusion pressure unfavorably. We still use sufentanil, awaiting further clarification of this issue.

Fentanyl, 5 μg/kg combined with less than 1% isoflurane in oxygen is an acceptable technique for anesthetic maintenance. Alternatively, sufentanil, 0.5 to 1 μg/kg load, followed by either incremental boluses (not to exceed 0.5 μg/kg/hr) or an IV infusion of 0.25 to 0.5 μg/kg/hr in combination with less than 1 percent isoflurane in oxygen may be used. The narcotic and the isoflurane dose are adjusted to yield the desired blood pressure. The sufentanil must be discontinued approximately 1 hour before the end of surgery, or the patient may not awaken promptly. If the patient has hypertension or tachycardia near the end of surgery, it is best to treat these with either labetalol or esmolol and not narcotics.

A volatile agent, preferably isoflurane, with little or no narcotic supplementation can also be used for maintenance of anesthesia. If isoflurane is used, the concentration should remain less than 1%. Hyperventilation in combination with less than 1% isoflurane generally results in stable intracranial dynamics.

Nitrous oxide may be used in an anesthetic regimen if it is deemed desirable. However, if the patient is suspected to have a pneumocephalus (recent intracranial surgery or trauma) or if there is a potential for air embolism, N_2O is contraindicated. N_2O will expand both the pneumocephalus and the air embolus. A tension pneumocephalus acts like an expanding mass lesion. A large air embolus can cause cardiovascular collapse (see Chapter 8).

Each of these anesthetic techniques produces an acceptable anesthetic state. However, the art of anesthesia dictates that the anesthesiologist learn to "read" the patient and not over- or undermedicate. This is frequently difficult for the novice and even occasionally difficult for the seasoned anesthesiologist. If a patient does not awaken promptly at the end of surgery, a relative excess of either volatile agent or narcotic is part of the differential diagnosis. The anesthesiologist must rationally evaluate this possibility.

Hyperventilation is an important adjunct to any neuroanesthetic technique. Hypocapnia decreases ICP prior to opening the dura, counteracts the vasodilation produced by the volatile anesthetic agents, and relaxes the surgical brain. Optimal hyperventilation during surgery would yield an arterial P_{CO_2} of 25 to 30 mm Hg. If increased ICP is a problem, it may be beneficial to reduce the P_{CO_2} to 20 to 25 mm Hg.

Muscle relaxation is also important during neurosurgery. Relaxation prevents patient movement at inappropriate times. It may decrease ICP by relaxing the chest wall, which decreases intrathoracic pressure and encourages venous drainage. To choose an agent for muscle relaxation, consider the length of the procedure and the impact of the drug on ICP (see Chapter 3).

A peripheral nerve stimulator is used to monitor neuromuscular blockade in all patients. Lesions that involve the motor cortex or any of its outflow tracts can cause muscle dysfunction on the contralateral side. When such a lesion is resected, the patient may be positioned with the lesion away from the anesthesia machine to allow more room for the surgical team and equipment. This means that the affected muscle groups, usually the patient's arm, are closest to the anesthesiologist and most convenient for neuromuscular monitoring. However, because of end-plate receptor proliferation, muscles that are functionally paretic are resistant to muscle relaxants. When a nerve stimulator is used on such a muscle, a much higher dose of relaxant is needed to produce the signs of neuromuscular blockade. The difference in sensitivity between normal and affected muscles can be quite large. Twitches can be completely absent in normal muscle, while the affected group shows all four twitches of the train of four. Hence, monitoring of these affected muscles can easily lead to an overdose of muscle relaxant.

The potential for overdose is partly advantageous because a deep level of relaxation is more likely to be maintained when a resistant muscle group is monitored. However, there does exist the problem of inability to reverse profound neuromuscular blockade in the normal muscles. This problem can be minimized by monitoring an unaffected muscle whenever possible. When this cannot be done, good judgment regarding the dose of relaxant must be used and constant vigilance for patient movement employed. At the end of the surgery, neuromuscular blockade is tested on an unaffected muscle prior to the administration of reversal agents and extubation.

A balanced salt solution is the fluid of choice for neurosurgical procedures. The volume of fluid administered should be minimized during the induction of anesthesia and then kept as low as hemodynamic stability and urine output will allow. When volume resuscitation is needed and the hematocrit does not dictate the use of blood, 500 to 1,000 ml of a colloid solution can be used effectively. (See Chapter 6 for a complete discussion of fluid therapy during neurosurgery.)

Emergence from anesthesia following supratentorial surgery should be smooth and gentle. When deciding to attempt a prompt awakening and extubation, consider the preoperative mental status, location of the surgery, extent of brain edema, and the quantity of intraoperative medication administered. A patient who was comatose preoperatively or who has undergone significant surgical manipulation for removal of a large, centrally located tumor is not a candidate for early extubation. Such a patient should remain intubated and be allowed to awaken slowly in the intensive care unit after a period of monitoring and continued ventilation. However, the majority of patients who undergo supratentorial surgery can be extubated in the operating suite upon the termination of surgery.

Special Problems

Stereotactic Surgery

With the advent of CT and MRI, the location of intracranial lesions can be pinpointed with great accuracy. This localization permits the biopsy and resection of lesions using a three-dimensional stereotactic approach.

Stereotactic surgery poses a special challenge to the anesthesiologist because of the equipment used to perform the stereotactic localization. The equipment consists of a platform that is attached to the patient's head and a localizing frame that rests on the platform. The platform and frame frequently obscure free access to the patient's airway.

The platform can usually be attached to the patient with minimal intravenous sedation and scalp infiltration with local anesthetics. Many patients undergoing brain biopsy can continue to have the biopsy with only monitored anesthesia care. However, some patients require general anesthesia.

Some patients requiring general anesthesia have a combination of facial characteristics and platform placement that allows access to the airway. If an anesthesia mask can fit over the mouth and nose, normal induction and intubation can be considered. Generally, the head and neck can be placed in the proper position for intubation. However, before any drugs are administered to the patient, the wrench needed to remove the stereotactic equipment must be physically present in case the equipment must be removed immediately.

Not all patients have facial characteristics and platform placement that allow for normal induction and intubation. Either they must be intubated while awake, or the frame must be removed and reattached after induction of anesthesia.

There are three methods for performing awake intubation in these patients. If there is access to the nose, a blind nasal intubation can be performed. This technique has been described abundantly in other publications. Not all patients can be successfully intubated with this technique, and bleeding is a frequent complication, which makes the subsequent use of the fiberoptic laryngoscope difficult.

For some practitioners, a fiberoptic technique is the method of choice. Two fiberoptic techniques have proved successful in these patients: the fiberoptic laryngoscope and the fiberoptic lighted stylet or lightwand. The preparation of the patient is the same for both techniques. An antisialagogue is administered, light intravenous sedation is administered, and a generous amount of topical anesthetic is applied to the nasal, oral, pharyngeal, and laryngeal surfaces. When the patient is properly prepared, intubation can be attempted.

A fiberoptic laryngoscope can be used to place the endotracheal tube either through the nose or through the mouth. The technique for fiberoptic laryngoscopy can be found in numerous sources and is not repeated here.

The lightwand is an inexpensive, easy alternative to the fiberoptic laryngoscope. The lighted stylet must be well lubricated before insertion into the endotracheal tube, and the proximal end of the tube must be cut so that the light of the stylet remains about 1 cm inside the tube tip. The distal 1 to 2 inches of the stylet and endotracheal tube are then bent into a rounded "J" curve of 90 degrees.

After the lightwand and the patient are ready, the patient slightly extends his head, opens his mouth wide, sticks out his tongue, which is held by the anesthesiologist or assistant, and is instructed to take slow deep breaths. The room is then darkened and the lightwand "lighted." The stylet and endotracheal tube are placed in the patient's mouth in the midline and allowed to follow the curve of the tongue into the oropharynx. The tip of the stylet should gently ride down the tongue over the epiglottis and engage the glottic inlet.

When the glottic inlet is engaged, an obvious glow of light, which extends down to the suprasternal notch, is seen in the midline. The stylet is then slightly advanced in the anterior direction and the endotracheal tube pushed off the stylet into the trachea.

If a dull transillumination is seen in the soft tissues of the neck on one side of the trachea, the tip of the endotracheal tube lies in the pyriform fossa. If the light suddenly dims or disappears, the tip is in the esophagus. In either case, the tip needs to be redirected. The stylet and endotracheal tube are redirected by withdrawing, gently rotating, and then readvancing it in short gentle passes until the trachea is located.

Once the endotracheal tube is presumed to be in the trachea, the patient is asked to speak. If he cannot speak and good air exchange is heard through the endotracheal tube, a sleep dose of thiopental (75 to 100 mg) is administered.

Management of patients for stereotactic surgery from the point of intubation on is no different than that for other supratentorial procedures.

Physiology of Intracranial Pressure

The skull is a semirigid structure that contains the brain, blood, and cerebrospinal fluid (CSF). The brain is 2 percent of body weight (1,400 g for a 70-kg person) and is composed of approximately 50% neurons and 50% glial cells. The normal cerebral blood volume is 3 to 7% of intracranial volume, or 40 to 90 ml. The total volume of CSF is approximately 140 ml, split evenly between the intracerebral and spinal compartments. The 70 ml of intracerebral CSF is again split evenly between the ventricular system and the cerebral subarachnoid space.

CSF is formed at a rate of approximately 30 to 35 ml/hr in adults. Certain drugs and pathologic conditions can alter CSF production-absorption kinetics and thus alter CSF volume and intracranial pressure. Drugs such as acetazolamide, ouabain, corticosteroids, spironolactone, furosemide, and vasopressin inhibit CSF formation. CSF production also decreases with decreasing body temperature. Halothane decreases both CSF production and absorption. Enflurane increases CSF production and decreases absorption. Isoflurane increases CSF absorption but leaves production at normal levels.

The ICP remains normal in the presence of an intracranial mass because of compensatory mechanisms. The expansion of non-CSF components results in displacement of CSF from within the cranium into the distensible spinal subarachnoid space. Some additional compensation may be provided by increased CSF reabsorption, which is pressure dependent up to an ICP limit of 30 mm Hg. When CSF volume buffering is exhausted, further spatial compensation must be achieved by a reduction in cerebral blood volume, or ICP will increase.

An exhaustible buffer system generates an intracranial compliance curve like that shown in Figure 7-2. Two areas of the curve are marked. The area between points 1 and 2 indicates the period of CSF and cerebral blood volume buffering. During this period, the increase in intracranial mass is compensated by displacement of CSF into the spinal subarachnoid space or by a reduction of cerebral blood volume. As buffering is exhausted (point 2), the genu of the curve is reached, and ICP increases with small increases in intracranial mass. Many neurosurgical patients may have a normal ICP but sit at or near point 2 of the curve. Even though ICP is normal, a very small increase in intracranial volume will increase ICP. As compensatory mechanisms fail, ICP rises, compressing vascular structures, inducing ischemia, shifting brain tissue, and producing brain death.

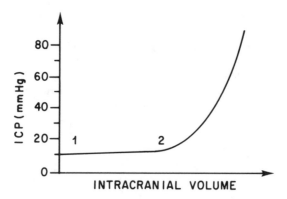

Figure 7-2   The intracranial compliance curve.

Therapy for increased ICP is multifaceted. One simple but often overlooked principle is assuring optimal venous drainage. Venous congestion of the brain increases cerebral blood volume and subsequently ICP. The optimal position of the head is midline with the head elevated 15 to 30 degrees.

Stimulation of the central nervous system can also have a detrimental effect on ICP. Unresponsive patients can experience pain and other stimulation of the central nervous system. This stimulation increases the oxygen consumption of the brain and thereby increases cerebral blood flow and cerebral blood volume. Drugs for deafferentation (analgesics, anxiolytics) must be used during painful procedures on comatose patients. A very light anesthetic is not optimal for a patient with increased ICP.

Preventive therapy is mandatory during respiratory care maneuvers (intubation, suctioning), since these maneuvers not only stimulate the central nervous system but also elicit reflexes such as bucking, which may impede venous drainage from the brain. Lidocaine, 1.5 mg/kg, and hyperventilation prior to suctioning can lessen the rise in ICP associated with airway care. Barbiturates and mannitol may occasionally be required.

General medical care, such as seizure prophylaxis, the treatment of hypoxia, and hyper- or hypotension, is also important in maintaining a normal cerebral blood volume and ICP. There are times when mild hypo- or hypertension is desirable, but in patients with increased ICP, normotension is the goal. If antihypertensive drugs are required to achieve normotension, care should be taken to avoid cerebral vasodilators, which will increase cerebral blood volume and ICP and at the same time decrease mean arterial pressure. Such an alteration in intracranial dynamics could prove fatal. A good choice for antihypertensive therapy is either labetalol or esmolol.

Acute therapeutic hyperventilation ($PaCO_2$ 20 to 25 mm Hg) has a rapid and generally successful influence on raised ICP. An acute reduction in $PaCO_2$ from 35 to 29 mm Hg lowers ICP 25 to 30% in most patients. A failure to respond to hyperventilation is a grave prognostic sign. Cerebral blood volume changes 1 to 1.5% (0.04 ml 100 g) for each 1 mm Hg change in $PaCO_2$ over a range of 20 to 80 mm Hg, or in an average brain of 1,400 g, roughly 0.56 ml per 1 mm Hg change in $PaCO_2$. Thus, hyperventilation from a $PaCO_2$ of 40 mm Hg to 20 mm Hg will decrease cerebral blood volume 10 to 15 ml. This is a small but very important volume when the patient is on the genu of the intracranial compliance curve.

The effect of prolonged hypocarbia on ICP is unclear. Hyperventilation influences cerebral blood volume by its effects on the pH of CSF. The pH of CSF returns to normal with persistent hypocapnia ($t_{1/2}$ of 6 hours). After 24 to 48 hours of hyperventilation there should be no active vasoconstriction. Some have suggested that chronic hyperventilation may have a sustained beneficial effect on brain water volume. Also, sustained hyperventilation should not be terminated until the underlying mass or edema has decreased in size, or a rebound increase in ICP will occur.

Hyperosmolar therapy extracts water from and reduces the volume of brain tissue. The latency from administration of osmotic agents to ICP reduction is several minutes, and a maximal reduction occurs at 20 to 60 minutes. Elevating the serum osmolarity by 10 mOsm/liter (to about 300 mOsm/L) reduces ICP in most patients. This can be achieved with mannitol, 0.25 mg/kg every 2 to 3 hours or 1 mg/kg less often. An acute elevation in serum osmolarity of 10 mOsm/L will extract about 100 to 150 ml of water. The upper limit for hyperosmolar therapy is 315 to 320 mOsm/L. A greater serum osmolarity is associated with a reduction in brain volume but is also associated with renal and neurologic dysfunction.

The loop diuretics furosemide and ethacrynic acid have also been used to control ICP. These agents act by brain dehydration, reduction of CSF formation, and reduction of cerebral edema. The onset of action for the loop diuretics is slower than that for osmotic agents. However, they are equally effective in reducing ICP.

Furosemide (0.7 mg/kg) administered 15 minutes after mannitol will potentiate the effect of mannitol. It does this by producing a large volume of hypotonic urine and thereby maintaining a favorable osmotic gradient for a longer time.

Case History

P.S., a 46-year-old right-handed female, was in her usual state of good health until 2 months prior to admission, when she began to experience intermittent anxiety and episodes of fainting accompanied by a sensation of vertigo. No tonic-clonic activity was noted to accompany these episodes, nor was there a loss of bowel or bladder continence. Over this 2-month period her family noticed subtle personality changes: she was less energetic, less talkative, and no longer interested in things which used to occupy her time. She denied headache, numbness, weakness, visual changes, and nausea or vomiting.

Her medical history was significant only for a remote cholecystectomy and a total vaginal hysterectomy. At the time of presentation she was not taking any medications.

On physical examination the patient was alert and oriented. Her speech was fluent, and her recent and remote memory were normal. Her affect,

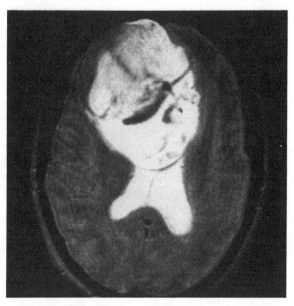

Figure 7-3   An MRI scan demonstrating a large, cystic, bifrontal mass with calcification and surrounding edema.

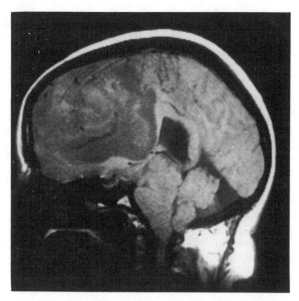

Figure 7-4   Sagittal MRI view of an extensive frontal mass.

however, was flat. All cranial nerves were intact and symmetrical, as were motor and sensory functions in all extremities. Results of cerebellar examination were normal, but her gait showed a slight circumduction of the left lower extremity. Cardiac and pulmonary examinations revealed no abnormalities. Her upper airway and neck mobility were normal.

The patient was evaluated by a neurologist who obtained an MRI scan (Figs. 7-3 and 7-4). She subsequently underwent a bifrontal craniotomy and tumor debulking. Findings at the time of surgery included a large, friable intracranial tumor which was moderately demarcated from the surrounding brain. The final pathologic diagnosis was anaplastic astrocytoma.

Suggested Reading

Adams RW, Cucchiara RF, Gronert GA, Messick JM, Michenfelder JD. Isoflurane and cerebrospinal fluid pressure in neurosurgical patients. Anesthesiology 1981; 54:97-99.

Artru AA. Effects of enflurane and isoflurane on resistance to reabsorption of CSF. Anesthesiology 1984; 61:529-533.

Artru AA. Isoflurane does not increase the rate of CSF production in the dog. Anesthesiology 1984; 60:193-197.

Bedford RF. Anesthetic management for supratentorial tumor surgery. J Neurooncol 1983; 1: 319-326.

Bedford RF, Morris L, Jane JA. Intracranial hypertension during surgery for supratentorial tumor: Correlation with preoperative computed tomography scans. Anesth Analg 1982; 61:430-433.

Bedford RF, Colley PS. Intracranial tumors: Supratentorial and infratentorial. In: Matjasko J, Katz J, eds. Clinical controversies in neuroanesthesia and neurosurgery. Orlando: Grune & Stratton, 1986:135.

Fishman RA. Brain edema. N Engl J Med 1975; 293:706–711.

Grosslight K, Colohan A, Bedford RF. Isoflurane anesthesia—risk factors for increases in ICP. Anesthesiology 1985; 63:533–536.

Messick JM, Newberg LA, Nugent M, Faust RJ. Principles of neuroanesthesia for the nonneurosurgical patient with CNS pathophysiology. Anesth Analg 1985; 64:143–174.

Shapiro HM. Intracranial hypertension: Therapeutic and anesthesiologic considerations. Anesthesiology 1975; 43:445–471.

Richard J. Sperry, M.D.

Posterior Fossa Surgery 8

Surgery in the posterior fossa can be a dramatic and dynamic experience. Constant vigilance on the part of the entire operating team and ongoing "real-time" communication with the neurosurgeon are essential for an optimal result.

The contents of the posterior fossa explain the drama of surgery on this area of the brain. The posterior fossa or infratentorial compartment is home to the brain stem. The major motor and sensory pathways, the primary cardiovascular and respiratory centers, the reticular activating system, and the nuclei of the lower cranial nerves are all concentrated in the brain stem. All these vital structures are contained in a tight space with little room to accommodate edema, tumor, or blood.

This chapter first presents the preoperative patient management and monitoring decisions for patients having posterior fossa surgery. Intraoperative and postoperative patient management are then discussed. Finally, an outline of intraoperative problems including air embolism is presented.

Preoperative Evaluation

The fundamentals of the preanesthetic visit for any surgical procedure have been abundantly discussed in the anesthesiology literature and should be followed for neurosurgery. Extra considerations for neurosurgical patients are outlined in the chapter on supratentorial tumors (see Chapter 7).

There are a few additional considerations in the patient with a posterior fossa mass lesion. First, these patients may have an unappreciated involvement of the brain stem. Hence, sedative premedication before their arrival in the operating room should be minimal, if administered at all, and prescribed judiciously. Involvement of the cardiovascular and respiratory centers may first become apparent with the administration of sedative medication. This is particularly true with respiratory depressants such as the narcotics. Respiratory depression induces hypercarbia and thereby increases the mass effect of the patient's lesion.

Sedative agents or respiratory depressants are best avoided before the time when the patient receives constant attention from the anesthesiologist. This general principle can be appropriately modified in the cases of posterior fossa exploration for aneurysm or cranial nerve decompression. In these cases, some preoperative analgesia and sedation may be desirable. However, prudence may dictate the administration of these drugs in the operating room holding area.

Position during surgery is the second consideration that must be addressed in patients with posterior fossa lesions. For various reasons the neurosurgeon may request that the patient be placed in the sitting position. This position places extra demands on the cardiovascular system (see Chapter 5). The patient's cardiovascular reserve must be evaluated adequately during the preoperative visit to determine whether he will tolerate the sitting position. If there are any objections, they should be raised with the neurosurgeon prior to the time of surgery.

Some authors suggest that uncontrolled hypertension, advanced age, and ASA physical status 3 or 4 all increase the risk of postural hypotension and are relative contraindications to the sitting position. Significant hypovolemia would be considered an absolute contraindication.

The potential for venous and paradoxical air embolism is another major consideration for patients who are placed in the sitting position. Venous air entrainment is a common event during surgery in the sitting position. The incidence of detectable air embolism is reported at between 20 and 40% of all cases. However, clinically significant air embolism is rare if appropriate monitoring is employed and if prompt measures are undertaken to halt the entrainment of air; hence the need for preoperative decisions regarding monitors and therapy for air embolism. Also, patients must be informed of the risks associated with air embolism as a part of obtaining informed consent.

The possibility of air crossing to the left side of the circulation from the right, creating a paradoxical air embolus, is real. The potential consequences of arterial air are so grave that everything possible must be done to prevent this complication. Known anatomic cardiac shunts or the presence of a ventriculoatrial CSF shunt, which would increase the total amount of air entering the right side of the heart, are absolute contraindications to the sitting position.

Technical aspects of the sitting position are discussed in Chapter 5. Further discussion of air embolism is presented later in this chapter under the heading Special Problems.

Monitoring

As for all patients receiving any anesthetic, neurosurgical patients should be given the routine monitors: temperature, probe, neuromuscular blockade, precordial or esophageal stethoscope, noninvasive blood pressure cuff, and continuous electrocardiographic (ECG) trace. For patients with ischemic heart disease, it may be beneficial to monitor simultaneously ECG leads II and V. Pulse oximetry is rapidly becoming accepted as the standard of care and should be used routinely.

In addition to the usual monitors, most neurosurgical procedures require an indwelling urinary catheter because of the length of many procedures and the occasional need to administer diuretics for brain relaxation.

An invasive blood pressure catheter and some form of end-tidal CO_2 monitoring are also highly desirable if not mandatory for all major intracranial procedures. Beat-to-beat blood pressure information is essential if the sitting position is used or if techniques such as induced hypotension are utilized. An arterial catheter also allows rapid determination of arterial blood gas tensions and electrolyte levels.

End-tidal CO_2 monitoring provides real-time information during hyperventilation and can serve as an early warning device for kinking of the endotracheal tube or a disconnection of the breathing system. The end-tidal CO_2 monitor is also an essential component of monitoring for venous air embolism.

Other monitors, such as pulmonary artery catheters, may be required for certain patients if their condition warrants. Also, if the sitting position is used, additional monitors should be employed. Foremost among these is precordial Doppler ultrasonography. The section on venous air embolism later in this chapter contains a full discussion of monitoring modalities useful for detecting this complication.

As in all situations when monitoring is used, one must guard against major patient management decisions as a reflex to isolated information. Monitors must never serve as a substitute for close patient observation and contact.

The decision to use a given monitor, especially an invasive one, must be made in light of the potential for morbidity associated with the monitoring system. Guidelines for the use of technology must never inhibit deliberate rational thought.

Anesthetic Management

Patients with posterior fossa lesions have the potential for developing obstruction of cerebrospinal fluid outflow at the level of the aqueduct of Sylvius or fourth ventricle. This obstructive hydrocephalus results from compression by the lesion. Thus, intracranial hypertension may result from even small, strategically placed lesions. Hence, these patients must always be considered to be at risk for developing increased intracranial pressure and must be treated appropriately.

The anesthetic management for posterior fossa procedures is essentially the same as that for supratentorial surgery. These anesthetic techniques are presented in Chapter 7 and are not repeated in this chapter.

Intravenous fluid administration during posterior fossa surgery should be limited to deficit and maintenance quantities of a balanced salt solution. Major volume resuscitation may be accomplished with blood, colloid, or crystalloid (see Chapter 6 for a complete discussion of fluid therapy during neurosurgery).

Emergence from anesthesia should, like induction, be as smooth and gentle as possible. Coughing against an endotracheal tube may precipitate intracranial bleeding. However, vomiting and pulmonary aspiration of gastric contents are real dangers in a patient who is not sufficiently alert to protect the airway. An adequate blood level of narcotic generally produces an awake patient who does not cough or strain to any significant degree. Alternatively, lidocaine, 1.5 mg/kg IV, decreases the amount of coughing and straining.

The decision to extubate a patient at the end of the procedure is not always an easy one. Generally, if a patient is alert preoperatively and the surgery is superficial and performed without much traction on the brain stem, it is assumed safe to extubate. However, deep-seated lesions or protracted surgery with frequent traction on the brain stem may place the patient in danger of apnea or a decreased sensorium with diminished airway reflexes. These patients should remain intubated and ventilated until they are out of danger.

Special Problems

Brainstem Stimulation

Historically patients with posterior fossa lesions were allowed to ventilate spontaneously during surgery. This was thought to allow for monitoring of the pontine respiratory centers for surgical encroachment. However, changes in blood pressure and the presence of arrhythmias are equally sensitive indicators of brainstem manipulation. Therefore, spontaneous ventilation during posterior fossa surgery can no longer be recommended.

Brainstem and cranial nerve stimulation can have dramatic effects. Profound hypertension results from stimulation of cranial nerve V, the periventricular gray area, the reticular formation, or the nucleus of the tractus solitarius. Significant bradycardia and escape rhythms result from stimulation of the vagus nerve. Hypotension can be a result of pontine or medullary compression. Ventricular and supraventricular arrhythmias can occur from stimulation of many brainstem structures.

Close attention to cardiovascular parameters during critical periods of surgery is essential to the patient's well-being. Not only will life-threatening conditions be diagnosed, but the surgeon may be informed of potential brainstem encroachment.

Air Embolism

Veins situated higher than the level of the right atrium have an intravascular pressure less than central venous pressure. The higher the vein is above the right atrium, the lower the intravascular pressure. At some elevation, veins will have a negative intravascular pressure. When a patient is tilted 65 degrees head-up, the pressure in the jugular bulb becomes subatmospheric. At this degree of head-up tilt or greater, the veins of the head and neck also have a subatmospheric pressure. If these veins are open to the atmosphere, they entrain air, causing a venous air embolus.

Once air enters the venous system, it can flow with the venous blood to the heart and subsequently to the pulmonary circulation. Venous air can occur as small or large bubbles. A capsule of platelets, lipid, and protein forms around the gas bubble. Additionally, gas exchange between the blood and the air bubble occurs readily.

Venous air can be entrained in either a slow or rapid fashion. Air entrained slowly, usually as a stream of small bubbles, is carried through the heart to lodge in the pulmonary capillary. This results in a functional decrease in the pulmonary capillary bed. Pulmonary artery and subsequently central venous pressures increase. If the pulmonary artery pressure increases enough, right ventricular failure may result and cardiac output will fall. However, a decrease in cardiac output is generally not seen until a large volume of air has been entrained, if it is entrained slowly.

Alveolar dead space increases with slow air embolization because of the decreased perfusion of the capillary bed. With constant ventilation the arterial Pco_2 increases and the arterial Po_2 decreases.

Rapid air embolism, frequently occurring as a series of large bubbles, often produces a swirling vortex of air in the superior vena cava, right atrium, or right ventricle. The increase in pulmonary artery pressure is initially less than with slow air embolism. However, a rapid air embolus can severely impede flow through the right heart, and subsequently cardiac output and blood pressure decrease.

Air embolism is most likely to occur during dissection of neck muscles, turning of the craniotomy flap, and dissection of a vascular tumor bed. Particular vigilance is required at these times.

A large air embolus can be a fatal event. In the first half of the 1960s, 93 cases of venous air embolism were reported in the literature. In the 40 untreated cases there was a 93% mortality rate! In those patients treated with various combinations of pressor drugs, left lateral positioning, and open cardiac massage, the mortality rate was less but still a significant 58%.

In 1969, a report came from the Mayo Clinic of 2,500 operations performed in the sitting position with no deaths attributable to venous air embolism. Thus, venous air embolism was initially regarded as a rare but devastating complication. However, our understanding of the true incidence of air embolism during procedures performed in the sitting position changed dramatically as sensitive monitors for venous air were employed.

In 1965, end-tidal CO_2 monitoring was introduced by Bethune and Brechner, followed in 1968 by the introduction of precordial Doppler ultrasonography by Maroon. With these sensitive monitors we soon learned that the incidence of detectable venous air embolism during procedures in the sitting position is 20 to 40%. The vast majority of these cases of air embolism are not clinically significant.

Monitoring for Air Embolism

Several methods are now available to monitor for air embolism.

Precordial Doppler Ultrasonography. The precordial Doppler is the most sensitive of the practical monitors and should be employed during all procedures in which air embolism is likely to occur. The Doppler generates an ultrasonic signal that is reflected by moving erythrocytes and moving cardiac structures. The reflected signal is received and processed to produce a characteristic rhythmic sound. When air, an excellent reflector, enters the Doppler detection field, a roaring noise is heard.

The Doppler can detect a bolus of air as small as 0.25 ml and is an excellent early warning system for air entrainment. However, with the Doppler there is no reliable way to quantitate the volume of air entrained.

The precordial Doppler is effective as an early detector only if it is placed to "listen" over the right side of the heart. The Doppler probe should be placed to the right of the sternum in the third to sixth intercostal space. Placement of the Doppler should be done after the patient is positioned, because the heart will move caudad when the patient is placed in the sitting position. Select the 2-Hz setting on the Doppler and check the position of the Doppler by injecting a rapid bolus of 10 ml of agitated saline through a central line (or if necessary a peripheral intravenous line). This rapid bolus produces a noticeable change in the Doppler sound if the Doppler is placed correctly. Hold the Doppler firmly in place by tight taping or some other mechanism.

The precordial Doppler is an excellent early warning device. The vast majority of the air detected with the Doppler is clinically unimportant. Detection of some air during a sitting procedure is to be expected and should not be cause for alarm. However, a continuous stream of air or frequent intermittent air should prompt a search for the source and elimination of further entrainment.

End-Tidal Carbon Dioxide Monitoring. End-tidal CO_2 monitoring is another sensitive indicator of venous air embolism. When air is trapped in the pulmonary capillary bed, alveolar dead space is created. If enough dead space is present, the diffusion gradient for CO_2 is increased. This causes an increased arterial P_{CO_2} value but a decreased alveolar P_{CO_2} value. Since the end-tidal P_{CO_2} represents alveolar P_{CO_2}, the end-tidal P_{CO_2} falls with an air embolus.

End-tidal CO_2 monitoring is less sensitive than precordial Doppler monitoring. The end-tidal Pco_2 begins to fall significantly when 0.25 to 0.5 ml/kg of air has been entrained into the pulmonary system.

The major advantages of end-tidal CO_2 monitoring are that it is easy to use, is noninvasive, and correlates closely with clinically significant air embolism. A disadvantage is that factors other than air embolism can affect an end-tidal CO_2 value. The most important of these is hypotension, which also increases the dead space in the lung.

End-Tidal Nitrogen Monitoring. End-tidal N_2 determination is another monitoring technique for air embolism. When a patient is connected to a breathing circuit and no air is utilized in the inhalation gas mixture, the nitrogen in the lungs is quickly eliminated. Normal end-tidal N_2 is therefore zero. When an air embolus occurs, nitrogen, a component of air, is excreted through the lungs, causing end-tidal N_2 to rise. End-tidal N_2 increases before end-tidal CO_2 decreases. However, end-tidal N_2 returns to normal before resolution of the air embolus. One chief advantage of end-tidal N_2 as a monitor for air embolism is the capacity to quantitate the amount of embolized air.

Pulmonary Artery Catheterization. The pulmonary artery catheter has been advocated as a technique to monitor for air embolism. It is true that the pulmonary artery pressure usually does increase with air embolism. However, the sensitivity of the pulmonary artery catheter is probably no greater than the end-tidal CO_2 monitor. Because of the risk associated with the use of pulmonary artery catheters and the fact that they provide little additional information, this author cannot recommend the pulmonary artery catheter as a monitor for air embolism.

Echocardiography. Echocardiography has been used in various forms to monitor for air embolism. An echocardiogram can be obtained from the precordial or subxyphoid area or via a transesophageal probe. Although echocardiography may be slightly more sensitive as a monitor for intracardiac air than the Doppler, it may interfere with the normal operation of the precordial Doppler. Also, echocardiography currently requires constant visual attention to detect intracardiac air. A case of vocal cord paralysis from the transesophageal probe has been reported.

One major advantage of echocardiography is that it is the only monitor available to detect air that crosses into the left side of the heart. Despite this advantage, this author believes that echocardiography is currently a research tool and should not be considered standard for the monitoring of air embolism.

Use of Nitrous Oxide

The use of N_2O as an anesthetic supplement during procedures in which air embolus is likely to occur has been controversial. Nitrous oxide is 34 times more soluble in blood than is nitrogen. It diffuses more rapidly into an air embolus than N_2 diffuses out. Hence, N_2O in the blood will increase the size of an air embolus, and the quantity of air causing morbidity or mortality will thus be decreased. The LD_{50} of air is 5.1 ml/kg in dogs and 0.5 ml/kg in rabbits. However, in rabbits breathing 75% N_2O, the LD_{50} is decreased to 0.16 ml/kg.

For a controversy to exist there must be opposing views. The arguments for the use of N_2O are that (1) less volatile agent will be used and so patients may have less cardiovascular depression and may awaken more quickly, and (2) since N_2O will increase the size of an air embolus, a smaller quantity of air will need to be entrained prior to identification and initiation of appropriate measures.

This author agrees that N_2O should be discontinued, if it is used at all, prior to skin incision. If it is necessary, it may be safely used early in the case until the patient is stabilized.

Positive End-Expiratory Pressure

Positive end-expiratory pressure (PEEP) has been suggested as a method to decrease the incidence of air embolism. The increase in intrathoracic pressure generated by PEEP would be transmitted to the cerebral veins and thereby decrease the entrainment of air. However, in animal models 10 cm H_2O PEEP is not always effective in accomplishing this goal.

There have been a few objections to the use of PEEP. It may decrease the mean arterial pressure and therefore cerebral perfusion pressure. Perkins and Bedford found that 10 cm H_2O of PEEP can reverse the normal left-to-right interatrial pressure gradient. This shift in the pressure gradient was postulated to increase the incidence of paradoxical air embolism. Subsequent work in pigs with a surgically created atrial septal defect demonstrated that a left-to-right pressure gradient may not always protect against paradoxical air embolism. This is so because a right-to-left pressure gradient develops at some point during the cardiac cycle, even when the mean pressure gradient is the opposite.

Central Venous Cannulation

The last issue relating to venous air embolism is the issue of central venous catheters. There is no question that air can be aspirated from a properly placed central venous catheter during episodes of air embolism in both humans and experimental animals. The aspiration of air has been conclusively shown to decrease the mortality from a lethal injection of air in animals and has been suggested as a contribution to resuscitation from air embolism in humans. Recently developed multiorificed catheters may even improve upon previous results.

However, the need for a central catheter during procedures in the sitting position is not compelling. With correctly functioning Doppler and end-tidal CO_2 equipment, air embolism can usually be diagnosed and halted prior to the entrainment of a significant amount of air. With this early warning system in place, it is rare to aspirate more than a few bubbles of air. The therapeutic benefit of central catheters has been significantly negated by these new monitors.

With a diminishing benefit, the risks of central venous cannulation become a significant factor. Eisenhauer and associates reported a 13.7% complication rate in 554 attempts at internal jugular vein cannulation. Although most of these complications were minor, there was a 4% rate of major complications (arterial puncture, pneumothorax, venous air embolism).

In light of a shrinking benefit-risk ratio for central venous catheters during episodes of air embolism, one should not view them as an absolute necessity and cry malpractice when they are not used. However, this author believes that some benefit can accrue from the use of a central venous catheter, and therefore a reasonable effort should be made to place one prior to a sitting craniotomy.

A small number of patients entrain a large quantity of air so quickly that other monitors do not serve as early warning devices, but rather merely confirm that something "bad" has occurred. Experimental evidence suggests that these patients will respond to air aspiration through a properly placed central catheter. Although the number of patients in this group is small, the risk of this occurrence is real and must not be ignored.

Another benefit of central catheters is that small amounts of air can be removed, thus decreasing the amount of air available for paradoxical embolization. Again, the number of patients who will benefit from this maneuver is small, but since it is impossible to predict who will or will not shunt air to the left side, all patients must be considered as potential beneficiaries.

As a result of the foregoing arguments, a reasonable effort should be made to place a central venous catheter properly in all patients about to have a sitting craniotomy. The term "reasonable effort" needs some clarification. If accessible arm or neck veins can be identified, then this author agrees with Michenfelder that a 10- to 15-minute attempt constitutes a reasonable effort. Anesthesiologists must know their skills well enough to determine the point at which patient risk is increasing more than patient benefit, and then quit if the attempt has been unsuccessful.

The issue of cannulation site (arm versus neck) has proponents on both sides. Although it is true that there is less risk associated with central venous cannulation through an antecubital vein, it is also true that antecubital catheters are frequently of a smaller diameter than catheters designed for the neck. In the case of massive air embolism a larger catheter placed in a jugular vein may be more beneficial, although its placement may increase the risk associated with central venous cannulation. This author prefers to use an antecubital vein but does not hesitate to move to a jugular vein if an antecubital vein is not available.

The last consideration for the placement of central catheters is where to locate the aspirating tip of the catheter. Early in the history of central vein cannulation for air embolism, it was assumed that the catheter tip should be localized in the mid right atrium. This early recommendation was based on intuition. In 1981, Bunegin et al. evaluated the catheter aspiration of air in an in vivo model of the human right atrium. They determined that it is critical to place the aspirating tip of the catheter in the upper quarter of the right atrium. Although the study by Bunegin et al. is important, it is an in vivo study, and extrapolation to humans must be done with caution.

The tip of a central venous catheter can be placed in the high right atrium with electrocardiographic guidance. Once access to the central circulation is obtained, fill the catheter with sodium bicarbonate (1 mEq/ml) or normal saline. Then electrically couple lead V of the electrocardiograph to the fluid inside the catheter. The tip of the catheter thus becomes an exploring electrode. Move the catheter until the p-wave becomes biphasic, indicating correct placement. Confirm the position of the catheter by injecting a rapid bolus of 5 to 10 ml of saline through the catheter to elicit the typical Doppler sound.

Therapy for Air Embolism

Finally, what should one do when faced with a significant air embolism? First, the surgeon should be notified and nitrous oxide discontinued, if it is being used. The surgeon should inspect the surgical field for an open vein. If an open vein is not found, a Valsalva maneuver or bilateral compression of the jugular veins for 5 to 10 seconds will increase the cerebral venous pressure and induce bleeding. Compression of the jugular veins will also halt ongoing air embolism. If air entrainment continues, the anesthesiologist should ask for an assistant. A second pair of hands will allow simultaneous jugular vein compression and central catheter aspiration.

If the blood pressure falls, additional therapy should be instituted. Ephedrine, 10 to 20 mg IV, and a bolus of fluid usually improves the blood pressure and propels the air into the pulmonary circulation. If this does not restore the blood pressure, the patient should be placed in the left lateral decubitus position with a 15-degree head-down tilt. This position may release an existing air lock and allow the cardiac output to increase.

Paradoxical Air Embolism

Paradoxical air embolism, air entering the left circulation, has been mentioned occasionally during the discussion of air embolism. Air may cross to the left side of the heart either through an intracardiac lesion or through other venous-arterial connections. Twenty to 30% of patients have a probe-patent foramen ovale that may become a gateway for paradoxical air. However, animal studies have demonstrated that air can cross from right to left with no demonstrable intracardiac lesion. Hence, all patients with venous air embolism are at risk for paradoxical air embolism.

The two main circulatory beds at risk are the coronary and the cerebral vascular beds. As little as 0.6 ml of air injected into the carotid artery of a cat decreases electroencephalographic amplitude and causes cerebral edema and increased intracranial pressure. Just 0.2 ml of air injected into a dog's coronary circulation results in myocardial damage.

Intraoperative diagnosis of paradoxical air embolism is very difficult. Echocardiography allows for visualization of left-sided air but is not always practical to use. Electrocardiographic changes may reflect coronary air. However, air is only one of many possible causes for ECG changes. Occasionally air bubbles may be visualized by the surgeon in the cerebral circulation.

The therapeutic options available to the anesthesiologist during paradoxical air embolism are very limited. The blood pressure and cardiac output should be supported if necessary. Effort should also be made to retrieve any venous air or to halt air entrainment that may be a source of ongoing paradoxical air embolism.

Paradoxical air embolism became a major concern in the late 1970s. Although the actual incidence of paradoxical air embolism is not known, seven cases of clinically significant paradoxical air embolism were reported through 1981.

Case History

G.G., a 54-year-old man, experienced a sudden loss of hearing in the left ear 4 months prior to admission. He was seen at this time by an audiologist who noted a 100 dB hearing loss on the left. A magnetic resonance imaging (MRI) scan showed a tumor in the left cerebellopontine angle, consistent with an acoustic neuroma (Fig. 8-1). The patient subsequently developed poor balance, which worsened greatly during the month prior to admission. He also experienced a metallic taste in his mouth. He did not have headache, nausea, vomiting, or numbness or weakness in the extremities or face.

The medical history was significant for poorly controlled hypertension, non–insulin-dependent diabetes mellitus, and gout. The patient had undergone a parathyroidectomy in the past for nephrolithiasis. His medications at the time of surgery were furosemide 40 mg daily, potassium chloride 20 mEq daily, and glyburide 10 mg each morning and 5 mg each evening.

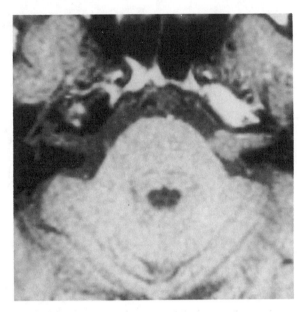

Figure 8-1 An MRI scan of a left acoustic neuroma. The tumor is rounded near the brain stem with a lateral tail along cranial nerve VIII.

On physical examination the patient had a blood pressure of 160/100 mm Hg. He was otherwise normal except for decreased hearing on the left with some bone conduction but no air conduction. His upper airway and neck mobility were normal. The glucose level was 288 mg/dl, potassium 4.3 mEq/L, and calcium 9.5 mg/dl.

The patient underwent a posterior fossa craniotomy in the sitting position for resection of an acoustic neuroma. He tolerated the seated position well, experiencing a few, but clinically insignificant, episodes of venous air embolism. His facial nerve was intact after the surgical procedure.

Suggested Reading

Artru AA, Colley PS. Placement of multiorificed CVP catheters via antecubital veins using intravascular electrocardiography. Anesthesiology 1988; 69:132–135.

Artru AA, Colley PS. The site of origin of the intravascular electrocardiogram recorded from multiorificed intravascular catheters. Anesthesiology 1988; 69:44–48.

Artru AA, Colley PS. Bunegin-Albin CVP catheter improves resuscitation from lethal venous air embolism. Anesthesiology Review 1985; 12:32–33.

Bedford RF. Perioperative venous air embolism. Seminars in Anesthesia 1987; 6:163–170.

Bunegin L, Albin MS, Helsel PE, Hoffman A, Hung T. Positioning the right atrial catheter: A model for reappraisal. Anesthesiology 1981; 55:343–348.

Colley PS, Artru AA. ECG-guided placement of sorenson CVP catheters via arm veins. Anesth Analg 1984; 63:953–956.

Cucchiara RF, Nugent M, Seward J, Messick JM. Air embolism in upright neurosurgical patients: Detection and localization by two-dimensional transesophageal echocardiography. Anesthesiology 1984; 60:353-355.

Gottdiener JS, Papademetriou V, Notargiacomo A, Park WY, Cutler DJ. Incidence and cardiac effects of systemic venous air embolism. Arch Intern Med 1988; 148:795-800.

Gronert GA, Messick JM, Cucchiara RF, Michenfelder JD. Paradoxical air embolism from a patent foramen ovale. Anesthesiology 1979; 50:548-549.

Marshall WK, Bedford RF, Miller ED. Cardiovascular responses in the seated position — impact of four anesthetic techniques. Anesth Analg 1983; 62:648-653.

Marshall WK, Bedford RF. Use of a pulmonary artery catheter for detection and treatment of venous air embolism: A prospective study in man. Anesthesiology 1980; 52:131-134.

Michenfelder JD. Central venous catheters in the management of air embolism: Whether as well as where. Anesthesiology 1981; 55:339-340.

Pearl RG, Larson CP. Hemodynamic effects of positive end-expiratory pressure during continuous venous air embolism in the dog. Anesthesiology 1986; 64:724-729.

Perkins NAK, Bedford RF. Hemodynamic consequences of PEEP in seated neurological patients. Implications for paradoxical air embolism. Anesth Analg 1984; 63:429-432.

Perkins-Pearson NAK, Marshall WK, Bedford RF. Atrial pressures in the seated position: Implication for paradoxical air embolism. Anesthesiology 1982; 57:493-497.

Toung TJK, Miyabe M, McShane AJ, Rogers MC, Traystman RJ. Effect of PEEP and jugular venous compression on canine cerebral blood flow and oxygen consumption in the head elevated position. Anesthesiology 1988; 68:53-58.

Zasslow MA, Pearl RG, Larson CP, Silverberg G, Shuer LF. PEEP does not affect left atrial–right atrial pressure difference in neurosurgical patients. Anesthesiology 1988; 68:760-763.

David J. Stone, M.D.

Anesthesia for Intracranial Vascular Surgery 9

Preoperative Assessment

Cardiovascular Evaluation

Volume Status

The majority of patients with aneurysmal subarachnoid hemorrhage are in the 40- to 60-year age range and often have no underlying medical problems. Many neurosurgeons have kept these patients on the "dry side" to avoid arterial hypertension that will increase the pressure across the wall of the aneurysm (or across the organizing clot of hemorrhage). These patients may receive diuretics and minimal fluid replacement in addition to undergoing a supine diuresis. Increased catecholamine levels cause vasoconstriction and decrease the functional intravascular space. This hypovolemia is unmasked when vasodilating (or simply sympatholytic) anesthetics are administered. For these reasons, anesthetists in the past needed to give large volumes of fluid before anesthesia could be safely induced.

Currently, neurosurgeons have become more liberal with fluids during the preoperative period to lessen the incidence and severity of vasospasm. A review of weight change, administered fluid, and patient appearance will give a rough idea of volume status, which will be further substantiated by blood pressure and pulse rate. Renal function and electrolyte status should be reviewed. Central venous and pulmonary capillary wedge pressure measurements are helpful, but not essential in every patient. Hypovolemia should be corrected before induction so that a sufficiently deep level of anesthesia for laryngoscopy and intubation can be achieved safely.

Hypertension

Patients without previous hypertension may become hypertensive in this setting because of increased catecholamine levels. Patients with increased intracranial pressure (ICP) may have reflex hypertension in an attempt to maintain cerebral perfusion pressure (CPP). The patient with an unclipped, ruptured aneurysm should have blood pressure reduced to normal levels as long as cerebral perfusion remains adequate. Vasospasm is a very difficult problem in these patients, because increased blood volume and pressure may be required to overcome the spasm without rerupturing the aneurysm. A pulmonary artery catheter may be useful to maintain optimal intravascular fluid status.

If ICP is normal, small intravenous increments of hydralazine, with or without propranolol, or a continuous infusion of nitroprusside may be used. Nitroglycerin may be used as an infusion, but hypertension may be refractory to it. Trimethaphan may interfere with neurologic evaluation by causing pupillary dilatation. Calcium blockers such as nicardipine may eventually be used to treat hypertension while preventing vasospasm, if studies in progress prove them to be useful.

If ICP is elevated, incremental doses of labetalol are useful, as this combined alpha- and beta-receptor blocker increases cerebral blood flow (and therefore cerebral blood volume and ICP) only minimally because of the paucity of alpha-receptors in the cerebral vasculature. Use of a pure beta-blocker, such as propranolol or esmolol, by infusion is acceptable. Oral administration of angiotensin-converting enzyme inhibitors (captopril, enalapril) will facilitate blood pressure control. It is critical to avoid wide swings in blood pressure, which may cause the aneurysm to rerupture.

Electrocardiographic Abnormalities

For reasons that are not understood, electrocardiographic abnormalities occur in more than half of patients with subarachnoid hemorrhage. These include changes in the morphology of the electrocardiogram, i.e., Q-T prolongation, abnormal S-T segments and T waves, appearance of U waves, as well as arrhythmias including ventricular tachycardia. While enzymatic and echocardiographic examinations have not revealed significant areas of infarction, pathologic examination has revealed microscopic areas of myocardial necrosis. This may be analogous to the "catecholamine myocarditis" seen in patients with pheochromocytoma who also have high catecholamine levels. This myocardial pathology does not appear to have much clinical significance with regard to myocardial function.

Neurologic Evaluation

Diagnosis

The patient often describes "the worst headache of her life," which is followed by meningeal signs due to blood in the CSF. Consciousness may be lost briefly because of an acute rise in ICP. Warning leaks occur in about half the patients and may be mild, so that it is extremely difficult for a busy primary care physician to distinguish a benign viral illness from a small subarachnoid hemorrhage. The diagnosis can be made from CT scan in most (90 to 95%) cases, and angiography then can be used for definitive anatomic diagnosis. In a small percentage of cases, the aneurysm cannot be located on the angiogram.

Although some clinicians may employ lumbar puncture in all patients without contraindications (especially increased ICP), others use lumbar puncture selectively in those in whom the diagnosis is not otherwise firmly established. Theoretically, lumbar puncture could precipitate rerupture by decreasing ICP and therefore increasing the pressure gradient across the wall (transmural) of the aneurysm [mean arterial pressure (MAP) minus ICP].

Aneurysms do not appear to be congenital, because they are found infrequently in pediatric postmortem examinations. They appear with time at vessel branch points. They are most commonly found around the circle of Willis and the bifurcation of the middle cerebral artery. Large aneurysms may produce focal symptoms that correspond to the local neuroanatomy involved. Aneurysms larger than 25 mm in diameter are often referred to as "giant aneurysms," but most range from 6 to 15 mm in diameter.

There are various numbering systems for classification of patient status with ruptured aneurysm. These systems grade patients on a scale of 0–1 to 4–5, with the higher numbers representing more severe neurologic dysfunction. It probably is most useful to realize that patients with minimal or no neurologic residual of subarachnoid hemorrhage do better than those who have severe focal signs, stupor, or coma. Neurologic findings may be caused by the mass effect of a large intracerebral hematoma. This will be obvious on CT scans and may require surgical drainage. Anesthesia follows the principles outlined for patients with intracranial masses (supra- or infratentorial). Hydrocephalus (communicating) may be caused by blood preventing free egress of CSF. This also will be found on the CT scan and may require shunting.

Vasospasm can be demonstrated angiographically in a majority of patients with subarachnoid hemorrhage, but is functionally significant in only a minority. Vasospasm peaks in incidence from about day 4 to day 12. Without employing angiography, its presence often is presumed from neurologic deterioration in the absence of further bleeding, mass effect, or hydrocephalus on the CT scan. Cerebral infarction may result. Treatment is considered in detail in Chapter 18.

Rebleeding is another source of morbidity and mortality. It is most likely to occur soon after the initial rupture. Preoperative rebleeding is discussed further in Chapter 18.

Timing of Surgery and Surgical Considerations

The timing of surgery for aneurysm clipping after subarachnoid hemorrhage has been a controversial issue in recent neurosurgical literature. Until recently, surgeons tended to wait several weeks to operate and were faced with better operating conditions and a lower mortality in the patients who received "late" surgery. However, this was largely due to the deaths of many patients earlier as a result of rebleeding, vasospasm, and medical complications. As neuroanesthesia and neurosurgery have advanced and early operating conditions have become more technically favorable, other neurosurgeons have advocated "early" surgery before rebleeding, vasospasm and other complications have taken their toll. Early surgery removes blood that may contribute to vasospasm and allows for more aggressive hemodynamic treatment of vasospasm if it occurs. A large cooperative study did not clearly settle the issue, and the neurosurgeon still must operate on a case-by-case basis. The neurosurgeon also must decide whether an unruptured aneurysm discovered on routine evaluation should be clipped.

The operative position of the patient largely depends on the location of the aneurysm and may involve any of the positions used in neurosurgery, occasionally even the sitting position. Special considerations of the sitting position are discussed in Chapter 8. Although the goal usually is to clip the aneurysm(s) at the base with a metal clip, other techniques may be employed, including direct thrombosis of the aneurysm, ligation of a proximal vessel, "trapping" the aneurysm with ligation of proximal and distal parent vessel, or reinforcement of the aneurysm wall.

Aneurysm surgery is exacting and often performed with an operating microscope. An absolutely still patient with stable hemodynamics is required to avoid aneurysmal rupture. Usually, hypotensive anesthesia is employed to facilitate aneurysm exposure and clipping as well as to decrease bleeding, should rupture occur. Spinal drains, hyperventilation, and mannitol may be employed to improve exposure. These issues are discussed in subsequent sections.

Pulmonary Evaluation

The patient with a subarachnoid hemorrhage who has an abnormal mental status may develop secretion retention and atelectasis because of lack of deep breathing and cough. Because chest physical therapy often results in hypertension, it is probably wise to employ a preoperative anticholinergic to reduce secretions and then a high tidal volume (12 to 15 ml/kg) intraoperatively to reduce atelectasis if there is a problem with oxygenation. Many clinicians have the impression that neurosurgical patients may develop ventilation-perfusion ($\dot{V}/\dot{Q}$) abnormalities in the absence of pulmonary parenchymal changes. These $\dot{V}/\dot{Q}$ changes may result from neurologic input to pulmonary blood vessels with subsequent changes in the distribution of pulmonary blood flow.

Premedications and the Preoperative Visit

This aspect of anesthetic care is especially important in patients scheduled to undergo intracranial vascular surgery, because it is essential for the patient to remain calm and normotensive in the preinduction period. Sedation is not employed if the patient is already stuporous or has a potential ICP problem. The patient who is wide awake should be adequately sedated. A small amount of narcotic is reasonable to reduce the discomfort of vascular cannula insertion. A benzodiazepine is a reasonable choice for sedation, e.g., diazepam (Valium) 5 to 20 mg PO, lorazepam (Ativan) 1 to 4 mg PO, or midazolam (Versed) 1 to 4 mg IM (or IV under skilled supervision). Other clinicians may choose to use barbiturates or other sedatives. If the patient is anxious on arrival at the operating room, 1-mg increments of IV midazolam are helpful. Some clinicians may pretreat with an antihypertensive if controlled hypotension is planned (see the section "Controlled Hypotension" later in this chapter).

     Although the mortality and morbidity of neurosurgery for an unruptured aneurysm are not high, surgery for ruptured aneurysm does involve a significant risk. Most reasonable people know that intracranial vascular neurosurgery carries such a risk. The anesthetist should not cause excessive worry for the patient, but the family should be made aware, if they are not already, that death or severe neurologic disability may occur as a result of the underlying disease, as well as from surgery and anesthesia.

Monitoring

Cardiovascular Monitoring

Blood Pressure

All patients should have intra-arterial monitoring of blood pressure. While some clinicians may prefer to induce anesthesia before insertion of an arterial cannula, most neuroanesthetists insert the cannula before induction in order to have a beat-to-beat monitor of blood pressure during the critical periods of laryngoscopy and intubation. Local anesthesia usually reduces the discomfort of insertion to a level that does not raise blood pressure unacceptably. On rare occasions, if insertion is difficult and/or the patient is anxious or uncooperative, anesthesia may proceed using the automated oscillometer (e.g., the Dinamap), preferably one with a "STAT" mode that provides blood pressures more frequently than one reading per minute. The arterial line subsequently can be inserted when the patient has been anesthetized.

Central Lines and Venous Access

In the majority of patients, central venous or pulmonary artery catheters are not necessary. However, they may be indicated when there is underlying cardiovascular disease or when the patient is to be operated on in the sitting position. Some clinicians routinely insert a CVP line to gain some estimate of volume status and to have central venous access for drug administration. However, it is critical to have adequate venous access for rapid blood and fluid administration in the event that there is rupture of the aneurysm (or arteriovenous malformation). A reasonable approach is to have at least two 18-gauge or greater intravenous lines that run well. Fortunately, massive and rapid hemorrhage is not common, but two lines also provide access for constant infusion in one line while the other is used for fluids, boluses of drugs, and blood administration.

Respiratory Monitoring

While the capnometer for measuring end-tidal CO_2 ($PetCO_2$) is not essential unless the sitting position is employed, it is a useful way of following carbon dioxide levels once the $PaCO_2$–$PetCO_2$ gradient has been established with a blood gas. Although I routinely employ immediate hyperventilation to improve surgical conditions, other clinicians may avoid it or wait until the dura is opened to avoid the theoretical risk that decreased ICP will cause aneurysmal rupture via increasing transmural pressure (MAP minus ICP). We also continue hyperventilation when hypotension is induced, while other clinicians may choose not to do so because of their concern that cerebral ischemia may result. In any case, it is useful to have a constant monitor of $PetCO_2$ levels. During controlled hypotension, pulmonary dead space may increase, resulting in an increase in the $PaCO_2$–$PetCO_2$ gradient.

Neurologic Monitoring

There are no routine intraoperative monitors of neurologic function. Some clinicians may employ the electroencephalogram as a monitor for cerebral ischemia (brain retraction, hypotension, hyperventilation, vasospasm are all potential causes). Others may wish to employ thiopental or isoflurane in doses that flatten the EEG in order to provide full brain protection. The surgical field obviously limits lead placement of routine scalp electrodes.

Induction of Anesthesia

After the placement of the arterial line and at least one dependable intravenous line, anesthesia can be induced. Thiopental generally is employed (4 to 5 mg/kg), unless the patient is hypovolemic or has cardiac dysfunction. Hypovolemia should be corrected appropriately before induction. The unusual patient with cardiac dysfunction should receive a careful induction with a reduced dose of thiopental plus narcotic and/or lidocaine, or even a pure narcotic induction if dysfunction is severe. The latter may delay awakening and necessitate postoperative ventilation and should be avoided if possible. An infusion of nitroprusside should be made up and immediately available, and blood should also be immediately available.

When the patient is asleep, as demonstrated by lack of eyelash reflex, the adequacy of mask ventilation is assured. An intubating dose of muscle relaxant is then given. A nondepolarizing relaxant allows enough time to establish a level of anesthesia sufficiently deep so that laryngoscopy and intubation will not produce severe hypertension with the possibility of aneurysm rupture. Any of the available nondepolarizers is acceptable (except gallamine, which produces unacceptable tachycardia at these doses). At this point, a narcotic is given to deepen the anesthesia. Doses are approximately 1.5 to 2.0 μg/kg for sufentanil or 10–15 μg/kg for fentanyl.

Limited experience with alfentanil during the induction phase suggests a dose of about 50 to 75 μg/kg. An advantage to alfentanil might be its quicker onset of action: while sufentanil and fentanyl require about 5 minutes to cause a 50% reduction in maximal spectral edge frequency, alfentanil causes a similar change in about one-third the time. (See Chapter 4 for discussion of spectral edge frequency and its utilization in pharmacokinetic studies.) Sufentanil has the theoretical advantage over fentanyl of a shorter beta (metabolism) half-life (140 minutes versus about 240 minutes), although these numbers have recently come into question.

Some clinicians may choose to use a dose of narcotic before anesthesia is induced. We have found that this may produce some chest wall rigidity and makes it more difficult to demonstrate the adequacy of mask ventilation. Pretreatment with narcotic is an excellent idea if a rapid-sequence induction is necessary because the patient presents a high risk of aspiration. Because aneurysm rupture is such a devastating complication, another option, though somewhat controversial, in the high-risk aspiration patient is the usual slow mask induction with *expert* cricoid pressure application and pretreatment with ranitidine or cimetidine, metoclopramide, and possibly Bicitra. Once paralysis is induced and proper cricoid pressure applied, the risk of aspiration is small, and the antacid and volume regimen described decreases the risk to very low levels.

Unless a rapid-sequence induction is chosen, the blood pressure response to laryngoscopy should be carefully observed so that if blood pressure rises to unacceptable levels, intubation can be delayed until anesthesia is deepened. A competent assistant is helpful during such inductions to observe blood pressure and administer necessary drugs quickly. A second, smaller dose of thiopental may be necessary to control blood pressure during laryngoscopy and intubation. The use of succinylcholine is acceptable if the aneurysm is unruptured and a rapid-sequence induction is necessary but we prefer a large dose of nondepolarizer (vecuronium, 0.15–0.25 mg/kg) in this situation.

Rupture during induction is an obvious disaster. Hypertension may occur as either a cause or a result and should be treated with thiopental and nitroprusside. Hypotension should be avoided to maintain CPP in the face of a possibly increased ICP. The surgeon then determines whether emergency clipping should be undertaken.

Maintenance of Anesthesia

Anesthetic Considerations

Once anesthesia has been safely induced, special concerns in aneurysm surgery include prevention of aneurysm rupture and provision of optimal surgical conditions as patient safety allows. Hypertension, especially abrupt increases in blood pressure, should be avoided. This usually requires deepening of anesthesia during periods of intense stimulation, i.e., head pinning initially, then incision, followed by turning of bone and dural flaps. This can be accomplished with a deep level of inhaled anesthesia (usually isoflurane) or with boluses of thiopental (2 to 4 mg/kg) or alfentanil (10 to 20 μg/kg) with or without IV lidocaine. Communication between surgeon and anesthesiologist or anesthetist is essential to ensure that the necessary depth of anesthesia is achieved.

To maintain hemodynamic stability, anesthesia is continued with a combination of nitrous oxide, isoflurane, and residual intravenous drugs (narcotic, thiopental). A pure nitrous-narcotic anesthetic may be chosen, but the addition of isoflurane may make sudden hypertension less likely, and we employ isoflurane so far as it is tolerated hemodynamically.

The following sections discuss special techniques which may be employed to increase the safety of aneurysm clipping by improving surgical access to and handling of the aneurysm.

Controlled Hypotension

Controlled hypotension, or hypotensive anesthesia, usually is employed to reduce the pressure across the aneurysm wall (and therefore lessen the likelihood of rupture), facilitate handling and clipping the aneurysm, and reduce bleeding should rupture occur. Pretreatment with captopril (3 mg/kg PO) or clonidine (0.05 mg/kg PO) reduces the amount of hypotensive agent required to achieve the desired level of blood pressure. Such pretreatment also may stabilize the hemodynamic course of the anesthetic, but this has not been studied in this setting. Although no comparative study of the drugs has been done, captopril appears to have a slight edge in clinical effectiveness.

At the University of Virginia, we employ hypotensive anesthesia for aneurysm surgery and use isoflurane in the vast majority of cases. Adequate anesthesia is assured, and there is a theoretical advantage of brain protection by isoflurane. Lam and his colleagues have shown that cerebral blood flow is minimally reduced at mean blood pressures of 50 mm Hg, and cerebral oxygen metabolism is reduced proportionately more than blood pressure. The latter effect may provide some protection against possible cerebral ischemia from hypotension, surgical retraction, and clipping of feeder vessels, if required.

Cardiac output is maintained during isoflurane-induced controlled hypotension. In normal subjects, the desired mean blood pressure is about 50 mm Hg ($\pm$ 5 mm) during dissection and clipping of the aneurysm. At times, the surgeon may request a mean blood pressure of 40 mm Hg, and this is well tolerated, even with continued hyperventilation. In chronically hypertensive patients, the elderly, and those with coronary and/or cerebrovascular disease, the anesthetist and surgeon should agree on an acceptable level of hypotension. Because this is surgery for a life- and brain-threatening problem, the anesthetist should be thoughtful but not excessively conservative in the application of hypotension if the surgeon is otherwise unable to safely approach and clip the aneurysm.

While isoflurane usually is adequate, I sometimes add small doses of labetalol (5-mg increments) to supplement the isoflurane if high levels are required (2.5% inspired). This is done to reduce the amount of anesthetic given and speed the patient's awakening at the end of the procedure. Labetalol possesses alpha- and beta-blocking properties and decreases blood pressure without significant dilatation of cerebral blood vessels. A small additional dose of narcotic sometimes is helpful, as well, in supplementing the isoflurane.

Nitroprusside is also commonly used to induce controlled hypotension. It is a direct arterial and venous dilator, and is given by continuous infusion at rates of 0.5 to 5 μg/kg/min. If higher doses are required, we recommend supplementation with another agent because of the possibility of cyanide toxicity at higher levels.

Nitroprusside has a rapid onset and offset, is very potent, and must be used with caution. As it is a cerebral vasodilator, it may increase cerebral blood flow and ICP, and at times its use will not improve operating conditions if the brain and blood vessels swell. This is more likely if there is a mass effect, if the brain parenchyma is inflamed (early surgery), or if the aneurysm is particularly large or otherwise surgically difficult. Recent data implies that nitroprusside is primarily a cerebral venodilator, thereby able to increase ICP with minimal CBF effect.

If, in fact, the aneurysm appears to represent a special surgical challenge, a thiopental infusion is useful in producing constricted vessels and a slack brain. It can be titrated, beginning with a dose of 2 mg/kg/hr. If more than 30 mg/kg is used, it is likely that awakening will be delayed, and even lower levels may delay awakening in conjunction with other administered drugs.

Other drugs may be used successfully for induced hypotension, but are employed infrequently in our practice. Nitroglycerin may be useful in the patient with coronary disease because it will dilate the free wall of coronary stenoses as well as producing venous and arterial dilation. Doses begin at 0.5 μg/kg/min followed by titration to effect. The major toxicity is vascular hypotension, although the propylene glycol diluent in some preparations may be a myocardial depressant. Nitroglycerin also adheres to the plastic of intravenous tubing, but the dose given is titrated to patient response. The main problem is that it is ineffective in producing hypotension in many patients.

Trimethaphan primarily is a ganglionic blocker that has some direct vasodilatory effect as well as histamine-releasing properties. The onset and offset are not as rapid as those of nitroprusside. The advantage of trimethaphan is that cerebral blood flow is not increased, but the use of isoflurane, which also has minimal effect on cerebral blood flow, has lessened the unique advantage of trimethaphan. Disadvantages include the possibility of patchy cerebral ischemia with hypotension and the production of unreactive, dilated pupils. The dose of trimethaphan is 1 mg/min to begin and then titrated to effect.

Hydralazine may be used for hypotension, but it is a cerebral vasodilator, and its delayed onset of action (10 to 20 minutes after the IV dose) and relatively slow metabolism make it more difficult to use than isoflurane or nitroprusside. It can be used to supplement hypotension in 2.5- to 5-mg IV boluses. If reflex tachycardia is produced, propranolol may be given in 0.25-mg IV doses.

Hypotension generally is begun as the surgeon approaches the aneurysm and continues until the aneurysm is clipped. At this time, blood pressure is allowed to rise to normotensive levels so that bleeding can be detected before the dura is closed. Care must be taken to avoid rebound hypertension. Some clinicians may choose to discontinue nitrous oxide during controlled hypotension because of its sympathetic nervous system stimulating effects, and may resume its use at this point. The addition of nitrous oxide raises the possibilities of ICP increase due to tension pneumocephalus or an increase in CBF.

Cerebrospinal Fluid Drains

The surgeon may decide to place a lumbar subarachnoid drain to remove CSF in order to produce a slack brain and better surgical exposure. Theoretically, an acute drop in pressure may increase the transmural pressure of the aneurysm (MAP minus ICP), especially as there may be some reflex increase in blood pressure. However, in practice, an increase sufficient to rupture the aneurysm is rarely, if ever, observed.

A catheter is placed through a needle inserted in the subarachnoid space by the surgeon or the anesthesiologist or anesthetist. The technique is similar to that used for continuous subarachnoid anesthesia. After it is established that the catheter is functioning, the flow is stopped to prevent an excessive transmural pressure increase. The surgeon will request that the drain be opened after the dura is opened. It is essential to label this catheter distinctly so that absolutely nothing can be accidentally injected into the subarachnoid space.

Mannitol

The pharmacology of mannitol has been reviewed thoroughly in previous sections. Mannitol is used in this setting to improve surgical conditions. We give 100 g of mannitol (500 cc of 20%) from the time of induction to skin incision, then give a second 100 g after skin incision. This is a large dose (2 to 4 g/kg), but in a single use will be effective without causing the metabolic disarray that large, repeated doses may cause.

Hyperventilation

Like spinal drains and mannitol, hyperventilation is used to slacken the brain. Again, there is the theoretical consideration of increased aneurysmal transmural gradient due to fall in ICP. However, we employ gradual hyperventilation immediately after induction to produce a $PaCO_2$ of 20 to 25 mm Hg. This can be followed with monitoring of end-tidal CO_2, although the gradient may increase if controlled hypotension results in increased pulmonary dead space. There also is a theoretical concern of brain ischemia if controlled hypotension is employed at mean blood pressures as low as 40 mm Hg, while the $PaCO_2$ is 20 mm Hg. Again, this has been successfully employed in our practice for many patients without evidence of ischemia.

Hypothermia

A decrease in temperature decreases $CMRO_2$, and theoretically provides some measure of brain protection. We have had no recent experience with hypothermia, even for giant posterior fossa aneurysm or arteriovenous malformations. When hypothermia is used, moderate hypothermia (31 to 32 °C) is employed, and can be produced with a thermal blanket circulating cold water. If IV fluids are not warmed, the operating room is cool, and gases are not humidified, many patients will experience a temperature drop to 34 °C without adjunctive measures. Deep hypothermia has a deleterious effect on clotting, immunity, and cardiac rhythm, and is rarely employed. Patients should be ventilated and intubated until temperature returns to 35 °C.

Intraoperative Aneurysm Rupture

If rupture occurs, mean blood pressure should be lowered to a level that allows the surgeon to visualize and gain control of the bleeding site. This may require a mean blood pressure as high as 50 mm Hg or as low as 20 to 30 mm Hg. Blood lost should continue to be replaced. The surgeon may have to clip a major artery proximal to the aneurysm or even compress one or both carotid arteries to find the aneurysm. Since hypotension may be severe and prolonged, it is reasonable to include agents that probably afford some degree of cerebral protection (thiopental, isoflurane) in the hypotensive regimen. It also is a good idea to get some help from one or more assistants if rupture occurs.

Pregnant Patient

The pregnant patient and fetus represent a special challenge in aneurysm surgery. Physiologic considerations include a full stomach situation, potential drug toxicities, and effects on uterine blood flow and fetal well-being. Although cesarean section can be performed at the time of aneurysm clipping, predelivery aneurysm clipping followed by delivery seems preferable.

These patients should receive an antiaspiration regimen of H_2 blocker, metoclopramide, and nonparticulate antacid before the induction of anesthesia. If indicated for airway considerations, a very careful intubation under sedation with local should be performed. A rapid-sequence intubation can be performed if special care is taken to blunt the hypertensive response to intubation. This might include fentanyl, 2 to 3 $\mu g/kg$ given several minutes before induction, followed by thiopental 5 mg/kg, lidocaine 1.5 mg/kg, and succinylcholine 1 mg/kg. We would not recommend pretreatment with a nondepolarizing relaxant, because it may result in excessive weakness in some patients, with subsequent aspiration. Furthermore, succinylcholine used alone seems to provide better intubating conditions. Succinylcholine should be avoided if rupture has occurred and/or if there is any neurologic deficit. Expert cricoid pressure is maintained and blood pressure carefully monitored.

Alternatively, a nondepolarizing relaxant can be used in an intubating dose. This generally provides adequate intubating conditions in an acceptably short time. Furthermore, if laryngoscopy produces an unacceptable rise in blood pressure, anesthesia can be deepened, while gentle mask ventilation is given with the maintenance of expert cricoid pressure. While the impact of aspiration is blunted by the antiaspiration drug regimen and cricoid pressure, aneurysm rupture is a devastating complication. Monitoring of fetal heart rate should be established before the induction of anesthesia.

Drugs frequently used during these procedures that are potentially toxic to the fetus include nitroprusside, mannitol, and beta-blockers. There is some controversy over the use of nitroprusside, but since it may cause fetal acidosis and cyanide toxicity, there is a strong relative contraindication to its use. Beta-blockers may cause fetal and neonatal bradycardia and hypoglycemia. Mannitol theoretically is worrisome in that it may cause fetal volume and electrolyte abnormalities. Our policy is to avoid mannitol if possible, but if it is needed for surgical exposure, we would administer a slightly lower dose than that usually employed (i.e., 0.5 to 1 g/kg).

Uterine blood flow is a major issue because of the effects of controlled hypotension and hypoventilation on the fetus. Isoflurane seems to be the ideal hypotensive agent in this situation, since it has little or no effect on uterine blood flow at levels of anesthetic that result in adequate hypotension (mean blood pressure 50 to 70 mm Hg). Monitoring the fetal heart rate should be a helpful guide to acceptable levels of hypotension. While we routinely hyperventilate other patients during hypotension, $PaCO_2$ probably should be kept above 30 mm Hg in the pregnant patient to avoid a reduction in uterine blood flow.

Emergence

After the aneurysm is clipped, the blood pressure is allowed to rise (not abruptly) to normotensive or mildly hypertensive levels so that bleeding can be detected and eliminated before dural closure. Labetalol is a useful drug to control blood pressure since the level of isoflurane is lightened toward the end of the case to allow awakening. If the patient was not neurologically impaired before induction and surgery has proceeded without difficulty, the patient should be extubated awake at the end of the case. If the patient was not fully awake before induction or if there have been surgical or anesthetic difficulties (e.g., rupture, excessive retraction, uncontrolled hypotension, vessel occlusion resulting in possible ischemia), it is prudent to leave the patient intubated through the transport stage. The patient then can be observed in the recovery area and extubated when awake there. During the time of actual emergence and transport, careful observation of blood pressure must be continued and blood pressure treated as indicated.

Arteriovenous Malformation

Arteriovenous malformations are congenital, intracerebral networks in which arteries flow directly into veins. The patient population generally is younger than those with aneurysms. They may present with bleeding or seizures, or less commonly with ischemia due to "steal" from normal areas or with high-output congestive heart failure.

The anesthetic problems are typically those of aneurysm surgery. Notably, arteriovenous malformations do not autoregulate their blood flow. The operation is likely to be longer and bloodier than that for aneurysm clipping. Surgery may be preceded by an attempt at embolization by the neuroradiologist in order to diminish the risk of surgery. The neurologic examination should be repeated after embolization to document new deficits that otherwise might be attributed to anesthesia and surgery.

Case History

S.L., a 48-year-old woman, had no history of medical problems. One month before admission she had seen her primary physician for severe headache, stiff neck, and mild fever and had been sent home with a diagnosis of "viral syndrome." She improved over the next few days until 1 day prior to admission, when she had a severe headache and briefly lost consciousness. Neurologic evaluation subsequently was notable only for a stiff neck and mild drowsiness. Computed tomography (CT) scan and cerebral angiography revealed rupture of an anterior communicating artery aneurysm. Lumbar puncture revealed bloody cerebrospinal fluid (CSF) with a minimally increased pressure. She was hospitalized in a quiet room and given codeine for headache and small doses of diazepam for sedation. Her arterial blood pressure was maintained in the normal range with as-needed dosing of intravenous hydralazine in 5-mg increments. Aneurysm clipping was scheduled for the third day after subarachnoid hemorrhage.

Suggested Reading

Artru AA. Cerebral metabolism and EEG during combination of hypocapnia and isoflurane-induced hypotension in dogs. Anesthesiology 1986; 65:602.

Artru AA. Partial preservation of cerebral vascular responsiveness to hypocapnia during isoflurane-induced hypotension in dogs. Anesth Analg 1986; 65:660.

Ausman JI, et al. Current management of cerebral aneurysms: is it based on facts or myths? Surg Neurol 1985; 24:625.

Boarini DJ, et al. Surgical treatment of aneurysms. Semin Neurol 1984; 4:280.

Ghignone M, et al. Anesthesia and hypertension: the effect of clonidine on perioperative hemodynamics and isoflurane requirements. Anesthesiology 1987; 67:3.

James DJ, et al. Hydralazine for controlled hypotension during neurosurgical operations. Anesth Analg 1982; 61:1016.

Kassell NF, et al. Treatment of ischemic deficits from vasospasm with intravascular volume expansion and induced arterial hypotension. Neurosurgery 1982; 11:337.

Lam AM, et al. Cardiovascular effects of isoflurane-induced hypotension for cerebral aneurysm surgery. Anesth Analg 1983; 62:742.

Newberg LA, et al. The cerebral effects of isoflurane at and above concentrations that suppress cortical electrical activity. Anesthesiology 1983; 59:23.

Newberg LA, et al. Cerebral protection by isoflurane during hypoxemia or ischemia. Anesthesiology 1983; 59:29.

Newman B, et al. The effect of isoflurane-induced hypotension on cerebral blood flow and cerebral metabolic rate for oxygen in humans. Anesthesiology 1986; 64:307.

Newman B, et al. Induced hypotension for clipping of a cerebral aneurysm during pregnancy: a case report and brief review. Anesth Analg 1986; 65:675.

Seyde WC, et al. Cerebral oxygen tension in rats during deliberate hypertension with sodium nitroprusside, 2-chloradenosine, or deep isoflurane anesthesia. Anesthesiology 1986; 64:480.

Woodside J, et al. Captopril reduces the dose requirement for sodium nitroprusside induced hypotension. Anesthesiology 1984; 60:413.

David J. Stone, M.D.

Anesthesia for Extracranial Vascular Surgery

10

Preoperative Assessment

Cardiovascular System

Coronary Artery Disease

The non-neurologic system of greatest interest to the anesthesiologist in this setting is the cardiovascular system, because it is the prime extracerebral site of intra- and postoperative morbidity and mortality. Coronary disease may be present in about half the patients who undergo carotid endarterectomy. The main factors to be considered are:

1. Is the angina stable?
2. Has the patient had a recent (within the last 6 months) myocardial infarction (MI)?

Other patients may have more ambiguous histories and raise the question of whether or not significant coronary disease is present. Even a careful history by a cardiologist may not be revealing, as evidenced by unexpectedly normal or abnormal coronary angiograms. Short of an angiogram, a thallium stress test utilizing exercise or dipyridamole (Persantin) is the best noninvasive screen for the presence of functionally significant coronary disease.

Dipyridamole acts by dilating arterioles in normal areas of myocardium, thereby producing a "coronary steal" from areas perfused by stenotic vessels. Normally, thallium is taken up in adequately perfused areas of myocardium. An old infarction will produce an area of no uptake that does not refill after the test. A poststenotic area at risk for ischemia will have reduced or absent uptake during the test but will refill when the stress has ended. Exercise dilates arteries in areas supplied by nonstenotic vessels by producing local metabolites (adenosine) that relax vessels and produce a "steal" effect. The accompanying tachycardia decreases blood supply by decreasing diastolic filling time, as well as increasing the demand for oxygenated blood.

If myocardium becomes dysfunctional during the test, stroke volume may fall and left ventricular pressures may rise, thereby contributing to decreasing coronary perfusion in diseased areas. Occasionally, the thallium test may produce false-negative results, and a normal test does not obviate the need for careful anesthetic management. The electrocardiographic stress test without thallium is too nonspecific and insensitive to be useful unless it is extremely abnormal. The coronary angiogram remains the "gold standard" for the presence of significant coronary artery disease and may be required on occasion to sort out an ambiguous situation.

If the anginal pattern has not worsened and symptoms do not occur at rest, the angina is considered to be stable. This distinction is important because patients with stable angina do not appear to have an increased risk from anesthesia and surgery, whereas patients with unstable angina do have a significantly increased risk. Careful questioning may reveal that the patient has reduced his activity or modified his drug regimen so that what initially appears to be stable angina may be, in fact, unstable.

While the more general question of whether coronary artery bypass grafting (CABG) should be performed before endarterectomy (or any vascular surgery procedure) has not been answered, it is clear that patients with unstable angina benefit from CABG regardless of whether or not other surgery is to be performed. Therefore, preoperative cardiologic consultation is recommended in the patient with suspected unstable angina to evaluate the patient for further therapy and diagnosis.

The patient with a recent (within the past 6 months) MI is a well-known special risk for anesthesia and surgery. Recent studies claim that with newer pharmacologic agents and monitoring techniques, this risk may be reduced from the roughly 15% incidence of MI (3 to 6 months after MI), 30% incidence (less than 3 months after MI), and 50% mortality after recurrent MI that has been repeatedly quoted in the literature. These patients are at high risk for ischemia and/or infarction, and cardiac consultation should be obtained even for asymptomatic patients who have had a recent MI in order to determine the need for further studies. The necessity and urgency of endarterectomy must be carefully reassessed because of the possibility that cardiac morbidity and mortality will outweigh the possible benefits of the operation.

In general, staged procedures are preferred in patients with combined coronary and carotid disease who require both operations, i.e., endarterectomy followed, days to months later, by CABG. In patients with unstable angina or severe left main coronary artery disease, "simultaneous" operations may be indicated with the endarterectomy performed before the institution of cardiopulmonary bypass. Angioplasty may prove to have a role in this setting.

It is important that patients' beta-blockers, calcium-blockers, and nitrates be continued through the day of surgery to avoid rebound ischemia. The combination of these drugs may predispose to intraoperative hypotension, and this should be kept in mind when the anesthetic plan is formulated. Dilators of large coronary vessels such as nitroglycerin or calcium blockers may be especially beneficial if alpha-agonists such as phenylephrine (Neo-Synephrine) are employed to increase blood pressure during surgery.

Myocardial Function

While myocardial dysfunction may be the result of coronary disease (either acutely or chronically as in "ischemic cardiomyopathy"), it must be separately evaluated; management may be quite different if heart failure is present, and there are many other causes of congestive heart failure. In patients undergoing vascular surgery, other likely causes include heart failure due to systemic hypertension, valvular heart disease (especially aortic stenosis and/or mitral regurgitation), and cor pulmonale due to chronic obstructive pulmonary disease.

Chronic systemic hypertension produces a thick-walled (hypertrophic), noncompliant left ventricle that progresses with time to a dilated chamber and biventricular failure. Aortic stenosis in this age group may be due to calcification of a bicuspid valve or degeneration of valve leaflets, resulting in aortic sclerosis. Classic signs of diminished carotid upstroke and low systolic and pulse pressures may be absent because of a markedly noncompliant vasculature. Mitral regurgitation may be caused by ischemia, mitral valve prolapse, left ventricular dilatation, endocarditis, or calcification of the mitral valve annulus. Both lesions may, of course, be rheumatic in etiology. Cor pulmonale occurs when the thin-walled right ventricle begins to fail when confronted with chronically high pulmonary vascular pressures. Many of these patients also have left-sided disease due to other causes.

Clinical signs and symptoms include dyspnea on exertion (or rest), paroxysmal nocturnal dyspnea, fatigue, edema, and orthopnea. In the patient with lung disease, it may be difficult to determine the relative contributions of cardiac and pulmonary disease to shortness of breath. Orthopnea and paroxysmal nocturnal dyspnea suggest a cardiac component. On physical examination, an S_3 gallop, murmur(s), and edema suggest cardiac (possibly cor pulmonale) disease. Chest radiography is useful for evaluation of cardiomegaly and elevated pulmonary arterial and venous pressures.

Further laboratory evaluation may include a test of ventricular function. A nuclear gated pool scan or echocardiography will assist in estimating ejection fraction (normally about 60 to 65%), as well as assessing wall motion. The echocardiogram may assist in the evaluation of valvular heart disease as well. If cardiac catheterization is done, ejection fraction and filling pressures will be available.

The most useful test is a careful evaluation of the patient's ability to exercise. If the patient can perform vigorous exercise without symptoms, it is clear that the anatomic lesion(s) is not causing a physiologic problem. However, inability to exercise may be due to other causes such as pulmonary, neurologic, rheumatologic, and vascular disease, and further noninvasive tests may be useful in planning the anesthetic, monitoring, and postoperative care. Severe valvular heart disease, especially critical aortic stenosis, may require prior or simultaneous repair. If doubt remains about the patient's function, it may be reasonable to insert a pulmonary artery catheter and make an evaluation of function from stroke volume (cardiac output/heart rate) and filling pressures (pulmonary capillary wedge pressure). The section on cardiovascular monitoring later in this chapter addresses this question in more detail.

Hypertension

A significant proportion of these patients have essential hypertension under varying degrees of control. Unless the endarterectomy is viewed as an emergency by the surgeon and neurologic consultants, time should be taken to bring blood pressure under reasonable control. Since hypertensive patients may require higher blood pressures to maintain cerebral blood flow (autoregulation curve shifted to the right) and may not possess effective autoregulation at all in diseased areas, care must be taken to avoid a rapid and excessive fall in blood pressure.

It is probably reasonable to attempt to achieve a systolic blood pressure less than 200 mm Hg and a diastolic blood pressure of 100 mm Hg or less. While these numbers would not generally constitute optimal blood pressure control to an internist in practice, they represent a practical compromise between good control and adequate perfusion. The actual means by which this is achieved is generally left to the primary physician or consultant. These drugs or carefully chosen substitutes should be continued through the perioperative period, i.e., on the morning of surgery and as soon as possible postoperatively. Uncontrolled hypertension may contribute to cardiovascular instability resulting in myocardial and cerebral ischemia as well as intracranial hemorrhage.

Cerebrovascular Function

A baseline of the patient's neurologic status should be recorded in the preoperative note. Although the anesthesiologist is not expected to perform a meticulous neurologic examination, he or she should be aware of general mental function as well as the gross status of the cranial nerves and motor function of the extremities. Patients who are actually having a stroke or who have had a stroke in the past 6 weeks are at an increased risk for perioperative neurologic problems, probably because of impaired autoregulation in the affected area.

Currently, endarterectomy during acute stroke is not generally recommended unless it has occurred acutely during or after angiography and is due to known acute carotid thrombosis. The angiogram may also reveal patients at high risk who have coexisting stenosis higher in the internal carotid (siphon area), extensive involvement distally into the internal carotid or proximally into the common carotid, slowed intracranial circulation time, and/or occlusion of the opposite internal carotid artery. At present, surgery on asymptomatic patients with $\geq 80\%$ diameter occlusions is controversial. Surgery on asymptomatic patients with lesser lesions as preparation for cardiopulmonary bypass or major vascular surgery currently is performed less frequently than in earlier years and is of unproven efficacy. Generally accepted indications for endarterectomy include hemispheric or monocular transient ischemic attacks, which are neurologic defects lasting less than 24 hours.

Chronic Obstructive Pulmonary Disease

Many of these patients have obstructive pulmonary disease as the result of heavy smoking that also has contributed to their vascular problems. Since carotid endarterectomy does not invoke major fluid shifts or an incision that impairs respiration, only the most severe respiratory cripple would be denied endarterectomy on a pulmonary basis. Consequently, preoperative pulmonary function tests are not routinely necessary. A room-air arterial blood gas determination (drawn sometime before the administration of respiratory depressant premedications) is useful to ascertain the patient's normal carbon dioxide level for the operation. Large amounts of secretions and bronchospasm are likely to be a problem in this group, and both can be blunted by the administration of glycopyrrolate. Although 0.2 mg IV will decrease secretions, a dose of 0.4 to 0.5 mg is required to inhibit bronchospasm maximally.

Steroids should be continued if the patient is taking them, and a preinduction dose of steroid (3 to 4 mg/kg IV hydrocortisone or 1 mg/kg PO prednisone) should be strongly considered in patients with a history of bronchospasm. Although some clinicians continue aminophylline through the operative period, the minimal additional bronchodilatation provided may not justify its toxicity. However, inhaled beta-2-agonists are quite useful and should be continued. They can be injected directly into the anesthetic circuit by an adapter, if necessary. Narcotics, intravenous lidocaine, and the potent anesthetic agents all act to diminish intraoperative bronchospasm as well. Preoperative and postoperative encouragement of deep breathing and coughing will help reduce the incidence of respiratory complications (atelectasis, pneumonia, exacerbation of bronchospasm). Incentive spirometry may be employed to reinforce deep breathing.

Renal System

Mild renal insufficiency may be due to chronic hypertension or even renal artery stenosis in this population of patients. Anesthetic management is minimally modified by this level of derangement in renal function. It might be reasonable to avoid large doses or combination doses of the older, nondepolarizing relaxants (curare, metocurine, pancuronium) so that satisfactory reversal can be obtained at the end of the operation. More severe renal failure can introduce the problems of volume status, platelet function, severe anemia, myocardial dysfunction, arrhythmias, and pericardial disease.

Diabetes

Diabetes is another common problem in this population because this disease predisposes patients to vascular disease. Patients whose diabetes is controlled by diet or oral hypoglycemics may develop severe hyperglycemia or, rarely, frank diabetic ketoacidosis when stressed by surgery. It is most critical not to precipitate the syndrome of nonketotic hyperosmolar coma, which has up to a 50% mortality. I prefer not to administer oral hypoglycemics on the day of surgery, but rather to manage fluids in the usual manner while checking blood glucose once or twice during the operation and two or three times during the following 24 hours. The issue of hyperglycemia and cerebral ischemia is addressed in Chapter 6, but it has become clear that it is essential to avoid hyperglycemia in endarterectomy patients, whether they are diabetic or not.

The perioperative management of insulin-dependent diabetes involves several basic approaches:

1. Administering some fraction of the morning insulin dose (usually one-half) and beginning glucose-containing fluids intravenously.
2. Administering an insulin infusion at 1 to 2 units/hr with intravenous glucose-containing fluids.
3. Withholding insulin, administering non-glucose-containing fluids (in patients with mild diabetes).
4. Using an artificial pancreas.

Whatever technique is chosen, it is critical to monitor glucose levels to avoid hypoglycemia and to keep glucose levels below 200 mg/dl as well, if possible.

Premedication

Sedation

It is optimal to have the patient as wide awake as possible after this relatively brief operation. For this reason, premedication is kept to a minimum. Many patients need no premedication. The anxious patient may receive a benzodiazepine such as diazepam (5 to 15 mg PO) or midazolam (1 to 3 mg IM). A narcotic will "take the edge off" the discomfort of line insertion and is strongly suggested if central cannulation is planned (morphine 5 to 12 mg IM). Although some practitioners successfully use heavier sedation preoperatively, I believe that drugs such as scopolamine or droperidol are best avoided in these patients since they may cause residual drowsiness, making neurologic evaluation difficult. If the patient is anxious in the induction area, a benzodiazepine may be give intravenously, e.g., midazolam in 1 mg increments.

Administration of Usual Medications

Antihypertensives and antianginal drugs should be continued up to and including the morning of surgery. It has been established that the beneficial effects of these drugs on blood pressure and cardiac ischemia outweigh possible negative inotropic effects. Diuretics and digoxin are variably administered on the day of surgery according to the clinician's judgment about volume status and potential for toxicity, respectively.

Special Considerations

Many of these patients have esophageal reflux, and some clinicians may choose to employ some combination of H_2 antagonist, nonparticulate antacid, and/or metoclopramide to reduce the impact of possible aspiration.

Monitoring

Cardiovascular Monitors

Blood Pressure

Because of the need to finely titrate blood pressure almost instantaneously and the value of arterial blood gases, an arterial line generally is employed. While the radial artery usually is cannulated, any of the acceptable sites may be used with appropriate precautions. It is best to insert the radial line on the side contralateral to the surgery so that the anesthetist has access to the site and so that there is no risk of an inserted shunt tip occluding pressure to that side. The arterial line should be inserted before the induction of anesthesia in most circumstances. As automated oscillometers (such as the Dinamap) become capable of more frequent blood pressure determinations, perhaps patients will eventually be monitored completely noninvasively when a capnometer is available and the arterial-to-end-tidal carbon dioxide gradient is established.

Electrocardiography

The electrocardiogram (ECG) is monitored to detect myocardial ischemia and disorders of rhythm. Because many of these patients have underlying heart disease, premature atrial and ventricular beats are even more common than usual. Sinus bradycardia or even asystole may occur when the carotid sinus is manipulated. Lead II is an excellent lead for detection and diagnosis of arrhythmias.

  The detection of ischemia with a single lead probably is best done with a lead that monitors the anterior wall of the heart, i.e., V_5 or its equivalent. The use of lead II alone may miss a large proportion of ischemic ECG changes. Both leads should be monitored, if possible, as is often done for cardiac surgery. If only one lead can be monitored, a modified lead V_5 may be easily produced by placing the left arm lead in the V_5 position (fifth intercostal space at the anterior axillary line) and monitoring lead "I." Ischemia may result in S-T elevation (especially coronary spasm, transmural ischemia or infarction) or S-T depression (subendocardial ischemia or infarction). Obtaining a baseline trace from the monitor may be useful, since the amplifier or oscilloscope may modify the baseline trace in worrisome fashion. Lesser changes in the ECG (S-T depression less than 1 minute, flattened T waves) may represent ischemia or merely be the result of drugs, changes in electrolyte status, stress, or the surgery itself.

Central Venous Pressure and Pulmonary Artery Catheters

Carotid surgery does not involve large fluid shifts or blood losses, but may be stressful because of marked swings in hemodynamics. A central venous pressure (CVP) line generally is not indicated unless the clinician desires access for drugs that should be given centrally (vasopressors, calcium). A pulmonary artery (PA; Swan-Ganz) catheter may be indicated in patients who have marked compromise of cardiac function. Indications include severe congestive heart failure, valvular heart disease which has progressed to cause symptoms, severe coronary disease such as unstable angina, recent myocardial infarction (within the last 6 months), or when combined endarterectomy-CABG is being performed.

The site of placement of the PA catheter poses a problem. Obviously, the internal and external jugular veins on the side of surgery cannot be cannulated. The opposite internal or external jugular vein may be used, but kinking due to position may occur. The antecubital veins are a relatively safe site because the complications of central venous puncture are avoided. If the catheter "hangs up" in the area of the axilla, manipulation of the arm, especially abduction, may allow for free passage into the thorax. Other sites include the subclavian or femoral veins.

The PA catheter will serve as a monitor of heart function and to a lesser extent of ischemia. The pulmonary capillary wedge pressure (PCWP) is used as an approximation of left ventricular end-diastolic pressure (LVEDP). The true "preload" which partially determines left ventricular function actually is the left ventricular end-diastolic volume. The LVEDP is altered by changes in compliance (changes in volume/changes in pressure), as well as by actual changes in preload. In fact, the PCWP is not a completely accurate measure of preload during anesthesia but serves as a useful clinical approximation. It is a useful monitor of the hydrostatic pressure exerted on the pulmonary capillaries and, therefore, of the likelihood of pulmonary edema.

When PCWP is interpreted along with cardiac output (CO) or stroke volume (CO/heart rate), the state of cardiac function can be assessed. Normally, PCWP is 5 to 12 mm Hg and stroke volume is 60 to 90 cc. The failing heart demonstrates a reduction in stroke volume, usually in spite of an increase in filling pressures. If cardiac function has not been completely evaluated preoperatively, this sort of analysis will give the clinician an understanding of the general functional capabilities of the patient's heart.

The PA catheter may function as an indicator of ischemia by demonstrating increasing filling pressures while stroke volume decreases. This will only occur when sufficient areas of the heart are involved so that global systolic and diastolic (less compliant) function are compromised. There also may be changes in the morphology of the wedge tracing, with V waves appearing because of compliance changes or ischemia-induced mitral regurgitation. It is not a sensitive monitor for lesser degrees of myocardial ischemia.

Echocardiography and Doppler Flow Studies

Two-dimensional (2-D) echocardiography employs high-frequency sound waves to examine the structures of the heart. In the cardiology suite it can be used to evaluate global myocardial function (ejection fraction), focal wall motion abnormalities (due to new ischemia or old infarction), valvular function, pericardial disease, and even the ascending aorta. In the operating room, some centers have begun to use intraesophageal 2-D echocardiography to evaluate focal wall motion, primarily. Echocardiography employed with a PA catheter allows for accurate detection of preload (ejection fraction =

stroke volume/left ventricular end-diastolic volume). Focal wall motion abnormalities are a more sensitive indicator of ischemia than ECG or PA pressure changes.

Doppler flow studies employ the Doppler shift principle (change in frequency as object moves with respect to a receiver) to determine cardiac output. The technology currently is evolving and probably will eventually allow for a noninvasive (relatively, if intraesophageal) monitor of cardiac output.

Respiratory Monitors

Capnometry is the measurement of carbon dioxide concentration during respiration, and capnography is the visual display of the tracing generated. Most of these devices employ the absorption of infrared light to determine carbon dioxide concentration. Flow-through or aspiration devices are used for the measurement. End-tidal CO_2 ($PETCO_2$) is measured because there usually is a good correlation with arterial PCO_2. The difference in these values should be established early in the case with an arterial blood gas determination so that the capnometric reading can be used for meaningful intraoperative monitoring. The gradient usually is 5 mm Hg or less, but patients with severe lung disease (and increased dead space) may have a baseline gradient of 15 to 20 mm Hg. This is due to areas of ventilation without perfusion (dead space) which tend to decrease the $PETCO_2$ and increase the $PaCO_2$.

There also are many causes of an increased gradient during surgery. These include marked falls in cardiac output, pulmonary emboli (including air), endobronchial intubation, and obstruction or leakage in the breathing system. The presence of CO_2 in exhaled gases also is excellent reassurance that the trachea, and not the esophagus, has been intubated. It is generally accepted that CO_2 levels should be kept around "normal" (for that patient) during carotid endarterectomy. This is discussed in the section on maintenance of anesthesia. If capnometry is unavailable, several intraoperative arterial blood gases probably should be obtained for the above purpose.

Neurologic Monitors

Electroencephalography

The electroencephalogram (EEG) may be employed as a monitor of cerebral ischemia, especially after carotid cross-clamping. When cerebral blood flow falls from its normal level of 50 cc/100 g brain tissue/min, the EEG generally is preserved until flow is reduced by about 50%. At this point, the EEG begins to decrease in frequency and amplitude until it becomes flat at about 60% reduction. From about 60 to 80% flow reduction, the flat EEG represents what has been referred to as the "ischemic penumbra." The electrical activity of the cell is absent, but the structural integrity of the cell remains and the ischemia is still reversible. At about 80% flow reduction, the cell membrane becomes leaky and cerebral infarction may follow. Thus, most patients who have EEG changes without flattening will not have resulting neurologic deficits, and even those with transient unilateral EEG flattening may not have areas of infarction.

The EEG wave frequencies are termed delta (0 to 4 Hz), theta (4 to 8 Hz), alpha (8 to 13 Hz), and beta (13 to 30 Hz). In general, light anesthetic states show an increase in beta activity. As anesthesia deepens, the EEG slows into the theta and delta range. Thiopental and isoflurane (2.5 MAC) can actually pharmacologically flatten the EEG.

The raw, 16-lead intraoperative EEG must be monitored by an electroencephalographer. For this reason, analyzed EEGs with simpler data interpretation have been developed for intraoperative use by the anesthesiologist. These employ fast Fourier transformation which converts the complex raw EEG waveform into the series of sine waves that mathematically make up the complex waves. The amplitude of the waves often is squared to represent power, a convention in radio engineering. The amount of power is analyzed at various frequencies (power-spectrum analysis). The resulting power at various frequencies can be represented as hills and valleys (compressed spectral array) or different colors (compressed density spectral array). If cross-clamping results in a sufficient decrease in blood flow, these EEG representations will demonstrate the frequency changes in the affected hemisphere, as would be seen in the more complex raw EEG.

Only a small proportion of eventual fixed neurologic deficits are caused by decreased flow during cross-clamping. Most deficits are caused by emboli generated by manipulation of the vessel or even by shunt insertion. Others may be caused by severe hypotension due to anesthetics. For many years, endarterectomies have been performed without shunting or EEG monitoring with good outcomes in the series published in the surgical literature. There may be a small percentage of endarterectomy patients who have a benefit in outcome from EEG monitoring. This benefit may be caused by shunt insertion by the surgeon when there is ischemia on EEG. At present, it should not be maintained that all endarterectomy patients must have EEG monitoring. In fact, surgical and anesthetic skills are far more important in outcome.

Other Monitors

If regional anesthesia is employed, the patient's neurologic examination can be used for ischemia detection during cross-clamping. This is not total assurance of reversibility as patients' deficits have remained after removal of the cross-clamp, probably on the basis of embolic deficits.

Carotid stump pressures have involved measuring intravascular pressures distal to the cross-clamp. These have been shown to be unacceptably unreliable. Xenon clearance can be used to accurately measure cerebral blood flow, but this is not generally available. Evoked potential and Doppler flow monitoring have not come into general use as neurologic monitors during carotid endarterectomy.

Induction and Maintenance of Anesthesia

Choice of Induction Agents

In patients free of coronary disease, hypertension, and congestive heart failure, a thiopental (4 to 5 mg/kg) induction is acceptable. The clinician may choose to blunt the tachycardic and hypertensive response to laryngoscopy and intubation in patients with hypertension and coronary disease. This may be accomplished with the administration of fentanyl (2 to 3 μg/kg) 5 minutes before the induction of anesthesia. Alternatives include the use of the rapidly acting beta-blocker esmolol (Brevibloc) in a dose of 0.5 mg/kg IV, or a small bolus of nitroprusside or nitroglycerin (50 to 100 μg). A slow induction using a nondepolarizing relaxant, mask ventilation, and adequate anesthesia with intravenous or inhaled agents will prevent excessive hemodynamic alterations. In the patient with carotid disease, it probably is wiser to accept a small amount of hypertension than to risk excessive hypotension. For example, if fentanyl pretreatment has been employed, the thiopental dose might be reduced to 3 to 4 mg/kg or even 2 mg/kg in a frail, elderly patient.

Patients with congestive heart failure may receive a high-dose narcotic induction for cardiac surgery or other procedures if ventilation can be provided postoperatively. Because the patient undergoing endarterectomy should be awake and breathing at the end of the procedure, the high-dose narcotic technique should be avoided if possible. A slow, controlled induction with mask ventilation usually can be performed with pentothal in 50-mg increments, lidocaine 1.5 mg/kg, and doses of narcotics that will not necessitate postoperative ventilation (fentanyl $\leq$12.5 μg/kg, or sufentanil $\leq$2.5 μg/kg). Alfentanil, which is a relatively new narcotic with fast onset and offset, is another option. It is about one-tenth as potent as fentanyl. Whatever technique is chosen, constant monitoring of blood pressure (and PA pressure, if available) in conjunction with the incremental administration of drugs should provide a safe induction.

Patients with bronchospastic disease should receive adequate anesthesia to prevent severe reflex bronchospasm. An inhalation induction may be inordinately long in these patients. A preinduction dose of glycopyrrolate (0.4 to 0.5 mg IV) is very useful in this regard, as is the use of intravenous lidocaine and narcotic in the induction regimen. Laryngotracheal application of lidocaine may aid tolerance of the tube, but can independently provoke some bronchoconstriction.

A patient with a suspected difficult airway should be handled in the same manner as for any operation. A careful awake intubation can provide very stable hemodynamics and minimal bronchial reactivity, if required, in patients with coronary disease or chronic obstructive pulmonary disease, respectively.

A classic rapid-sequence intubation generally is chosen for patients at risk for aspiration. However, this may result in unacceptable hemodynamic swings. The patient should receive adequate pharmacologic protection against aspiration. Once a nondepolarizing relaxant has taken effect and expert cricoid pressure is applied, it is unlikely that a significant aspiration will occur, even though positive pressure ventilation is given by mask. Using this method, drugs can be given a little more slowly, and if laryngoscopy produces a brisk hemodynamic response, intubation should be delayed until anesthesia is deepened. In each individual case, the clinician must weigh the risk of aspiration against the risk of hemodynamic changes and proceed accordingly.

Relaxants

There are no strong recommendations that can be made in the choice of relaxants. The trachea can be intubated with succinylcholine unless there is a neurologic contraindication, but a nondepolarizing relaxant allows for time to establish a deeper level of anesthesia, if necessary. Vecuronium probably produces the most stable hemodynamics. Because the operation usually is not excessively long, the combination of pancuronium with curare or metocurine probably should be avoided to ensure ease of reversal at the end of the case. If renal insufficiency is present, the older nondepolarizers (curare, metocurine, pancuronium) might be difficult to reverse if an intubating dose has been given. Patients on phenytoin (Dilantin) will be resistant to all the nondepolarizing relaxants except atracurium.

Succinylcholine should be avoided for at least 6 months in patients who have had a neurologic deficit (i.e., stroke). If there is doubt about the use of succinylcholine, it is probably best to use a nondepolarizing relaxant after careful evaluation of the airway. Notably, in stroke patients, the "twitch" monitor of neuromuscular blockade should be placed on a normal limb because an affected limb will be relatively resistant to blockade. This would predispose to an overdose of relaxants and possible difficulty in reversing them.

Maintenance of Anesthesia

General anesthesia can be maintained with inhalation agents, with a nitrous oxide–narcotic technique, or by a combination of agents titrated to maintain the desired heart rate and blood pressure. The nitrous oxide–narcotic technique has the potential advantage of quick awakening by the patient as long as the dose of narcotic is appropriately limited. However, some patients may become unacceptably hypertensive and tachycardic. The potent inhaled agents will control blood pressure at the cost of a slight delay in awakening. Some patients will not tolerate anesthetizing doses of these gases because of underlying myocardial dysfunction. However, the potent agents usually can be added to a nitrous oxide–narcotic base as required to control blood pressure. Blood pressure probably should be maintained at normotensive levels or slightly (10 to 20%) above usual systolic or mean blood pressure.

Among the potent inhaled agents, isoflurane has the theoretical benefit of brain protection. In fact, many patients cannot tolerate a very high dose of isoflurane, halothane, or enflurane and maintain the desired blood pressure. A recent study found that isoflurane does not provide brain protection for focal ischemia, although an accompanying editorial found several flaws in the study. Although carotid cross-clamping does not produce a strict model of focal brain ischemia, it certainly is a somewhat similar situation. Furthermore, isoflurane may cause coronary steal by dilating small arteries and shunting blood flow from areas of the heart supplied by stenotic areas. This also is an area of some controversy. Investigators at the Mayo Clinic have found that patients receiving isoflurane do seem to receive some brain protection since they tolerate lower cerebral blood flows without resulting ischemia. Thus, at present, it is not certain that one potent agent can be strongly recommended over the others for this operation.

The desirable level of arterial carbon dioxide has been a controversial point in the past. Hypercarbia will dilate cerebral vessels but may produce a steal effect if only normal vessels dilate. Hypocarbia theoretically would constrict normal vessels and shunt blood into diseased areas. However, studies have found that this effect is unpredictable and that hypocarbia appears to worsen ischemic stroke. For these reasons, there has been a recent consensus that $PaCO_2$ levels close to normocarbia are desirable.

Regional Anesthesia

Regional anesthesia can be produced by separate block of C_2, C_3, and C_4, or more easily by a single block at C_4 as described by Winnie. The C_4 level is identified at the top of the thyroid cartilage, and the needle is inserted in the interscalene groove in a slightly caudal direction to avoid epidural or spinal puncture. The local anesthetic (10 to 15 ml of chosen solution) is injected when a paresthesia is obtained or the transverse process is encountered. In the latter case, the needle is backed up a millimeter or two before injection. Risks include spinal or epidural injection, vertebral artery injection with instant severe seizures, and recurrent laryngeal and phrenic nerve palsies, which will be significant if the opposite nerve was injured previously. Local anesthesia can be performed by the surgeon via a field block.

The advantage of regional anesthesia is the resulting ability to monitor the patient neurologically after carotid cross-clamping. It is successfully employed at many institutions. At other hospitals, there may be resistance to the technique by patients, surgeons, and anesthesiologists. Regional anesthesia does not allow for the control of airway and ventilation afforded by general anesthesia. There is the theoretical concern that the brain protection of anesthetics is lost. Like most debates in the area of regional-versus-general anesthesia, there is no clear-cut difference in outcome, and the choice is made by the preferences of patient, surgeon, and anesthesiologist and the skill of the latter.

Special Considerations During Surgery

Incision of the artery and manipulation of the carotid sinus may result in bradycardia, hypotension, or both. This vagal response can be blocked with anticholinergics or by local injection of a dilute lidocaine solution. If severe bradycardia and/or hypotension occur(s), the surgeon should be informed so that the situation can be rectified.

At the time of carotid cross-clamping, the blood pressure should not be significantly below normal. Frequently, phenylephrine is used as a bolus (25 to 100 μg) or drip (20 to 100 μg/min) to raise blood pressure to the desire level. Unfortunately, this may constrict coronary arteries and contribute to myocardial ischemia. One study found that patients receiving phenylephrine had a higher rate of myocardial infarction. However, it is effective, does not cause tachycardia, and is commonly used for this purpose. The concurrent use of nitroglycerin may afford some protection with regard to coronary constriction. An excessive rise in blood pressure probably increases cerebral blood flow to a minimal degree.

Some clinicians will give a bolus of thiopental just before the carotid is cross-clamped. This is given to protect the brain from possible ischemia. However, it makes it difficult to maintain the desired blood pressure. Some will even begin a thiopental infusion to ensure that adequate levels are maintained (or continue an infusion that has been employed as part of the anesthetic). The results of this practice are not clear at present and cannot be recommended or criticized.

If cross-clamping produces ischemic EEG changes, some surgeons insert a shunt to bypass the occluded area. Other surgeons decide to put in a shunt preoperatively because of anatomic risks. Finally, there are surgeons who never insert shunts. Differences in neurologic morbidity between these practices are not large but, in fact, cross-clamping without shunting has given the best results in the past. Newer surgical studies may yield different results. In any case, this is clearly the surgeon's decision.

Emergence

The anesthetic is designed for prompt emergence. Ideally, the patient is awake and extubated in the operating room, where a brief neurologic examination can be performed. If neuromuscular blockade is adequately reversed but the patient is still asleep, deep extubation can be performed if there are no contraindications, such as esophageal reflux or a difficult airway. If neurologic compromise is suspected, the patient should not be extubated while deep. A rare patient will have airway obstruction due to bilateral hypoglossal nerve damage after endarterectomies have been performed on both sides.

It is important to avoid extremes of blood pressure during this time. Labetalol, a combined alpha- and beta-blocker, is an effective way to reduce blood pressure while avoiding tachycardia. It can be given in 5-mg intravenous increments. Nitroglycerin or nitroprusside infusions (begin at 0.25 μg/kg/min and titrate) also can be used for rapid blood pressure control. Details of recovery room management can be found in that chapter.

Extracranial-Intracranial Bypass

This operation, which anastomoses a branch of the superficial temporal artery with the middle cerebral artery, was designed to bypass high carotid occlusions inaccessible to endarterectomy. Unfortunately, a large cooperative study found no benefit to the operation, and it will be performed infrequently in the future.

This population of patients has the same underlying medical problems as those for endarterectomy. Special considerations include maintaining slight hypercarbia to dilate cerebral vessels and facilitate the anastomoses. Large changes in thoracic pressures transmitted to the brain may cause a "brain bounce" which makes surgery more difficult. For this reason, small tidal volumes may be employed at higher than normal frequencies. Positive end-expiratory pressure may be used to maintain lung expansion. Some anesthetists have successfully used high-frequency ventilation for this purpose.

Case History

J.M., a 62-year-old male, was scheduled for right carotid endarterectomy. Recently, he had several transient ischemic attacks referable to the right cerebral cortex, but no history of stroke. His medical problems included angina for which he was taking atenolol, 50 mg/day; nifedipine, 10 mg four times a day; and nitroglycerin paste, 1 inch three times a day. He had dyspnea when he walked up one flight of stairs, but no orthopnea, paroxysmal nocturnal dyspnea, or edema. He had smoked two packs of cigarettes a day for 40 years. He also had hypertension for which he was taking HCTZ 50 mg per day.

Physical examination was notable for blood pressure of 160/95 in both arms, an S_4 gallop on cardiac examination, and an increase in anteroposterior lung dimensions with a global decrease in lung sounds. Complete blood count, clotting studies, and chemical analysis were notable for potassium of 3.2 mEq/L and creatinine of 2.1 mg/dl. Electrocardiography revealed left axis deviation and nonspecific ST-T wave changes. The chest film was read as "hyperexpanded lung fields with normal heart size."

Suggested Reading

Beaupre PN, et al. Does pulmonary artery occlusion pressure adequately reflect left ventricular filling during anesthesia and surgery? Anesthesiology 1983; 59:3A.

Becker LC. Is isoflurane dangerous for the patient with coronary artery disease? Anesthesiology 1987; 66:259.

Breslow MJ, et al. Changes in T-wave morphology following anesthesia and surgery: a common recovery room phenomenon. Anesthesiology 1986; 64:398.

Eagle KA, et al. Dipyridamole-thallium scanning in patients undergoing vascular surgery: optimizing preoperative evaluation of cardiac risk. JAMA 1987; 257:2185.

Ferguson GG. Intraoperative monitoring and internal shunts: are they necessary in carotid endarterectomy? Stroke 1982; 13:287.

Goldman L. Cardiac risks and complications of noncardiac surgery. Ann Intern Med 1983; 98:504.

Grotta JC. Current medical and surgical therapy for cerebrovascular disease. N Engl J Med 1987; 317:1505.

Levy WJ, et al. Automated EEG processing for intraoperative monitoring. Anesthesiology 1980; 53:223.

Messick JM, et al. Correlation of regional cerebral blood flow (rCBF) with EEG changes during isoflurane anesthesia for carotid endarterectomy: critical rCBF. Anesthesiology 1987; 66:344.

Michenfelder JD, et al. Isoflurane when compared to enflurane and halothane decreases the frequency of cerebral ischemia during carotid endarterectomy. Anesthesiology 1987; 67:336.

Nehls DG, et al. A comparison of cerebral protective effects of isoflurane and barbiturates during temporary focal ischemia in primates. Anesthesiology 1987; 66:453.

Plum F. Extracranial-intracranial arterial bypass and cerebral vascular disease. N Engl J Med 1985; 313:1221.

Rao TLK, et al. Reinfarction following anesthesia in patients with myocardial infarction. Anesthesiology 1983; 59:499.

Relman AS. The extracranial-intracranial arterial bypass study: what have we learned? N Engl J Med 1987; 316:809.

Slogoff S, et al. Does perioperative myocardial ischemia lead to postoperative myocardial infarction? Anesthesiology 1985; 62:107.

Sundt TM, et al. Correlation of cerebral blood flow and electroencephalographic changes during carotid endarterectomy. Mayo Clin Proc 1981; 56:533.

Teplick R. The anesthetic management of the hemodynamically unstable patient. ASA Annual Refresher Course Lecture 113, 1986.

Winnie AP, et al. Interscalene cervical plexus block: a single-injection technique. Anesth Analg 1975; 54:370.

Bruce A. Mannes, M.D., and Richard J. Sperry, M.D.

Neuroendocrine Disease and Pituitary Surgery 11

The pituitary gland has been called the master gland of the endocrine system. This system regulates metabolism at a cellular level within the body and accomplishes this function with messenger compounds known as hormones. The pituitary gland regulates the production and secretion of several hormones. When this regulatory mechanism malfunctions, significant endocrine pathophysiology may develop, requiring medical or surgical intervention.

This chapter discusses the anesthetic implications of neuroendocrine disease. The normal anatomy and physiology of the pituitary gland are discussed, and the common pathophysiologic conditions that follow pituitary dysfunction are described. Because neuroendocrine disease is found in many patients who present for anesthesia and surgery, neuroendocrine disease is discussed at some length. Finally, the anesthetic management of pituitary surgery is considered.

Normal Anatomy

The pituitary gland lies in the sella turcica of the sphenoid bone. It consists of two lobes, the anterior adenohypophysis and the posterior neurohypophysis. The gland varies in weight between 0.5 and 0.6 g, is larger in females, and is largest in multiparous women.

Within the sella, the gland is separated from the optic chiasm superiorly by the diaphragm sella (composed of dura mater). The diaphragm is pierced by the pituitary stalk with its arachnoid covering. The stalk maintains a connection between the hypothalamus and pituitary. The pituitary is bordered laterally by the cavernous sinus and its contents: cranial nerves III, IV, V_1, VI, and the cavernous portion of the internal carotid artery.

Because of the close proximity of the pituitary gland to surrounding neurovascular structures, many potential surgical complications exist. Surgical trauma can induce significant arterial and venous bleeding, which can produce difficult operating conditions and significant blood loss. Cranial nerve palsy can also result from surgical trauma.

Physiology

The function of the pituitary gland is controlled by the hypothalamus. The anatomic division of the pituitary is also a functional division. Each division secretes its own hormones.

Anterior Pituitary (Adenohypophysis)

The hormones secreted by the anterior pituitary are classified as either acidophilic or basophilic, based on cellular staining characteristics.

Acidophilic Hormones

Growth Hormone (GH). This hormone promotes the growth of all tissues and organs by specific metabolic effects: (1) increasing the rate of protein synthesis, (2) increasing the mobilization of free fatty acids, and (3) decreasing the rate of glucose utilization and uptake by cells while increasing glycogen storage. The diminished cellular uptake of glucose produced by GH stimulates the pancreas to release insulin. A condition known as pituitary diabetes exists when the pancreas is unable to manufacture sufficient insulin to meet the demands of hyperglycemia resulting from an excess of GH.

Secretion of GH is controlled by growth hormone releasing factor (GH-RF) and growth hormone inhibiting factor (GH-IF) that are released by the hypothalamus. GH is a stress hormone, and stressful conditions such as surgical and anesthetic stimulation, anxiety, physical exertion, and hypoglycemia promote its release. Obesity and increased levels of free fatty acids decrease GH release.

Medications also affect GH release. Dopamine agonists increase GH serum levels and corticosteroids suppress GH release, which may be partially responsible for the growth plateau noted in children who receive steroids for prolonged periods.

Prolactin (Prl). This hormone is responsible for supporting growth and development of breast tissue in preparation for breast feeding. Secretion of Prl is also controlled by the hypothalamus.

Increased levels of Prl have been noted during surgical procedures. The release of endogenous opioids may be responsible for this increase. Medications such as the dopamine receptor antagonists also increase the serum Prl level. The list of these medications important to anesthesiologists includes metoclopramide, alpha-methyldopa, reserpine, and the phenothiazines.

Basophilic Hormones

Gonadotrophins (GN). There are two specific gonadotrophins released by the pituitary: luteinizing hormone (LH) and follicle-stimulating hormone (FSH). These hormones play a major role in the reproductive years when they stimulate growth and maturation of the reproductive organs.

Adrenocorticotrophic Hormone (ACTH). ACTH stimulates the adrenal cortex to produce and secrete corticosteroids. Absence of ACTH produces atrophy of the adrenal cortex. The zona glomerulosa, which produces mineralocorticoids (aldosterone), is minimally affected by the absence of ACTH. Hypophysectomy has little effect on electrolyte balance owing to continued release of aldosterone from the adrenal cortex.

The serum ACTH level is controlled by the hypothalamus, which secretes corticotrophin releasing factor (CRF). Serum cortisol completes the control loop by inhibiting CRF release. Normally there is a biphasic (diurnal) release of ACTH that is frequently lost with pituitary disease.

Thyroid-Stimulating Hormone (TSH).   TSH accelerates the formation of thyroid hormone and the uptake of iodine by the thyroid gland. TSH is released from the pituitary gland after stimulation by thyrotropin releasing factor (TRF). TRF is released from the hypothalamus in response to low circulating levels of thyroid hormone.

Posterior Pituitary (Neurohypophysis)

Two hormones, vasopressin (ADH) and oxytocin, are released from the posterior pituitary. ADH and oxytocin are both synthesized in the hypothalamus and transported to the neurohypophysis for release.

Antidiuretic Hormone (ADH or Vasopressin)

ADH is formed in the supraoptic nuclei of the hypothalamus. The role of ADH is to regulate both the osmotic pressure in extracellular fluid and the blood volume. ADH exerts its effect in the kidney where it increases the permeability of the renal collecting ducts to water. This results in the conservation of free water by the excretion of a concentrated urine.

ADH release is regulated by the osmoreceptors in the hypothalamus. When these receptors detect a rise in plasma osmolarity to greater than 280 mOsm/L, ADH is released, increasing free water absorption in the kidney and thus returning osmolarity to normal. Many additional factors modulate the release of ADH. By far the most potent stimulus for release of ADH is hypotension related to blood loss. The serum ADH level is also increased during surgical stimulation.

Oxytocin

Oxytocin is produced in the paraventricular nuclei of the hypothalamus. The release of oxytocin is independent of ADH. Oxytocin is a potent substance that augments uterine contractions and contributes to breast milk letdown.

Pituitary Tumors

Pituitary neoplasms comprise approximately 15% of all intracranial tumors. The majority are pituitary adenomas that are histologically benign and originate in the anterior pituitary. Pituitary carcinomas and metastatic disease to the pituitary have been reported, but they are uncommon. Nonendocrine tumors are also found. Many of these tumors are incidental findings at autopsy; however, others are of clinical significance and produce conspicuous problems for the patient.

Prolactin-secreting adenomas represent the most common functioning pituitary lesion. They represent 30% of all pituitary adenomas. Female patients present with galactorrhea, amenorrhea, and complaints of infertility; males most frequently complain of impotence. Headache, visual disturbances, and elevated intracranial pressure are more common in males, because they present with larger tumors (often > 10 mm) at the time of diagnosis.

Tumors that secrete excess GH produce a condition known as acromegaly, in which GH affects all tissues and organ systems to produce enlarged bodily structures. Most affected are the bones and soft tissues of the hands, feet, and face. The enlarged facial structures of these patients may make them difficult to intubate. Excess GH can cause coronary artery disease, hypertension, and cardiomyopathy. Hyperglycemia is also a frequent finding reflecting a GH-induced glucose intolerance.

Cushing's syndrome describes a group of disease states that have in common excess production of ACTH and hypercortisolemia. ACTH-producing pituitary tumors (adenomas), ectopic ACTH-producing tumors (oat cell lung tumors), and adrenal hyperplasia are included.

Cushing's disease describes abnormal ACTH production from a pituitary source, either tumor or hyperplasia. The clinical features of this condition all relate to an increase in ACTH production and hypercortisolemia. Hirsutism, abdominal striae, obesity, easy bruisability, acne, and moon facies are the traditional signs seen with Cushing's disease. Hypertension and diabetes mellitus may also be present clinically; muscle weakness (proximal) and osteoporosis may be present but go undetected.

Panhypopituitarism

Panhypopituitarism results from large tumors that destroy either normal pituitary or hypothalamic tissue or exert pressure on vascular structures and interrupt the blood supply to these organs. These patients show signs of anterior pituitary deficiency, but may or may not demonstrate diabetes insipidus from ADH deficiency. Adrenocortical hormones are necessary for the renal excretion of water, and diuresis may begin only after steroid replacement. These patients are susceptible to hemodynamic instability during periods of stress and to hypoglycemia.

In the setting of acute pituitary failure, hypothyroidism is uncommon. The long serum half-life of thyroxine (T_4) may prevent symptoms of thyroid failure. If steroid replacement has been instituted in patients suspected of pituitary failure, thyroid function must be evaluated.

Pituitary Apoplexy

Pituitary apoplexy is a condition produced by hemorrhagic infarction and necrosis of a pituitary tumor. This normally occurs in large tumors that either outgrow or compress their blood supply. Hemodynamic instability and hypotension are frequently seen and may require aggressive intervention.

Surgical Treatment of Pituitary Tumors

Medical and surgical therapy exist for both functional and nonfunctional pituitary tumors. Harvey Cushing introduced the oronasal midline rhinoseptal transsphenoidal approach to the pituitary in 1910 (Fig. 11-1). In 1962, Hardy helped to repopularize the procedure with the introduction of the surgical microscope and microsurgical dissection techniques. These advances simplified tumor removal by making it easier to distinguish tumor from normal gland.

Transsphenoidal surgery offers several advantages over the intracranial approach. First, statistically there is less morbidity and mortality because of decreased

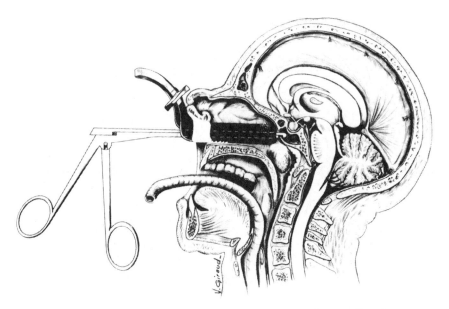

Figure 11-1 The transsphenoidal approach to the pituitary. (From Wilkins, Robert, and Rengachary, eds. Neurosurgery. New York: McGraw-Hill, 1985. Used with permission.)

blood loss and less manipulation of brain tissue. Second, there is less chance of inducing panhypopituitarism and a lower incidence of permanent diabetes insipidus.

For large tumors (>10 mm), tumors of uncertain type, and tumors that have substantial extrasellar extension, the transsphenoidal approach is inadequate. Such cases require an intracranial approach.

Preoperative Evaluation

The preoperative evaluation is the foundation on which the anesthesiologist builds an appropriate anesthetic plan. Included in this evaluation should be a thorough history and physical examination. Current medications, known allergies, and previous experiences with anesthetics should also be ascertained. The special considerations for neurosurgical patients are discussed in Chapter 7.

Monitors

Intraoperative monitoring should be commensurate with the underlying pathology and the procedure planned. Basic monitoring should include electrocardiography, automated blood pressure cuff, pulse oximetry, temperature probe, esophageal or precordial stethoscope, and urinary catheter. Capnography is another excellent physiologic monitor that should be considered standard. Invasive blood pressure monitoring should also be used for both transsphenoidal and intracranial operations. This allows for rapid and sequential measurements of blood chemistries and blood gases in addition to real-time blood pressure measurement.

Anesthetic Management

The basics of anesthetic management for patients with an intracranial mass (presented in Chapter 7) should be followed for pituitary surgery. Rather than repeat the discussion here, only a few special considerations for pituitary surgery are presented.

Intraoperative evoked potentials have been used to monitor the integrity of the optic nerves and chiasm during pituitary surgery. Technical difficulties have decreased its clinical usefulness. However, if evoked potentials are to be monitored, the anesthetic technique should not include a high concentration of volatile anesthetic agent. The volatile agents all increase the latency and decrease the amplitude of evoked potentials. A narcotic-based anesthetic with a very low concentration of volatile anesthetic agent is best.

In patients with a subarachnoid communication to the atmosphere (CSF rhinorrhea), there is a potential for air to enter the subarachnoid space. These patients should not receive nitrous oxide as a part of their anesthetic management. Nitrous oxide will expand subarachnoid air and potentially create a tension pneumocephalus.

As for all neurosurgical procedures, neuromuscular paralysis is an important adjunct during anesthesia for pituitary surgery. Microscopic dissection is possible only if the patient is absolutely still. Neuromuscular relaxation is particularly important if a narcotic-based anesthetic is used since these patients have a greater tendency to move during surgery, even if the anesthetic depth is appropriate.

Significant blood loss is a possibility during pituitary surgery because of the proximity of the operative site to the cavernous sinus and carotid artery. Intravenous access should be adequate to handle brisk hemorrhage.

Air embolism is also a risk if the cavernous sinus is entered. Most authorities recommend that a precordial Doppler be placed over the right heart and that end-tidal CO_2 monitoring be employed (see Chapter 8 for a discussion of air embolism). If end-tidal N_2 monitoring is available, this is one instance when it could prove very useful. A rent in the cavernous sinus can lead to significant hemorrhage and hypotension. Hypotension decreases the end-tidal CO_2 tension and thus confuses the diagnosis of air embolism by a similar decrease in end-tidal CO_2 tension.

Large pituitary tumors with extrasellar extension may require craniotomy rather than the transsphenoidal approach. This creates the potential for additional blood loss and the need for significant brain retraction. Blood products should be available along with both a loop and osmotic diuretic. The diuretic is a must if the patient presents with increased intracranial pressure.

During transsphenoidal procedures, local anesthetic solutions containing epinephrine are frequently used by the surgeon along the path where the retracting speculum is placed. Total spinal blocks have been reported if the anesthetic mixture penetrates the cribriform plate and the arachnoid. Also, when cocaine is used topically as a vasoconstrictor, the potential for catechol-generated arrhythmias exists.

Special Problems

Hormonal Supplementation

Most clinicians believe that intraoperative steroid supplementation in the patient with pituitary disease is the standard of care. The reasons include the uncertainty that a diseased pituitary will respond to surgical stress, and the manipulation and/or removal of anterior pituitary tissue involved in the surgical procedure, which may disrupt existing hypothalamic-pituitary-adrenal function.

There are many ways to supplement a patient with glucocorticoids. One method is to give 100 mg of hydrocortisone IV on induction of anesthesia, followed by a 50- to 100-mg IV bolus every 6 hours. Constant infusions have also been used. For example, 100 mg of hydrocortisone is placed in 500 ml of solution and infused at between 50 and 75 ml/hr (10 to 15 mg/hr).

Thyroid replacement is seldom indicated in the euthyroid patient while in the operating room. This is because of the long half-life of thyroxine (7 days). If needed, 500 μg of thyroxine can be administered intravenously.

Diabetes mellitus may require intraoperative treatment to regulate the serum blood glucose, especially when the patient is administered supplemental glucocorticoids. Regular insulin administered intravenously and titrated to the desired blood level is an easy, acceptable management.

Diabetes Insipidus

Diabetes insipidus (DI) from transsphenoidal surgery typically results from either local edema at the surgical site or trauma to the posterior pituitary. This problem develops in some form in about 40% of all patients and is usually transient, lasting less than 7 days. The initial manifestation of DI is polyuria in the postoperative period. The urine volume is typically 150 to 200 ml/hr but may exceed 1 to 2L/hr. DI most commonly occurs within 12 to 24 hours of the operation, but cases have been reported to develop intraoperatively. Early diagnosis and treatment are essential to prevent fluid and electrolyte imbalance.

The diagnosis is made by measuring the urine output and the osmolality of serum and urine. Polyuria with a low urinary specific gravity and osmolality combined with a high serum osmolality suggest DI. Other conditions that need to be considered are mannitol or glucose diuresis and fluid overload.

The goal of therapy is to restore normal fluid and electrolyte balance. This requires the accurate measurement of all intake and daily weights. Trends in serum sodium level (which is greater than 140 mEq/L in DI) and serum and urine osmolality help to guide fluid replacement.

Medical therapy for DI consists of intravenous fluid replacement and exogenous ADH or vasopressin administration. If serum hypernatremia is present as a result of persistent water losses, the fluid deficit may be calculated. The calculation for an 80-kg patient who has a normal percentage of body water and a current serum sodium level of 160 mEq/L follows:

> **Normal total body water (TBW)**
> 80-kg male × 60% water weight = 48 L TBW
> **Normal total body sodium**
> Serum Na+ 140 mEq/L × 48 L = 6,720 mEq total body Na+
> **Current total body water**
> Serum Na+ 160 mEq/L / 6,720 mEq = 42 L TBW
> **Calculated fluid deficit**
> 48 L − 42 L = 6 L

Fluid replacement should begin with one-half of the deficit using a free water solution. The patient's status should then be reevaluated in 1 to 2 hours.

Vasopressin, or exogenous ADH, can be administered subcutaneously, intramuscularly, or by nasal spray. Active preparations include an aqueous short-acting form (4 to 6 hours) given subcutaneously, an oil-based long-acting form (24 to 48 hours) given either intramuscularly or subcutaneously, and desmopressin (DDAVP) nasal spray administered twice a day. All preparations come mixed as units per milliliter. A normal dose range of aqueous vasopressin is 0.1 to 0.3 ml of a 20 U/ml solution, and for oil-based vasopressin, 0.25 to 0.5 ml of a 5 U/ml solution. The dose of vasopressin is titrated to patient response. As urine output decreases and serum sodium normalizes, the exogenous ADH is tapered to avoid water intoxication and hyponatremia.

Preoperative DI is commonly managed by nasal administration of DDAVP spray twice a day. However, in the immediate postoperative period, patients have nasal packing, which precludes the use of nasal spray.

Case History

M.L., a 45-year-old female, had a 19-year history of amenorrhea and a recent serum prolactin level of 458 ng/ml. She also had a 2-year history of fatigue and a recent decrease in visual acuity. She denied galactorrhea, weight loss, change in appetite, heat or cold intolerance, insomnia, or a change in peripheral vision.

Her medical history was significant only for a remote bilateral tubal ligation and an appendectomy. At the time of presentation she was not taking any medications.

No significant abnormalities were found on physical examination. Her visual fields were full to confrontation, and all cranial nerves were intact

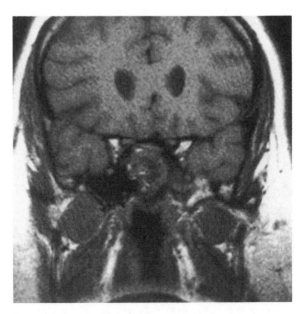

Figure 11-2   An MRI scan of a cystic pituitary adenoma.

and symmetrical. There was no discharge from her nipples. The upper airway and neck mobility were normal.

A magnetic resonance imaging (MRI) scan was obtained, which showed a cystic sellar and infrasellar mass (Fig. 11–2). The mass extended into the sphenoid and ethmoid sinuses.

The patient underwent a transsphenoidal hypophysectomy and excision of tumor from the paranasal sinuses. Pathologic study showed a pituitary adenoma. Postoperatively she had a brief period of diabetes insipidus which cleared after 3 days. On postoperative day 4 her serum prolactin level was 11.5 ng/ml.

Suggested Reading

Abboud CF, Laws ER. Clinical endocrinological approach to hypothalamic-pituitary disease. J Neurosurg 1979; 51:271–291.

Black PM, Zervas NT, Candia GL. Incidence and management of complications of trans-sphenoidal operation for pituitary adenomas. Neurosurgery 1987; 20:920–924.

Hays RM. Antidiuretic hormone. N Engl J Med 1976; 295:307–322.

Laws ER. Pituitary surgery. Endocrinol Metab Clin North Am 1987; 16:647–665.

Matjasko J. Perioperative management of patients with pituitary tumors. Seminars in Anesthesia 1984; 3:155–167.

Shucart WA, Jackson IJ. Management of diabetes insipidus in neurosurgical patients. J Neurosurg 1976; 44:65–71.

David J. Stone, M.D.

Anesthesia for Spinal Cord Surgery 12

Laminectomy

Laminectomy may be performed for disk disease, chronic bony spinal cord compression, neoplasm, or abscess. Disk problems generally occur in the lower cervical and lumbar levels and cause symptoms of root compression, although a central disk may rarely cause cord or cauda equina compression. Osteophytic projections in the cervical area (spondylosis) or spinal stenosis in the lumbar area may compress the cord. Resections of intramedullary cord tumors and arteriovenous malformations as well as meningiomas and neurofibromas are required below the foramen magnum, but are less common than their intracranial equivalents. Extradural cord compression may be produced by primary lymphomas or metastatic disease. These latter laminectomies may involve major blood losses. Epidural abscess may be caused by local disease (e.g., osteomyelitis) or spread of systemic infection (e.g., tuberculosis). If tuberculosis may be present, appropriate filters should be used between the anesthetic machine and the disposable tubing circuit.

Preoperative Considerations

Many patients presenting for disk surgery are young and healthy and require only a basic preoperative evaluation. On the other hand, patients with cervical spondylosis and lumbar spinal stenosis are frequently elderly and require the special considerations of the geriatric patient. In general, these include reduced reserve in the cardiac, pulmonary, and renal systems; altered drug responsiveness and metabolism; and frequently, the presence of underlying diseases and consequent polypharmacy. It is important to evaluate these patients individually, since physiology is a more important consideration than chronology. The status of coagulation must be evaluated carefully in patients with malignant spinal cord compression and arteriovenous malformations. All patients should have an evaluation of baseline neurologic status.

Positioning

The supine position is employed mainly for anterior fusion procedures of the cervical spine, such as the Cloward procedure. Some surgeons may use the sitting position for cervical spine surgery to improve exposure by reducing venous congestion and arterial pressure. Problems with the sitting position are discussed in more detail in Chapter 8. The lateral or semiprone position may be used for spinal surgery. Most commonly, though, the prone position is employed for spinal surgery at all levels.

Incorrect positioning may cause restriction of respiratory movements and obstruction of the inferior vena cava. The latter may cause hypotension because of decreased venous return to the heart, as well as excessive venous bleeding due to distended epidural and lumbar veins. Therefore, it is important to ensure that the abdomen is not compressed. It is also essential to avoid points of excessive pressure, especially around the eyes and genitals. I induce general anesthesia on a stretcher and then carefully move the patient onto the operating table with plenty of able help or have the patient comfortably position himself after an awake neurolept intubation. Devices supporting the neck (e.g., collars) should never be removed without the consent of the surgeons. If cervical spine instability is known or suspected, the surgeons should be present to assist in positioning. Further details on positioning are found in Chapter 5.

Intraoperative Management

Regional anesthesia may be employed for a first-time operation in the lumbar area. Disadvantages include potential respiratory compromise and difficulties in airway management in the prone position if general anesthesia becomes necessary. Regional anesthesia is strongly discouraged in the obese patient or the patient with significant pulmonary disease. If regional block is performed and anesthesia becomes unsatisfactory during the procedure, the surgeon is in an appropriate anatomic position to carefully add local anesthetic to the operated area. I do not commonly employ regional anesthesia for this procedure, but would do so at the patient's request if, in my judgment, it was not contraindicated. I do not employ intraspinal narcotics unless the patient can be appropriately monitored after the procedure, i.e., in the intensive care unit (ICU) or step-down unit.

If there is no anticipated difficulty in airway management, anesthesia can be induced while the patient is supine on a stretcher prior to being turned into the prone position on the operating room table. Neurologic contraindications to succinylcholine should be kept in mind. Care must be taken to continue some element of monitoring (at least an esophageal stethoscope) through the period of turning. One problem of turning the patient is hypotension, which probably results from venous pooling in the legs and abdomen after anesthetics have reduced the low and high pressure baroreflex control of peripheral vascular resistance. Such hypotension can be reduced by wrapping the legs, turning the patient slowly, and maintaining a light level of anesthesia with nitrous oxide and a narcotic. If the patient is particularly fragile from the standpoint of cardiovascular disease, extreme age, obesity, or multiple medical problems, an arterial line will greatly assist in monitoring the turn to the prone position.

Another complication of turning is displacement of the endotracheal tube. In all neuroanesthetics, the tube must be securely fixed. Not only can the tube slip out of the mouth, it can (more commonly) be displaced downward on turning and result in an endobronchial (usually right) intubation or cause bronchospasm due to carinal or bronchial irritation. I have seen extremely severe bronchospasm after the prone position is assumed; if the patient is predisposed to bronchospasm, all care should be given to prevent this. This would include avoidance of downward tube displacement; administration of anticholinergics, steroid, and inhaled beta-2-agonist before induction; and inclusion of adequate narcotic in the anesthetic before turning. It may be difficult or even hazardous (from a blood pressure standpoint) to employ a deep inhalational anesthetic to prevent bronchospasm during turning.

If the airway presents difficulties, the anesthetist may choose to employ one of the intubation techniques involving sedation and local anesthesia. These are described later in this chapter in the section on cervical spine trauma. In addition to the causes for difficult intubation that may be found in any patient, patients undergoing cervical spine surgery may be unable to extend the neck sufficiently for successful direct laryngoscopy. Some patients may note that neck movements produce symptoms of cord or root compression or vertebral artery insufficiency. The anesthetist must judge whether sedated intubation with topicalization is indicated. If cerebral insufficiency, any cord symptoms, or severe root symptoms are produced on neck movement, an intubation technique that moves the neck minimally should be employed.

Patients with rheumatoid arthritis have multiple problems, including diminished cervical movement, potential for subluxation at the C1-C2 interface, inability to open the mouth widely, diminished mandibulohyoid distance due to impaired mandibular growth, and a complex rotation of the larynx that can make direct visualization of the cords difficult. Fiberoptic bronchoscopy is extremely useful in these patients.

Some anesthetists employ sedated intubation with topicalization so that the patient can comfortably assume the prone position while avoiding undue pressure on key anatomic areas. If the surgeon is going to pin the head in the supine position for cervical laminectomy, there is no reason to do this. It also might be argued that if sufficient systemic analgesia has been employed to facilitate intubation, the patient is not going to be bothered by 15 seconds of pressure on a usually sensitive area.

Many surgeons employ a local anesthetic with epinephrine to topicalize the area of incision. The dose of epinephrine should be reviewed so that it is less than 2 μg/kg to avoid cardiac arrhythmias. Muscle relaxation may be required to facilitate surgical dissection and to ensure that there is no patient movement that could result in cord damage during surgery. Some surgeons employ a chymopapain injection during surgery to reduce disk material. There is a significant incidence of anaphylactic reactions to chymopapain (1 to 2%), and these patients should probably receive prophylaxis with an antihistamine (H_1 with or without H_2) and steroids. If anaphylaxis occurs, the key drug is epinephrine (50 to 500 μg IV boluses as required). Additional steroids, antihistamines, and volume are also indicated. Prominent manifestations include hypotension caused by vasodilation, skin signs, and bronchospasm. Airway edema may occur, and the patient should not be extubated if there is angioedema until the swelling is markedly reduced.

Patients with metastatic disease who undergo laminectomy present a special problem because of their frequently debilitated state and the extensive blood loss associated with these procedures. Surgery is undertaken when maximum radiation has been given and failed or when required to prevent or treat fracture-dislocation. Preoperative evaluation may reveal pulmonary involvement from tumor, radiation, drugs, or infection; pancytopenia; tolerance to narcotics; pericardial or myocardial involvement by tumor; dehydration; and various degrees of neurologic dysfunction. Bleeding may be severe and sudden and ranges from about 2,000 to 5,500 ml, depending on approach. The placement of an arterial line and two large-bore intravenous catheters is recommended. Central venous or pulmonary artery catheters may be indicated in individual patients according to their cardiovascular status preoperatively. Coagulation should be assessed and abnormalities corrected. Cell savers for recycling lost blood cannot be used for fear of hematogenous spread of the tumor. This concern with blood loss is in contrast to laminectomy for benign disease in which about half a unit of blood (250 ml) is usually lost.

Although patients may be extubated while deep or awake after lumbar laminectomy (some anesthetists extubate them while still prone after muscle strength and respirations are adequate), patients should be extubated awake after cervical laminectomy, so that there is no requirement for neck manipulation to maintain the airway.

Spinal Cord Trauma

Preoperative Evaluation

Neurologic Status

The results of the neurologic examination depend on the level of the spinal cord involved by the trauma. Levels from T2 to T12 cause paraplegia but leave the upper extremities and diaphragm intact. Levels from C5 to T1 cause a varying degree of upper extremity paralysis as well. The diaphragm is innervated by cervical roots 3 to 5, and their involvement causes various degrees of ventilatory impairment immediately, but patients with an intact C5 level may retain enough function to survive without ventilation.

It is essential to avoid neck motion and further cord damage in these patients. In some cases, the patient's neck may already have been completely stabilized with a halo. For the anesthesiologist, this represents a fundamental change in airway management that normally employs cervical flexion and extension at the atlantoaxial (C1–C2) joint to achieve the desired "sniffing position." Flexion is even more deleterious than extension, but both should be avoided if possible, even in what appears acutely to be complete quadriplegia, as the latter state may go on to show variable degrees of improvement.

The cord itself is not usually severed, but is injured by factors such as compression from bone or foreign body, hematoma, edema, and ischemia. Currently, no pharmacologic treatment (steroids, mannitol, naloxone, thyroid-stimulating hormone) or physical measure (local hypothermia) has been clearly shown to be more beneficial than simply maintaining spinal cord perfusion with volume and vasoactive drugs. Steroids are routinely employed in some centers. Spinal cord blood flow is controlled in fairly similar fashion to cerebral blood flow. As with head injury, severe hypercarbia should be avoided to prevent increases in intraspinal pressure that may result in ischemia.

The surgical treatment of these injuries is somewhat controversial. If there is clear-cut cord compression by bone or hematoma, most surgeons agree that decompression is necessary. Other surgeons take a more aggressive approach to early internal reduction and fixation, at least in part, to accelerate rehabilitation. Whether the local surgeons practice early fixation or not, the anesthesiologist is faced with the problem of anesthetizing the patient for other procedures, in any case.

Cardiovascular Status

A certain amount of cardioaccelerator and vasoconstrictor tone is lost as a result of cord injuries that involve T1 to L1 levels. This may result in so-called spinal shock hours to weeks after the injury in patients with injury to levels above T6. Not only do these patients pool volume in the periphery, they have unopposed parasympathetic tone, resulting in bradycardia and an inability to increase the chronotropic or inotropic state of the heart. The tendency to bradycardia is remarkable upon such stimuli as suctioning or endotracheal intubation and can be prevented with atropine, 0.6 to 1 mg IV.

Shock in this setting may have other etiologies, such as hemorrhage, pericardial tamponade, tension hemopneumothorax, or low blood pressure due to a vascular injury, especially a tear of the aorta. The trauma team must be involved in this investigation. As a rule, the hypotension of spinal shock is associated with relative bradycardia, while that of hemorrhage is associated with tachycardia. However, hemorrhage may coexist with spinal cord injury, resulting in blood loss without tachycardia.

Both forms of shock can be approached initially with fluids while preliminary evaluation proceeds. However, the patient with spinal shock will not handle large fluid challenges well because of an inability to increase heart rate and contractility. The Swan-Ganz (pulmonary artery) catheter may be used in this setting to avoid fluid overload. Spinal shock should be managed in part with doses of intravenous atropine and vasopressors to avoid the administration of large amounts of fluid. Some authors feel strongly that inotropes (dopamine) should be used rather than pure vasopressors.

Hemorrhagic shock, by contrast, requires aggressive replacement of blood and crystalloid and surgical measures to stop the bleeding. Sorting these out in practice can be quite difficult, which is why the pulmonary artery catheter is useful. The patient with spinal shock is especially likely to have hypotension during anesthetic induction and maintenance and must be treated with special care at those times. The rapid administration of a large dose of a cardiovascular depressant, such as thiopental, should be avoided.

The trauma patient may also have suffered a myocardial contusion resulting in cardiac dysfunction and dysrhythmias. Although electrocardiography and enzyme studies are unsatisfactorily nonspecific, two-dimensional echocardiography or a nuclear study may show areas of focal wall motion abnormalities otherwise inexplicable in a young, previously healthy patient. Treatment is directed toward the resulting abnormalities in heart rhythm and contractility.

Respiratory Status

The degree of respiratory compromise depends on the level of spinal injury as previously discussed. However, even injury to levels below those involved in diaphragmatic innervation will affect respiratory function, because the abdominal muscles are essential to a forceful cough. Even when secretions can be removed from large central airways by suction, the weak or nonexistent cough of these patients predisposes them to hypoxemia and recurrent atelectasis because of the accumulation of secretions in peripheral airways. Table 12-1 lists the innervation of the principal respiratory muscles.

In addition to diaphragmatic and cough mechanism dysfunction, other pulmonary disorders may occur. Although underlying pulmonary disease is somewhat

Table 12-1 Innervation of the Muscles of Respiration

Sternocleidomastoid (CN XI, C2-3)	Accessory inspiratory
Trapezius (CN XI, C3-4)	Accessory inspiratory
Diaphragm (C3-5)	Inspiratory
Scalenes (C4-8)	Inspiratory
Intercostals (T1-12)	Inspiratory and expiratory
Abdominal (T7-T12, L1)	Expiratory

uncommon in this generally young population, many are smokers with baseline problems of cough, secretions, and bronchospasm, and others may have asthma or, less commonly, other underlying pulmonary disorders.

Patients with spinal cord injuries sometimes suffer pulmonary contusion, which is essentially a bruised area of lung resulting in an area of very low $\dot{V}/\dot{Q}$ distribution, resulting in hypoxia. It also represents an area that is a good potential culture medium for pneumonia-producing bacteria. The chest wall above the contusion may be unstable, resulting in difficulty reexpanding the injured area of lung. This occurs when several adjacent ribs are broken in more than one place, resulting in a flail chest that does not expand with the remainder of the chest wall during inspiration. There is no specific treatment, but the patients should receive oxygen, positive airway pressure, and ventilation as required. A spinal cord injury above this level obviates the issue of pain control. In patients with pain, the use of intercostal nerve blocks, intrapleural administration of local anesthetics, transcutaneous nerve stimulation, and/or systemic analgesics, administered as patient-controlled analgesia, if possible, assist in control of pain and allow for deeper, more effective breathing. The use of epidural local anesthetics or narcotics may not be advisable in the context of acute spinal injury.

Other pulmonary problems in this setting include aspiration, neurogenic or cardiogenic pulmonary edema, inhalation injuries, fat embolism, and adult respiratory distress syndrome (ARDS) due to many causes, including sepsis. Neurogenic pulmonary edema can follow spinal as well as intracranial trauma, and probably involves increased capillary permeability as well as increased pulmonary venous pressures.

Preoperative evaluation should include an appreciation of these superimposed problems, as well as the current level of dysfunction caused by the spinal cord injury. Bronchospasm, if present, should be treated with theophylline, beta-2-agonists, anticholinergics, and steroids. Secretions should be handled with adequate hydration, suction, and a preoperative anticholinergic. If the spine is unstable, chest physical therapy may be contraindicated. Emergency surgery may have to be performed on patients in less than optimal pulmonary condition. Blood gases should be available, as well as devices for supplying intraoperative positive end-expiratory pressure. If lung compliance is severely diminished, many ventilators on anesthetic machines will not deliver adequate pressures for ventilation, and a modern ventilator from the ICU may be needed. Anesthesia can be provided intravenously in such a case.

Other Systems

In trauma patients, other systems may be involved with the underlying disease or associated injuries. Head trauma is discussed in detail in Chapter 16. Injuries to the maxilla, skull base, and mandible in association with cervical spine trauma may produce great difficulties in airway management. For instance, the patient may have a basilar skull fracture that is a strong relative contraindication to nasal intubation and a mandibular injury that makes it impossible to open the mouth. Maxillary fractures may result in airway obstruction when the free-floating fragment falls backward in the supine position and occludes the airway. Occasionally, these airways may need to be managed with cricothyroidotomy or tracheostomy. Cervical spine injuries may be associated with injuries to the larynx and may present as various degrees of vocal dysfunction or airway obstruction.

Cardiac tamponade, tension pneumothorax, and rapid bleeding into the pleural space(s) must be considered possible causes of hypotension. An aortic tear is an extremely serious injury that requires angiography for diagnosis and to guide surgical repair. It is usually suspected when mediastinal widening is seen on the chest film.

Intra-abdominal injuries may be acutely responsible for hemorrhage that can be detected by peritoneal lavage or computed tomographic (CT) scan. The CT scan will also detect retroperitoneal bleeding, which is frequently caused by pelvic fractures. Fractures, especially of the pelvis and femur, may account for a large amount of blood loss. Overall, injuries that are life-threatening because of hemorrhage, aortic rupture, or cardiac tamponade or are brain-threatening take precedence over less acute problems.

In the chronically injured patient, calcium and renal function should be checked, because the former may rise as a result of immobilization and the latter may be impaired due to chronic and recurrent infections.

Intraoperative Considerations

Anesthesia Induction and Maintenance

Airway Management. The induction of anesthesia in patients with cervical spine injury requires special precautions. In some patients neck immobility is assured by a halo, but others may require assistance by the surgeons to maintain neck immobility during intubation.

In general, intubation with careful topicalization and sedation is preferred, but in children and in uncooperative adults, a rapid-sequence intubation with the surgeon immobilizing the neck is preferable to having a thrashing patient who injures himself further in resisting intubation. I suggest such an intubation be performed only by a skilled, experienced practitioner who has able assistance and the immediate availability of cricothyroidotomy. The use of an anticholinergic is highly recommended to reduce secretions and improve visualization.

Nasal intubation is contraindicated in the presence of significant coagulopathy and relatively strongly contraindicated in the presence of basilar skull fracture. In some patients, it is impossible to pass an adequately sized tube (at least No. 6 ID in women, No. 7 ID in men) through the nose.

Nasal topicalization may be achieved with 4% cocaine (up to 3 mg/kg), with a combination of 3% lidocaine and 0.25% Neo-Synephrine (up to 3 mg/kg lidocaine), or with the initial introduction of Neo-Synephrine nose drops to dilate and vasoconstrict the nasal mucosa. Then, a lesser concentration of lidocaine (1 to 2%) is used to topicalize the nose and nasopharynx. The lower concentration allows for the safe use of more lidocaine for further topicalization of the pharynx, larynx, and trachea.

Lidocaine can be introduced deeply into the nose with the plastic cannula of a 16- or 18-gauge intravenous line, or long Q-Tips (three or four) can be saturated with lidocaine and placed until they touch the posterior wall of the nasopharynx. This can be comfortably accomplished with a slow, twisting motion. Once in place, further lidocaine can be dripped in along the wooden sticks, which are slowly pulled out in stages to topicalize the entire mucosa. When three Q-Tips can be introduced, a No. 7 ID endotracheal tube can usually be successfully passed into that nostril either directly or through a soft nasal airway guide.

If the cricothyroid membrane is accessible, laryngotracheal anesthesia can be supplied with the translaryngeal administration of local anesthetic through the cricothyroid membrane. If a cervical collar or other device is in place, it should not be removed without consulting the responsible surgeons. Inject 2 to 4 cc of 1 to 2% lidocaine through the cricothyroid membrane with a 23-gauge needle after air is aspirated to ensure that the needle is within the lumen of the airway.

Blind nasal intubation is accomplished by listening to the patient's breathing sounds through the tube until a position of maximal sound volume is achieved, which presumably should represent a tip position just above the vocal cords. The tube can then be passed into the trachea during an inspiration when the vocal cords open. It is advisable to bend the tube to give it some anterior curvature before it is passed. This can be done by placing the tube tip in the adaptor to form a circle of the tube or by placing a stylet in the tube in the shape desired and removing the stylet before tube placement.

Often, the tube passes into the esophagus rather than the trachea. If there is no cervical spine problem, the neck can be manipulated with extension and rotation to help guide the tip into the trachea. This cannot be done when there is any question of potential injury to the cervical cord. The fiberoptic bronchoscope is probably the preferred way to initiate nasal intubation in these situations. If fiberoptic bronchoscopy is planned, the transtracheal injection is not necessary, since it does present a small risk (bleeding, mainly), and the lidocaine can be injected through the bronchoscope when the cords are visualized. Use of the fiberoptic scope is more difficult after bleeding and edema result from unsuccessful blind attempts. Successful use of the scope requires practice. Fiberoptic intubations require some time and should not be relied upon when an airway is immediately necessary.

Blind nasal intubation may be facilitated by the Endotrol endotracheal tube in which tension on a loop near the proximal end pulls the endotracheal tube tip anteriorly. Gorback has described a technique of blind nasal intubation in which the cuff is inflated to bring the tip anteriorly and then deflated after the tip is passed 2 cm into the larynx. Berry has described the use of a stylet in blind nasal intubation. In brief, the stylet is formed into a C-shape and passed into the tube after the tube has been introduced into the pharynx. The stylet will then bring the tube tip anteriorly when the tube is slid off, hopefully into the trachea.

Oral intubation can be accomplished with the fiberoptic scope, light-wand stylet, direct laryngoscopy, or blindly with the aid of a curved Macintosh laryngoscope blade. The mucosal surface of the tongue can be topicalized with 10% lidocaine spray. However, this does not blunt the discomfort of the laryngoscope blade pressure.

Glossopharyngeal blocks as described by Woods and Lander can blunt this pressure response. Inject 2 cc of 1% lidocaine with epinephrine through a 25-gauge needle just at the point where the anterior tonsillar pillar approximates the base of the tongue on both sides. This block allows the laryngoscope to be comfortably placed in usual fashion and, when the cords are visualized, they can be topicalized with an "LTA" kit or with 4 to 5 cc of 1% lidocaine. Superior laryngeal nerve blocks topicalize the supraglottic area and are accomplished with 2 cc of 1% lidocaine given through a 25-gauge needle through the lateral portion of the thyrohyoid membrane. Thorough topicalization can allow a reasonably comfortable intubation with minimal sedation.

Narcotics blunt discomfort at the cost of a less responsive patient who may protect the airway poorly. Fentanyl can be used in slow 1- to 2-cc increments and has the advantage of rapid and specific reversal with naloxone (which should be available). In addition to fentanyl, droperidol can be used (1.25 to 5 mg IV) to give additional sedation without further respiratory depression. While some practitioners prefer a benzodiazepine, the action of these drugs is unpredictable (some patients are quickly oversedated), and the respiratory depression is not reversible with naloxone. The inclusion of a narcotic is extremely helpful in blunting gag and cough responses. As noted previously, the use of an anticholinergic (glycopyrrolate, 0.4 to 0.5 mg IV) is nearly essential to decrease the secretions that reduce visibility and increase airway irritability.

During direct oral laryngoscopy, the head should be stabilized by the responsible surgical service. If the cords or even the arytenoid (corniculate) cartilages cannot be visualized, a blind technique can be employed. A curved-blade laryngoscope is inserted to raise the epiglottis, and an endotracheal tube with a curved stylet is passed blindly through the cords. Because the clinician does not see the tube pass through the cords when employing blind techniques, it is optimal to confirm endotracheal intubation with a fiberoptic examination or analysis of end-tidal CO_2 because all the commonly used clinical signs (i.e., bilateral breath sounds and chest movement) may be unreliable.

The light-wand stylet can be used to facilitate blind oral intubation. The room must be darkened, so use of a pulse oximeter is even more strongly recommended than for other techniques, because the patient's color is not observable. When the light is seen brightly in the midline, the tube is inserted another 2 cm and then slipped off the stylet into the trachea.

A retrograde intubation can be performed if other methods fail and there is no urgency to the situation. The cricothyroid membrane area is topicalized with 1 to 2 cc of 1% lidocaine injected with a 23-gauge needle. Either an epidural (17-gauge) or central venous (16-gauge) needle is then inserted through the membrane and the epidural or central venous catheter inserted into the larynx to be coughed up through the cords by the patient. Nasal or oral intubation is then accomplished by sliding the endotracheal tube over the stretched-out catheter. The tube may be held up at the glottis, and this may be helped by rotating the tube or slackening the catheter.

If intubation cannot be performed, a cricothyroidotomy is indicated if an airway is needed urgently. This is best performed by an experienced surgeon, but may be done by the anesthesiologist if necessary. The cricothyroid membrane is incised, and a small endotracheal or tracheostomy tube is inserted. There is a risk of laryngeal damage, but this is a life-saving procedure to be used when other measures fail or are impossible (severe facial trauma). Although some surgeons perform cricothyroidotomies electively, most choose to perform a formal tracheostomy if time permits, but even in the best of hands it is extremely difficult to perform a tracheostomy quickly enough to deliver oxygen to the brain of a hypoxic patient.

Anesthesia Induction. As previously noted, there may be compromise of the cardiovascular system due to spinal shock, cardiac trauma, or hypovolemia; thus anesthesia must be induced carefully. The use of atropine is strongly recommended before intubation and is helpful in an already intubated patient to reduce secretions, bronchospasm, and reflex bradycardia. If rapid-sequence intubation is chosen, ketamine (0.5 to 2 mg/kg) is a reasonable induction agent. Elevated intracranial pressure is a relative contraindication to its use, because cerebral blood flow is generally increased by ketamine. Thiopental should be used with caution because of its potential to cause severe hypotension. Etomidate may be a useful drug, but experience with its use is limited. Carefully chosen doses of midazolam or alfentanil are options as well. The key to avoiding problems is giving the chosen drugs slowly and observing carefully for cardiovascular response.

Anesthesia can be maintained with ketamine or narcotics alone or with nitrous oxide. A potent anesthetic agent such as isoflurane can be added if tolerated. Fluid and blood replacement should be exacting to avoid both overload and hypovolemia. The pulmonary artery catheter will reveal increasing pulmonary capillary wedge pressures that persist after a volume bolus when the left heart is volume overloaded. At that point, fluids are restricted and diuretics given, if judged necessary. Temperature is carefully monitored since these patients lose thermal regulation because of their autonomic dysfunction. Warmed fluids, heated, humidified gases, warming blanket, head covers, and an increase in the operating room temperature all help.

Succinylcholine generally should be avoided since a hyperkalemic response may develop that is not prevented with pretreatment with nondepolarizing relaxants. The use of succinylcholine may be acceptable in the acutely injured patient (up to 24 hours after injury). I suggest that succinylcholine not be used in these patients, even long after the injury has passed. Any of the nondepolarizing drugs is acceptable. Pancuronium has the advantage of sympathetic stimulation in these patients.

Autonomic Hyperreflexia.   After the period of spinal shock has ended, the deafferented spinal cord may produce a group of deleterious reflexes known as autonomic hyperreflexia. When areas are stimulated below the level of the lesion, the affected cord segments respond with neural transmission, resulting in muscular (hyperreflexia, rigidity, spasm) and autonomic (hypertension) responses. Normal cord segments compensate for the hypertension with bradycardia and vasodilation. With cord levels above T 7, this compensation may not be adequate to prevent hypertension severe enough to cause intracranial hemorrhage. The patient may be sweaty, nauseated, and agitated and complain of headache. Cardiac arrhythmias and block may occur. Pain, bladder or bowel distention, or surgical stimulation may all trigger this reflex. The reflex can be blunted by general, spinal, or epidural anesthesia.

General anesthesia does not block the reflex if the level of anesthesia is too light, but care must be taken to avoid hypotension with deep anesthesia. Epidural anesthesia is difficult because it is impossible to know the effect of a test dose if the spinal cord injury level is high enough to cause autonomic hyperreflexia. Therefore, extreme care should be taken to avoid a high spinal level if the dura has been inadvertently punctured. Spinal anesthesia may be technically difficult, and the patient must be carefully watched for hypotension and bradycardia. A continuous technique with a subarachnoid catheter can be considered and has the advantage of slower dosing in small increments to avoid an excessively high level. Spinal headache will not be a problem in the already bedridden patient. Drugs to treat hypertension (hydralazine, nitroprusside) should be available to treat autonomic hyperreflexia if it occurs.

Other Considerations.   After control of the airway has been established, ventilation should be controlled with large tidal volume breaths (10 to 15 ml/kg) to avoid hypercarbia and atelectasis. Care should be taken to avoid hypotension caused by decreased venous return when mechanical ventilation is begun.

Patients with chronic spinal cord injury should be moved carefully to avoid fractures of weakened bones. Areas of pressure should be checked for and relieved.

Postoperative Recovery and Intensive Care

The general principles of recovery and intensive care are outlined in the chapters devoted to those subjects. This section specifically addresses the problems of the patient with spinal cord injury.

Respiratory Status

Problems of the respiratory system are key in the management of these patients. Because general anesthesia reduces postoperative vital capacity by about half, the patient with respiratory impairment because of a high cord lesion may require postoperative ventilation. Patients who have an acute injury affecting the cervical segments should clearly be left intubated and ventilated. As noted previously, lesions below C5 should not affect the diaphragm but they will importantly affect the expiratory muscles necessary for generating a forceful cough. This is why these patients are so susceptible to retention of secretions with resulting atelectasis and lobar collapse. After thoracic or upper abdominal surgery, vital capacity (and functional residual capacity) is reduced for days and the patient with borderline preoperative lung function may require more prolonged mechanical ventilation.

In general, a patient with chronic injury who is operated on for a single problem is less likely to have difficulty than an acutely injured patient operated on for multiple traumatic injuries. We often employ spinal anesthesia for orthopaedic and urologic injuries in chronic patients so that the patient's ability to ventilate himself has been demonstrated throughout the case. In the multiply injured patient, there is little question about continuing postoperative intubation and ventilation.

In chronically injured patients with major procedures or in acutely injured patients with lower levels and minor procedures, the best way to proceed may be less clear. In this instance, it is reasonable to bring the patient to the recovery area while intubated and to wean the patient slowly from support while monitoring oxygenation and ventilation. Some sedation may be necessary to allow the patient to tolerate the tube and pain above the level of the injury. This may delay weaning and even necessitate resumption of mechanical ventilation, but the process cannot be rushed.

As noted, the critical problems in these patients are loss of ventilatory capacity due to cervical injury and loss of forceful cough due to expiratory muscle weakness. Even lower cord lesions affect the abdominal muscles (T7 to T12, L1) and therefore cough. Loss of ventilatory capacity limits the patient's ability to expel CO_2 and to cough, since coughing is less effective from low lung volumes. Secretions pool because suction does not remove them from the noncentral airways (see next section for cardiovascular response to suctioning). If not contraindicated by an unstable injury, chest physical therapy (percussion, vibration, postural drainage, cough amplification) will bring secretions to the central airways where they can be suctioned. While bronchoscopic treatment of major atelectasis can usually be avoided in other populations, bronchoscopic removal of plugs and secretions is very helpful in this group because they suffer from recurrent lung collapses, which cause severe $\dot{V}/\dot{Q}$ abnormalities and hypoxemia.

Treatment of pneumonia, ARDS, pulmonary edema, and chronic management of the airway are discussed in Chapter 18.

Cardiovascular Status

Spinal shock and autonomic hyperreflexia have been previously discussed. Autonomic hyperreflexia may appear postoperatively as general or regional anesthesia is wearing off.

During the spinal shock period, bradycardia is a recurrent problem. Asystole in response to stimuli, such as suctioning, may also occur because of an unopposed vagal reflex in patients who have lost all or most of the cardioaccelerator input (T1 to T6) of their sympathetic nervous system. The reflex can be blunted with the administration of atropine (0.4 to 1 mg IV), which blocks the vagus. Atropine is also useful in that it reduces secretion volume (but not viscosity) and is a bronchodilator. Hypoxemia should be carefully avoided because it exacerbates the reflex. A small dose of intravenous narcotic or intravenous or intratracheal (1 to 1.5 mg/kg) lidocaine will make suctioning more comfortable for the patient. I have had patients who have required temporary pacemaker insertion so that they could safely tolerate suctioning.

Genitourinary Status

An indwelling Foley catheter is generally left in place during the acute phase, to be replaced eventually by intermittent catheterization. These patients consequently have recurrent urinary tract infections leading to renal dysfunction from tubulointerstitial nephritis and amyloidosis.

Other Problems

Other problems include deep venous thrombosis, which can be prevented with elastic stockings, external pneumatic compression, and physical therapy; upper gastrointestinal bleeding, which can be minimized with antacids, H_2 blockers, or sucralfate; contractures; psychological problems; and osteoporosis and pressure sores resulting from immobility.

Correction of Spinal Deformities

Spinal deformities generally fall into the province of the orthopedic surgeon, but are discussed briefly here.

Preoperative Evaluation

Respiratory Status

Patients with spinal curvature severe enough to require surgery often have reduced lung volumes because of the chest wall deformity. If neuromuscular disease is present, respiratory function may be limited on this basis as well. Although there are grading systems for the degree of skeletal deformity, the anesthesiologist is primarily interested in the functional result, which can be examined with arterial blood gases and pulmonary function tests, including vital capacity and peak inspiratory and expiratory pressures.

If vital capacity is less than 40% of the predicted level, postoperative ventilation is required. Although patients with higher vital capacities may not require postoperative ventilation, they must be judged on an individual basis. For instance, low peak inspiratory and expiratory pressures indicating respiratory muscle weakness may lead one to prophylactically ventilate the postoperative patient who had a borderline preoperative vital capacity. The arterial blood gas is useful for gauging the degree of resting hypercarbia that may be present, as well as for evaluating the alveolar-arterial oxygen gradient.

Preoperative measures include the teaching of a deep breathing and cough regimen, which may include incentive spirometry, elimination of infection, treatment of bronchospasm, removal of secretions, as well as informing patients what they can expect and how they can help themselves.

Cardiovascular Status

The low lung volumes of chest wall deformity may result in pulmonary hypertension and cor pulmonale. Hypoxemia may contribute to pulmonary hypertension and result in polycythemia as well. Patients with underlying muscular dystrophy may have an associated cardiomyopathy with the problems of cardiac muscle dysfunction, arrhythmias, and heart block. There is a high incidence of mitral valve prolapse in these patients.

Because exercise tolerance is often not helpful in evaluating the hearts of these patients, echocardiography may be indicated to screen for myocardial and valvular abnormalities.

Neurologic Status

A screening examination should be performed by the anesthesiologist to document grossly any degree of preoperative neurologic impairments, e.g., baseline mental retardation, neuropathies, myopathy, and spinal cord dysfunction.

Anesthesia Induction and Maintenance

The two outstanding problems of these operations are blood loss and neurologic injury (about 1%). The induction of anesthesia is notable for the avoidance of succinylcholine in patients with neurologic deficits and the probable higher incidence of malignant hyperthermia in patients with muscular dystrophies. An arterial line and two intravenous catheters are placed, and many anesthetists place a central venous pressure monitor as well to aid in determination of intravascular volume. The patient is carefully turned prone onto the chosen frame, with care taken to assure that the abdomen lies free and there are no pressure points.

Hypotensive Anesthesia

In order to minimize blood loss and provide better surgical conditions, some degree of controlled hypotension is often employed. If a wake-up test is planned, deep levels of anesthesia cannot be used for hypotension, and specific hypotensive agents are added to a nitrous-narcotic anesthetic. Patients may be pretreated with propranolol, captopril (3 mg/kg PO), or clonidine (0.05 mg/kg PO).

Moderate hypotension (mean blood pressure 60 mm Hg) is the goal, and sodium nitroprusside (SNP) is the most commonly used drug in this setting. After pretreatment with one of the above drugs, which moderate the sympathetic and/or angiotensin response to hypotension, tolerable doses of SNP (0.25 to 8 μg/kg/min) usually result in the desired blood pressure. Small increments of labetalol (starting with 2.5 mg IV), a combined alpha- and beta-blocker, help if the SNP doses required are unacceptable. A more detailed discussion of controlled hypotension can be found in Chapter 9.

Other Measures to Reduce Blood Loss or Exogenous Transfusions

Good positioning is the key to avoid vena caval compression and excessive blood flow through epidural veins. Recently desmopressin (DDAVP) has been found to reduce blood loss in Harrington rod cases. This is a modified form of vasopressin that improves the function of what are presumably normal platelets in this setting. The dose is 0.3 μg/ kg and must be given over 20 to 30 minutes to avoid hypotension.

The patient may donate his own blood preoperatively for intraoperative administration. Hematocrits in the mid-20s are tolerable so long as intravascular volume and cardiac function are normal. Lost blood may be recycled in the Cell Saver for transfusion. If blood loss is severe, blood should be given as indicated, because the risk of death from hemorrhagic shock is still more unacceptable than the extremely unlikely acquisition of AIDS or hepatitis B, although non-A, non-B hepatitis is a not-uncommon sequela of transfusion.

Monitoring

There are two main techniques for monitoring spinal cord function during these operations: the wake-up test and somatosensory evoked potentials (SSEPs). The wake-up test does just that, and the patient demonstrates movement of the lower extremities. Many still consider it the gold standard of intraoperative spinal cord monitoring. The SSEP involves stimuli to sensory nerves in the lower extremities and recordings from the scalp. These are found in the cerebral recording with the help of a computer and evaluated for amplitude and latency. Details of evoked potential monitoring are given in Chapter 4.

To perform the wake-up test, the patient is informed preoperatively that it will occur, that he will be asked to move his legs, and that he will feel little or no pain. Preoperative sedation should be minimal, and the anesthetic is performed with nitrous oxide and a narcotic that is short-acting in moderate doses (fentanyl, sufentanil, alfentanil). The trachea may be sprayed with lidocaine to help the awakened patient tolerate the tube, which should be very securely taped in place to avoid dislodgement during the "wake-up." The surgeon should give about a 45-minute warning so that no further narcotic or relaxant is given before the test.

When the surgeon is ready for the test, the relaxant is reversed and the nitrous oxide turned off. The patient is asked to move his feet and toes and is watched carefully to avoid injuring himself. Once motion has been demonstrated, anesthesia can be reinduced with thiopental and continued with inhalation agents. The wake-up test is not a true monitor in the sense that it is not continuous, but it does provide assurance that damage has not been done up to the time of the test. The wake-up test should be used with caution, if at all, in patients with bronchospastic disease, emotional disorders, or mental retardation.

The main problem with SSEPs is that they may remain normal while motor function is lost. Motor potentials are being developed to deal with this problem. The SSEPs may also become abnormal (false positive) when no damage has been done to the spinal cord. Since inhaled and intravenous agents may affect the tracing, the monitoring neurologist should be informed of their use. With conventional SSEP monitoring, deep inhalational anesthesia unacceptably alters the tracing, but a new spinal epidural recording technique may allow for use of deep inhalational anesthesia. The reference containing the opposing opinions of Grundy and Michenfelder regarding the use of the wake-up test and SSEPs in this setting is enlightening.

Postoperative Care

As noted earlier, patients with severe compromise of respiratory function should be ventilated postoperatively. Borderline patients can be brought to recovery or the ICU with the tube in place and evaluated on an individual basis with the help of arterial blood gas determinations. Patients with muscular dystrophies may be extraordinarily sensitive to sedation and are best left intubated until their prolonged wake-up is accomplished. Blood loss needs to be monitored.

Postoperative lung expansile maneuvers are begun, which may simply involve chest physical therapy, cough, and deep breathing. Incentive spirometry may be used to help the patient take deep breaths to expand atelectatic areas and take good coughs. In the uncooperative patient, mask continuous positive airway pressure (5 to 15 cm H_2O) will expand the lungs without the patient's help. It should not be used until the patient is wide awake in order to avoid aspiration. Patients with chest wall deformity and/or muscular weakness may be a group in which intermittent positive pressure breathing is helpful. This technique gives the patient a gas volume limited by the peak pressure generated.

Operations for Pain

Operations for pain are done uncommonly and involve surgical interruption of pain pathways. They are usually performed in patients with terminal disease, because the effect of cordotomy diminishes with time. Interruption of the anterolateral tract in the high cervical or thoracic areas requires a laminectomy and general anesthesia, and the previously noted principles of anesthesia for laminectomy apply. After high cervical operations, there may be impairment of respiration and circulation because of the nerve roots involved. Hypotension may occur even after unilateral cordotomy. Cordotomy can also be performed with a percutaneous stereotactic technique that does not require general anesthesia.

Case History

J.R. was a 28-year-old male injured in a motorcycle accident. He had no history of medical problems except a 10-year history of smoking two packs of cigarettes a day. He also drank 6 to 12 cans of beer a day. Admission work-up in the emergency room revealed a sensory level at C6, with weakness of the biceps muscles on motor examination. Spinal films revealed fracture and subluxation (an incomplete dislocation) of the spinal column at C6–C7. Blood pressure was initially 80 systolic with a pulse rate of 60; it rose to 100 systolic with the administration of 1 L normal saline and infusion of phenylephrine at 40 μg/min. The patient's neck was stabilized in the field with a cervical collar and later by the surgeons with a cervical halo. The patient was fully alert with a patent airway. Further work-up was notable for several rib fractures on the left with an underlying infiltrate probably representing a pulmonary contusion. The patient was scheduled for open reduction and internal fixation on the second day after admission because the fracture-dislocation had not been adequately reduced by halo traction.

Suggested Reading

Benumof JL. Anesthesia for thoracic surgery. Philadelphia: WB Saunders, 1987.

Berry FA. The use of a stylet in blind nasotracheal intubation. Anesthesiology 1984; 61:469.

Colice GL. Neurogenic pulmonary edema. Clin Chest Med 1985; 6:473.

Ebert TJ, et al. Fentanyl-diazepam anesthesia with or without N$_2$O does not attenuate cardiopulmonary baroreflex-medicated vasconstrictor responses to controlled hypovolemia in humans. Anesth Analg 1988; 67:548.

Fox DJ, et al. Comparison of intubation techniques on the awake patient: the Flexilum™ surgical light (lightwand) versus blind nasal approach. Anesthesiology 1987; 66:69.

Freedman WA, Grundy BL. Are the sensory evoked potentials useful in the operating room? Monitoring of sensory evoked potentials is highly reliable and helpful in the operating room. J Clin Monit 1987; 3:38.

Gorback MS. Inflation of the endotracheal tube cuff as an aid to blind nasotracheal intubation. Anesth Analg 1987; 66:917.

Grande CM, et al. Appropriate techniques for airway management of emergency patients with suspected spinal cord injury. Anesth Analg 1988; 67:714.

Gronert GA, Theye RA. Pathology of hyperkalemia induced by succinylcholine. Anesthesiology 1975; 43:89.

Kafer ER. Respiratory and cardiovascular functions in scoliosis and the principles of anesthetic management. Anesthesiology 1980; 52:339.

Kallos T, Smith TC. The respiratory effects of Innovar given for premedication. Br J Anaesth 1969; 41:303.

Keenan MA, et al. Acquired laryngeal deviation associated with cervical spine disease in erosive polyarticular arthritis. Anesthesiology 1983; 58:441.

Kobrinsky NL, et al. 1-desamino-8-D-arginine vasopressin (desmopressin) decreases operative blood loss in patients having Harrington Rod surgery. Ann Intern Med 1987; 107:446.

Levy JH. Anaphylactic reactions in anesthesia and intensive care. Boston: Butterworths, 1986.

Mackenzie CF, et al. Assessment of cardiac and respiratory function during surgery on patients with acute quadriplegia. J Neurosurg 1985; 62:843.

Mackenzie CF, Drucker TB. Cervical spinal cord injury. In: Matjasko J, ed. Clinical controversies in neuroanesthesia and neurosurgery. New York: Grune and Stratton, 1986.

Michenfelder JD. Are the sensory evoked potentials useful in the operating room? Intraoperative monitoring of sensory evoked potentials may be neither a proven nor an indicated technique. J Clin Monit 1987; 3:45.

Pathak KS, et al. Effects of halothane, enflurane, and isoflurane on somatosensory evoked potentials during nitrous oxide anesthesia. Anesthesiology 1987; 66:753.

Patil VU, et al. Fiberoptic endoscopy in anesthesia. Chicago: Year Book, 1983.

Schonwald G, et al. Cardiovascular complications during anesthesia in chronic spinal cord injured patients. Anesthesiology 1981; 55:550.

Smith DS. Anesthetic management of patients with spinal cord injury. American Society of Anesthesiologists Annual Refresher Course Lecture 521, 1987.

Sutherland GR, Sibbald WS. Blunt traumatic myocardial injury. Crit Care Clin 1985; 1:663.

Tindal S. Anesthesia for spinal decompression in metastatic disease. Anesth Analg 1987; 66:894.

Woods AM, Lander CJ. Abolition of gagging and the hemodynamic response to awake laryngoscopy. Anesthesiology 1987; 67:220A.

Adrian J. Hobbs, M.B., and Joseph A. Stirt, M.D.

Pediatric Neuroanesthesia   13

Pediatric neuroanesthesia requires the knowledge and skills of two subdisciplines of anesthesia, pediatric anesthesia and neuroanesthesia. Pediatric anatomy, physiology, and pharmacology differ from those in the adult, the differences being most pronounced in neonates.

Anatomic and Physical Differences

Central Nervous System

The brain at birth comprises 10% of total body weight. It doubles in weight within 6 months and triples in weight by 1 year. Twenty-five percent of the adult complement of brain cells are present at birth, and the most rapid growth of axons, dendrites, glial cells, and blood vessels occurs in the first year. The infant cerebral vasculature is fragile with poor supporting structures, especially at the venous end. Thus, surges of arterial pressure or venous obstruction can cause intracerebral hemorrhage, which may extend into the ventricles and cause an intraventricular hemorrhage.

The cranial fontanelles close early in life. The posterior fontanelle closes in the perinatal period, and the anterior fontanelle at 10 to 16 months. However, even prior to closure of the fibrous fontanelles, the cranium is relatively rigid and will not accommodate rapid intracranial expansion without a compromising pressure rise. Slow volume increases are accommodated by expansion of the fontanelles and separation of the suture lines. Palpation of the fontanelles can be used clinically to assess intracranial pressure in infants.

The concept of the cranium as a closed box with a fixed volume is the keystone of neuroanesthesia. An increase in the volume of one of its components must result in the decrease in volume of the other components, a pressure rise, or herniation of the contents through the foramen magnum.

The components of the cranium are neurons and glial tissue (70%), extracellular fluid (ECF) (10%), cerebrospinal fluid (CSF) (10%), and cerebral blood volume (CBV) (10%).

Examples of compartment expansion include neurons and glial tissue— tumors; ECF—edema secondary to tumor, trauma, or hypoxia; CSF—obstructive

Table 13-1 Cerebral Blood Flow and Cerebral Metabolic Rate for Oxygen ($CMRO_2$) in the Infant, Child, and Adult

Patient	Cerebral Blood Flow (ml/100 g/min)	$CMRO_2$ (ml O_2/100 g/min)
Neonate	40	2.3
Child (3–11 yr)	100	5.0
Adult	50	3.0

hydrocephalus, CSF overproduction; and CBV—hypertension, hypoxia, hypercarbia, and some anesthetic agents. The ECF, CSF, and CBV can all be manipulated by the anesthesiologist to counteract volume expansion of the other components.

Cerebrospinal fluid production and circulation commences during the eighth intrauterine week. The choroid plexuses in the temporal horns of the lateral ventricles, the posterior portion of the third ventricle, and the roof of the fourth ventricle are the main sites of production. A small contribution also comes from the meningeal and ependymal vessels of the brain and spinal cord. Neonatal CSF production is approximately 20 ml/hr. The CSF system is a dynamic one. Cerebrospinal fluid flows from the lateral ventricles through the foramina of Munro to the third ventricle, thence along the aqueduct of Sylvius into the fourth ventricle, where it exits via the lateral foramina of Luschka and the midline foramen of Magendie into the cisterna magna and then throughout the cranial and spinal subarachnoid spaces, where it is reabsorbed through the arachnoid villi.

Cerebral blood flow (CBF) varies according to the metabolic demands of the brain. Products of metabolism, including adenosine and hydrogen ions, mediate local flow. Therefore, any global cause of acidosis (hypoxia, ischemia, or hypercarbia) will cause vasodilatation, an increase in cerebral blood flow, and increased CBV.

As in the adult, CBF = CPP/CVR (where CPP = cerebral perfusion pressure and CVR = cerebral vascular resistance) and CPP = MAP − ICP* (where MAP = mean systemic arterial pressure and ICP = intracranial pressure). Maintaining an adequate CPP, especially in the compromised brain, is a guide to having adequate cerebral perfusion.

Cerebral blood flow and cerebral metabolic rate for oxygen ($CMRO_2$) in the infant and pediatric patient vary directly with the number of neurons present (Table 13-1). In the infant the ischemic threshold is lower than in the adult. The electrical threshold is in the range of 15 to 20 ml/100 g/min and structural damage occurs with flows of 10 ml/100 g/min or less.

As in the adult, mental activity increases regional CBF, but does not increase overall CBF and $CMRO_2$. Seizures and hyperthermia increase global CBF and $CMRO_2$.

Hyperthermia increases CBF by 7 to 15%/°C because of the increased neuronal metabolic rate. Treatment should be aimed at hypothalamic suppression of the pyrexia and the avoidance of shivering, which will raise the oxygen requirement of the body as a whole.

Seizures involve widespread neuronal discharge resulting in a raised global cerebral metabolic rate and CBF. If substrate demand cannot be met (more likely with

* Note that when CVP is greater than ICP, CVP is used.

prolonged seizure duration), loss of neuron function occurs. The use of muscle relaxants abolishes clinical signs of seizures but does not reduce the increased $CMRO_2$. In the infant, ictal hypertension may cause an intracerebral hemorrhage.

Autoregulation of CBF occurs over a lower range of blood pressures than in the adult. Extrapolation from animal data suggests the range 30 to 100 mm Hg (see Table 13–2 for systemic blood pressures). Autoregulation is impaired by cerebral hypoxia and ischemia (e.g., birth asphyxia or respiratory distress syndrome), head trauma (associated in children with hyperemia and therefore increased CBV), peritumor brain edema, and volatile anesthetic agents. When impaired, CBF varies with mean arterial pressure. An awake intubation in a vigorous neonate may exceed the limits of blood pressure autoregulation and precipitate a periventricular hemorrhage.

PaCO₂. As in the adult, $PaCO_2$ exerts a profound effect on CBF. Normal term infants have a $PaCO_2$ in the range of 30 to 35 mm Hg, increasing to the adult value of 35 to 45 mm Hg in the first year. As previously discussed, children run a higher CBF than adults. This suggests that the CO_2 response curve is displaced in an upward direction. The CBF changes approximately 2 ml/100 g/min for each 1 mm Hg change in $PaCO_2$. Thus, an increase in $PaCO_2$ from 35 mm Hg to 55 mm Hg will double CBF in the infant, and changes over the physiologic range of 20 to 80 mm Hg may produce a fourfold change. The term neonate will increase his minute ventilation in response to hypercarbia, whereas the preterm infant does not and is therefore at more risk.

PaO₂. The response to PaO_2 varies throughout the first year of life. Fetal PaO_2 is about 30 mm Hg and may fall to as low as 15 mm Hg during birth. Total oxygen carriage is sufficient because of the high perinatal hematocrit, the presence of hemoglobin (Hb)F and the low levels of red cell 2,3-diphosphoglycerate (DPG), which results in a left-displaced oxygen dissociation curve that has a higher oxygen carrying capacity (1.25 times) than HbA at a similar partial pressure. In infants, CBF increases when an oxygen partial pressure of 25 mm Hg is reached. In the older infant (3 to 6 months), CBF increases rapidly when PaO_2 falls below 50 mm Hg. Administering 100% oxygen to a neonate reduces CBF by 33% (a 12% decrease is seen in adults).

Therapeutic Measures to Control ICP

Positioning. A 30-degree head-up tilt with the head and body in line to avoid kinking the jugular veins avoids venous back pressure, reducing the CPP.

Table 13-2 Pediatric Cardiovascular Norms

Age	Heart Rate (beats/min)	Blood Pressure (mm Hg)	
		Systolic	Diastolic
Preterm neonate	120–180	44–60	30
Term neonate	100–180	55–70	35
1 yr	100–140	70–100	60
3 yr	85–115	75–110	70
5 yr	80–100	80–120	70

Fluid Restriction and Dehydration. Following an insult the extracellular fluid compartment expands. Loop diuretics, e.g., furosemide (1 mg/kg) cause initial venodilatation, which reduces CVP, and rapid diuresis. Osmotic diuretics, e.g., mannitol (0.25 to 1.0 g/kg), cause a transient increase in the circulating blood volume and hence increased cerebral blood flow before the diuresis occurs. Repeated osmotic diuretic therapy may cause serum hyperosmolality (320 mOsm/L), which predisposes to renal tubular necrosis.

Drugs. Barbiturates act in a dose-dependent manner by reducing the cerebral metabolic rate ($CMRO_2$), which means a reduced substrate demand and so a reduced CBF, CBV, and hence a reduction in ICP. A bolus dose of sodium pentothal (4 to 6 mg/kg) at induction and smaller bolus doses (1 to 2 mg/kg) during maintenance of anesthesia or in the critical care setting work well to reduce ICP rises during especially stimulating procedures; however, care must be taken in the volume-depleted patient that CPP is not compromised by the coincident blood pressure drop.

     Glucocorticoids reduce focal edema (e.g., around a tumor) and also reduce CSF production. They have no proven use in the management of lesions producing global edema.

Ventilation. Controlling $PaCO_2$ by ventilation allows rapid alteration of CBF and hence CBV. Reducing the CO_2 to 20 mm Hg probably gives the maximum effect. Prolonged hyperventilation (12 hours) allows time for readjustment of the CSF bicarbonate concentration; therefore, moderate hyperventilation ($PaCO_2 = 30$ mm Hg) is used, reserving maximal hyperventilation for critical ICP rises.

Respiratory System

Upper Airway

The following features of the upper airway in infants and children must be considered:

     1. Infants are obligate nose breathers until the age of 6 months. The nasal passages comprise 45% of airway resistance at birth. Secretions and nasogastric tubes significantly increase the work of breathing. The insertion of an oral airway relieves the problem. In the older child, adenoidal tissue may create a similar problem.

     2. The tongue is relatively large and may obstruct the airway. Subluxation of the mandible or insertion of an oral airway may relieve obstruction. A straight-bladed laryngoscope facilitates laryngoscopy.

     3. Milk teeth are shed at 6 to 8 years of age; loose teeth may be dislodged and inhaled.

     4. The epiglottis is often long and floppy and difficult to pick up. The larynx is higher (C4) and more anterior (because of the relatively large tongue) than in adults.

     5. The cricoid ring (the only complete cartilaginous ring of the trachea) is (until puberty) the narrowest point in the trachea. Oversize endotracheal tubes, or poorly fixed tubes that piston up and down the airway, will cause edema, postoperative stridor, and possibly respiratory obstruction. One millimeter of circumferential edema in a neonatal trachea reduces the airway diameter by 60% and increases the resistance eightfold.

     6. The neonatal trachea is 4 cm long, which predisposes to endobronchial intubation. As in adults, this tends to be the right mainstem bronchus; therefore, left axillary auscultation is essential after initial and final positioning of the patient. Indeed, purposeful endobronchial intubation (while continuously auscultating the left axilla)

allows the tube length that results in ablation of breath sounds to be noted and the endotracheal tube to be withdrawn 2 cm so that it lies in the correct position. Remember that flexion or extension of the neck will move the tube down or up the trachea (flexion, down; extension, up), possibly causing endobronchial intubation or extubation. Table 13-3 contains a chart of endotracheal tube sizes and lengths at various ages.

Endotracheal tube size and length can also be calculated using the following formulas:

$$\frac{\text{Age (yr)}}{4} + 4 = \text{internal diameter of tube (mm)}$$

$$\frac{\text{Age (yr)}}{2} + 12 = \text{tube length to teeth}$$

Lower Airway

The following differences in the lower airway of the infant and child must be considered:

1. Neonatal oxygen consumption is approximately 7 ml/kg/min (adult value is 3 ml/kg/min), the tidal volume is 6 ml/kg/min, of which the dead space is 2 ml/kg/min (similar to adult values); however, the rapid respiratory rate (30/min) allows higher alveolar ventilation of approximately 150 ml/kg/min (adult 70 ml/kg/min), but at the cost of an increased work of breathing.

2. The infant lungs are poorly compliant, but the chest wall, air passages, and diaphragm are very compliant; the result is airway closure occurring within normal tidal volume ventilation, i.e., closing volume (CV) approximates functional residual capacity (FRC), and causes a ventilation-perfusion mismatch that predisposes to hypoxemia. This problem is compounded by (a) a supine patient where the abdomen splints the diaphragm (especially if the stomach contains air), (b) a prone patient if the abdomen is not allowed to hang free, and (c) general anesthesia in the spontaneously ventilating patient. The use of a small amount of positive end-expiratory pressure (PEEP) will increase FRC and prevent the CV from encroaching upon it. At about 6 years of age, the CV is exceeded by the FRC. Ideally children younger than this should have controlled respiration. All children with raised ICP and all infants require controlled ventilation.

Table 13-3 Endotracheal Tube Size and Length

Patient Age (yr)	Internal Diameter (mm)	Length to Teeth/Gums (cm)	
		Oral	Nasal
Premature	2.5 to 3.0	10.5	13.5
Neonate	3.5	12	14
1	4.0	13	15
2	4.5	14	16
4	5.0	15	17
6	5.5	17	19
8	6.0	19	21
10	6.5	20	22
12	7.0	21	23

Cardiovascular System

Table 13–2 shows the changes in heart rate and blood pressure with age. The infant cardiac ventricles are relatively noncompliant and so have a fixed stroke volume (approximately 1 ml/kg). A bradycardia is indicative of a low cardiac output, whereas an increased cardiac output requires a tachycardia.

Within the age ranges shown in Table 13–2, the systolic blood pressure trend (provided an excessive dosage of inhalational agents is not being used) is a good guide to the volume status of the infant, as it has a poorly developed baroreceptor response.

Hematology

Table 13–4 shows the change in pediatric blood volume with age.

The hematocrit, 47 to 60 at birth, falls to 28 to 35 at 3 months of age as a result of the cessation of HbF production and its shortened life span. Tissue oxygen delivery may be unchanged because the oxygen dissociation curve shifts to the right as the concentration of HbA and 2,3-DPG rises.

For infants, the hematocrit should be kept above 30, whereas for older children 25 is the lowest acceptable limit. One formula to estimate the allowable blood loss before commencing blood transfusion is:

$$\text{Maximum allowable blood loss} = \frac{(\text{Patient hct} - 30) \times \text{EBV}}{\text{Patient hct}}$$

For blood losses of between 10% of the EBV and the maximum allowable blood loss, a colloid (e.g., 5% albumin) is used to expand the circulation. Likewise, hypotension of possible hypovolemic origin is best managed with a fluid challenge of 10% of the EBV.

Where the blood volume has been replaced, the clotting status and platelet count needs to be ascertained and replacements given as necessary.

Remember:

1. Hypothermia predisposes to coagulopathies.
2. Neonates have a transient platelet dysfunction due to low platelet serotonin.
3. Neonatal vitamin K-dependent factors will be low if vitamin K was not given at birth, predisposing to prolonged surgical bleeding or spontaneous hemorrhage.

Table 13-4 Estimated Blood Volume (EBV) vs. Age

Age	Blood Volume (ml/kg)
Premature	100
Neonate	90
6 wk	80
>2 yr	70

Fluids

Traditional pediatric maintenance fluid requirements are calculated as follows:

1. For the first 10 kg = 100 ml/kg/day (4 ml/kg/hr)
2. For the next 10 kg, add 50 ml/kg/day (2 ml/kg/hr) to the above
3. For weight above 20 kg, add 25 ml/kg/day (1 ml/kg/hr)
4. For example, a 23-kg child requires $(4 \times 10 \text{ kg}) + (2 \times 10 \text{ kg}) + (1 \times 3 \text{ kg}) = 63$ ml/hr.

For neurosurgical procedures use two-thirds of the calculated maintenance requirement and reassess after 1 hour.

If the blood-brain barrier (BBB) is intact (and this is an important assumption when mannitol is used to lower ICP), restricting crystalloid administration will help prevent expansion of the ECF if salt solutions are used, and expansion of the intracellular fluid (ICF) volume if dextrose solutions are infused. In this instance, colloid solutions can be used to provide volume. If the BBB is not intact, then both colloid and crystalloid will extravasate into the ECF and increase ICP.

Neonates and infants often require the infusion of 5% or 10% dextrose solutions to prevent hypoglycemia. When they are used, the plasma glucose level should be monitored to prevent hyperglycemia, which in the ischemic brain is associated with neurologic damage.

Temperature Regulation

Infants and children have twice the surface area/weight ratio of adults. Heat is lost by conduction, convection, radiation, and evaporation. Infants less than 3 months of age do not shiver, but rely on stores of brown fat. Both shivering and brown fat metabolism increase oxygen requirement and may cause hypoxia and metabolic acidosis, thus increasing ICP. General anesthesia, hypoglycemia, intracranial hemorrhage, hypoxia, and prematurity inhibit the metabolic response to cold. Hypothermia also decreases surfactant production, affects coagulation, and prolongs drug action (notably muscle relaxants). However, mild hypothermia reduces cerebral substrate requirement and has been used to good effect, provided controlled rewarming, avoiding shivering, is carried out. The neutral temperature for a term infant is 31°C, an unacceptable long-term working environment.

Methods to prevent hypothermia include:

1. Warm operating room (at least 75°F [24°C])
2. Surgeons ready
3. Warming mattress on the operating table
4. Overhead radiant heater during induction
5. Warmed anesthetic gases (36°C) and intravenous fluids
6. Wrapping noninvolved extremities, trunk, and/or head in heat-reflecting foil
7. Using warmed skin preparation and drapes
8. Warmed wraps at end of surgery
9. Warm incubator for transfer to recovery unit.

Preanesthetic Management

Preoperative Assessment

Throughout the assessment it is important to (1) establish a rapport with the patient and his parents in order to reduce preinduction anxiety not only in the patient but also in the parents, who will subconsciously communicate their anxiety to the child; (2) decide on premedication, if used at all; and (3) decide on the options for a smooth induction of anesthesia (intravenous, inhalational, intramuscular, or rectal).

Take a preoperative history of birth problems, developmental milestones, previous anesthetics, family problems associated with anesthesia, other medical problems (history of asthma, croup, or recent upper respiratory tract infection), allergies, medications, and the status of teeth. Assess whether the patient has or will have a full stomach at induction. The emergency trauma patient must be treated as having a full stomach, and the child with raised ICP may have delayed gastric emptying and also be at risk.

Note the neurologic history, with emphasis on developmental delays, behavior changes, seizures, vomiting, or headaches. The Glasgow Coma Scale (Table 16-1) allows objective reproducible testing.

Make a physical assessment of respiratory and cardiovascular systems, the airway for ease of intubation, and the extremities for vascular access and circulatory volume status (important if vomiting has been severe). An upper respiratory tract infection is a contraindication to nonurgent surgery as increased secretions may cause a stormy induction, with bronchospasm and breath holding, and predispose to postoperative respiratory tract infections.

Perform a neurologic assessment for signs of raised ICP, e.g., tense fontanelles, hydrocephaly, or lassitude in the infant; pupillary, motor, or cognitive deficits in older children. Most important is the change in the level of consciousness over a period of time; the Glasgow Coma Scale provides an easily reproducible scoring system, and over a period of time the trend in the patient's status can be appreciated.

Review the physical (weight and blood pressure) and laboratory work-up. Baseline values of hematocrit, urea and electrolytes, and urinalysis are helpful. Serum and urinary osmolalities provide a good indication of volume status and also indicate the presence of antidiuretic hormone (ADH) secretion or diabetes insipidus. A blood sample for typing and cross-matching is usually required. Further work-up, e.g., clotting studies, depends on the procedure and the patient status.

Review the neurodiagnostic procedures with special reference to possible raised ICP.

Oral Intake

The last milk or solid meal should be at least 6 hours preoperatively. A clear liquid or 5% dextrose drink at 10 ml/kg is allowed 3 hours preoperatively for children under 6 months of age, 4 hours preoperatively for children under 3 years of age.

Premedication

If raised ICP is suspected or proven, a narcotic or sedative premedicant is avoided because of the risk of hypoventilation causing hypercarbia, an increased cerebral blood flow, and hence increased ICP.

An antisialagogue (glycopyrrolate, 10 μg/kg PO or IM, or atropine, 20 μg/kg PO or IM) provides good prolonged action if secretions will be a problem (e.g., the prone patient). Intramuscular injections may cause crying and raise ICP, so should be avoided in those at risk.

If ICP is not a concern, use promethazine (1 mg/kg PO) or chloral hydrate (100 mg/kg PO) for infants; an alternative is diazepam (0.3 mg/kg PO), which provides good sedation in the anxious patient.

Generally, children under 6 months of age will tolerate separation from their parents well; between 6 months and 6 years of age they will usually need either preoperative sedation or the parents present at induction. Older children tend to be more independent, but nevertheless are often very anxious and may benefit from premedication.

Anesthetic Management

Monitoring

Basic monitoring consists of a precordial/esophageal stethoscope, electrocardiography (ECG), noninvasive blood pressure measuring device, temperature probe, and pulse oximeter. Children have a higher oxygen consumption than adults, and hypoxia causes a rise in ICP. An end-tidal CO_2 monitor allows for rapid adjustment of ventilation of normo- or hypocapnic requirements. End-tidal CO_2 is usually 3 to 4 mm Hg lower than arterial carbon dioxide tension.

When air embolism is a risk (any operation where the operative site lies above the heart, and especially if venous sinuses or sinusoids may be opened, e.g., posterior fossa surgery or cranial reconstruction), a precordial Doppler and an end-tidal CO_2 monitor are indicated. The precordial Doppler is an extremely sensitive and early indicator of air embolism, detecting even small bubbles present in injected drugs. The end-tidal CO_2 monitor will detect significant air embolism by a sudden reduction in its reading due to ventilation of nonperfused lung zones. Remember the possible risk of a patent foramen ovale leading to arterial air embolization, with disastrous results if the bubble rests in the cerebral or coronary circulation.

Once detected, the response to air entrainment must be rapid:

1. Tell the surgeon, who will either flood the wound with saline or pack it with wet swabs.
2. Administer 100% oxygen to prevent nitrous oxide from enlarging existing bubbles.
3. Lower the head of the table and/or compress the neck veins to reduce the wound-atrium gradient and prevent further entrainment. The application of PEEP will have a similar effect but may lower an already low blood pressure.
4. If a right atrial catheter is in situ, attempt air aspiration through it.
5. If possible, a left lateral position will hold air in the right atrium and aid air aspiration.
6. Institute resuscitative measures as required, remembering that a pulmonary artery air lock may be difficult to disperse, necessitating prolonged resuscitation.
7. Depending on the extent of air embolism, avoid the reintroduction of nitrous oxide, and continue the anesthetic with a volatile agent.

Direct blood pressure monitoring is useful when blood loss or centrally mediated blood pressure disturbances are likely. In the newborn, umbilical artery catheterization may be used; otherwise, a 24-gauge catheter can usually be placed in the radial, dorsalis pedis, or posterial tibial artery of small infants, or a 22-gauge femoral line can be inserted. In older children, a 22-gauge or 20-gauge catheter is placed peripherally as mentioned above.

Central venous pressure monitoring is indicated if large blood loss or air embolism is expected. The percutaneous approach to the internal jugular, subclavian, or femoral veins can be used. If raised ICP is a consideration, the internal jugular is avoided to prevent compromising cerebral venous runoff.

Urinary catheterization is necessary for prolonged procedures, when diuretics will be used, or when large volume shifts are anticipated.

A nerve stimulator is useful for long procedures in order to produce a stable degree of neuromuscular blockade, to ascertain that reversal is possible at the end of the procedure, and to document adequate reversal in the patient who is slow to wake up.

Positioning

As for any surgical procedure, general patient protection measures must be carried out. The eyes must be securely taped closed or the lids sewn shut (tarsorrhaphy), and the pressure points must be adequately padded. Once the patient is positioned, especially when prone, the face should be inspected visually for pressure points, the lung fields checked for bilateral air entry, and the endotracheal tube secured. The endotracheal tube should be taped to the side of the mouth that is uppermost to keep secretions from loosening the tape. A generous amount of benzoin is applied to the skin to provide good fixation. Remember that it is the total skin-tape and tape-tube interface that is important and not layering the tape upon itself.

Ten degrees of head-up tilt aids venous runoff and helps lower ICP, but it also predisposes to venous air entrainment. Rotation of the head to one side may kink the jugular veins and reduce venous runoff; instead, rotate the whole body.

Severe neck flexion for posterior surgery may kink or dislodge the endotracheal tube. RAE tubes are preformed and less likely to be dislodged; spiral reinforced endotracheal tubes are better still, but have a thicker wall section, often necessitating the use of a smaller tube.

The sitting position is often used for posterior fossa surgery in older children. As mentioned above, the risk of air entrainment is high because of the gradient between the operative site and the right atrium and the large number of venous sinusoids that the surgeon will cut through. A quoted incidence of air embolism of 30% in these patients speaks for the use of a non–nitrous oxide technique.

The prone position is frequently used for young children. Endotracheal tube fixation as described above is of paramount importance, and an antisialagogue is advisable to reduce secretions.

Induction

Important considerations for anesthetic induction are:

1. Does the patient have raised ICP?
2. Does the patient have a full stomach?
3. How old is the patient? Will he cooperate?

The aim is for smooth induction of anesthesia without crying, struggling, breath holding, or other events that will raise ICP, at the same time allowing rapid control of the airway.

Induction Methods

Intravenous Induction.   The method of choice, provided venous access is possible, is intravenous induction. Eutectic local anesthetic mixtures can make venipuncture painless (they take 1 hour to work), and in the drowsy child little distraction is needed. Remember that restlessness may be caused by hypoxia in the acutely ill patient. For the combative child it must be decided whether the rapid insertion of an intravenous cannula and a fast intravenous induction will raise the ICP more than a gaseous induction with the attendant risks of coughing, breath holding, and laryngospasm, and also the propensity that all volatile agents have for raising ICP, thus necessitating early assistance of ventilation.

For the acute trauma case with a head injury, a full stomach must be assumed and a rapid-sequence induction is indicated in the pediatric patient, with initial preoxygenation followed by cricoid pressure as the induction agents (lidocaine 1.5 mg/kg, thiopental 4 to 6 mg/kg, and succinylcholine 1.5 mg/kg for neuromuscular blockade) are being given. Once intubation and verification of proper endotracheal tube placement has been performed, cricoid pressure is released and hyperventilation instituted as required. Succinylcholine does cause raised ICP secondary to increased cerebral metabolic rate. This effect can be blocked by pretreatment with a small dose of nondepolarizing neuromuscular blocking agent, or in the elective patient whose airway has been assessed as normal, by avoiding succinylcholine and using a nondepolarizing agent with controlled mask hyperventilation prior to intubation.

Inhalation Induction.   Inhalation is an acceptable method of induction provided that raised ICP is not a concern. This is a useful method, as induction can be performed with the child feeling secure cradled in the parent's arms. This is the method of choice for all children with upper airway anomalies, because it allows laryngoscopy, assessment of the airway, and intubation before the patient is paralyzed.

Rectal Induction.   Methohexital (30 mg/kg) with the patient sitting on the parent's lap provides a smooth, if longer (5 to 10 minutes) induction phase in small children. It is important to monitor the child carefully for airway obstruction or hypoventilation.

Intramuscular Induction.   Ketamine in the dose range of 3 to 10 mg/kg provides sedation up to dissociative anesthesia at the higher dose range. It is contraindicated if raised ICP is suspected, because it causes increased cerebral blood flow and raised intracranial pressure. Ketamine abolishes airway reflexes, so the airway must be closely observed. Methohexital 10 mg/kg IM can also be used for the uncooperative child.

Muscle Relaxants

Depolarizing muscle relaxants cause a transient rise in ICP that can be blocked by pretreatment with a nondepolarizing neuromuscular blocking agent. Nevertheless, nondepolarizing agents are preferred.

The characteristics of nondepolarizing agents are as follows:

1. Pancuronium (0.1 mg/kg) causes vagolysis and sympathetic stimulation, properties that are unwanted in the elective case but have a place in the trauma victim.

2. Metocurine (0.3 mg/kg) has a weak ganglion-blocking and histamine-releasing action; except in the atopic individual, these effects cause little or no disturbance to the pediatric cardiovascular system.

3. Tubocurarine (0.6 mg/kg) is a more powerful ganglion-blocking agent and also releases histamine. It also has little hemodynamic effect in the pediatric patient, but ganglion blockade may raise intracranial blood volume and histamine release may increase cerebral blood flow.

4. The two intermediate-duration agents, atracurium and vecuronium, are suitable for either an intermittent bolus technique or use as an infusion that allows a stable level of neuromuscular blockade to be attained and monitored with a nerve stimulator. Vecuronium has almost no cardiovascular side effects, whereas atracurium in intubating doses may cause histamine release and a mild, transient fall in blood pressure. This may be minimized by administration in divided doses over several minutes.

Maintenance

Maintenance usually consists of nitrous oxide, oxygen, and a small increment of isoflurane to achieve MAC anesthesia. Isoflurane is the volatile agent of choice because of its minimal effect on ICP when hyperventilation is established. When air embolism is a risk, an air/oxygen/isoflurane technique is used. An initial bolus of a short-acting narcotic agent (fentanyl) or intermittent doses of the ultra-short-acting alfentanil are given to cover the stress of intubation, skin incision, and raising the periosteum. Increments of the induction agent can also be used to ameliorate the surgical stress response. Once the cranium is open and the dura incised, the anesthetic requirement drops as the brain itself has no sensory innervation. Nitrous oxide, oxygen, and a small amount of isoflurane provide adequate anesthesia.

For operations on or near the brain stem, the ECG and blood pressure need careful monitoring for surgically induced disturbances. Treatment is cessation of the surgical stimulus.

Controlled Hypotension

An improvement in the surgical field can often be produced by correct patient positioning, improving venous runoff. When arterial pressure needs to be reduced to decrease wall tension in arteriovenous malformations or to reduce arterial spurting in major craniofacial reconstruction, controlled hypotension has a place. The volatile anesthetic agents, ganglion blockers (trimethaphan, pentolinium), alpha-blockers (phentolamine), or vasodilators (nitroglycerin, sodium nitroprusside, hydralazine) have all been used. However, they all raise ICP and so are contraindicated in patients with raised ICP until the dura is open. Reflex tachycardia is frequently a problem, necessitating the addition of a beta-blocker, but also allowing reduced dosage of the hypotensive agent.

Severe Hemodilution

Severe hemodilution is accepted as being a hematocrit of 20% at the end of a procedure. Oxygen transport is maintained by improved flow characteristics and elevated cardiac output and aided by the reduced oxygen requirement of the anesthetized patient. An arterial cannula is essential to allow frequent hematocrit and acid-base estimation.

Reversal of Anesthesia

The objective of anesthesia reversal is an awake, responsive, pain-free, normocarbic, nonhypoxic patient whose neurologic status can be easily monitored in the recovery ward.

Volatile agents need to be discontinued sufficiently early to allow elimination. Tracheal and oropharyngeal toilet is performed prior to reversing the neuromuscular blockade in order to avoid coughing and straining on the endotracheal tube. Lidocaine (0.5 mg/kg IV) just prior to reversal has an antitussive effect. A nerve stimulator indicates the ability to reverse the blockade and documents adequate reversal. Once blockade is reversed, the patient is placed in a sitting position as cardiovascular parameters allow and taken to the recovery room breathing supplemental oxygen. There, a full neurologic assessment is performed, and the patient is observed for any deterioration in vital or neurologic signs.

If ICP is still elevated at the end of surgery, or postoperative edema is expected, the insertion of an ICP bolt and a postoperative period of elective ventilation allows for stabilization. Any rise in ICP can be treated with hyperventilation, small doses of induction agents (while ensuring that cerebral perfusion pressure does not fall), and diuretics. Background sedation can be provided by narcotic and benzodiazepine infusions with small boluses being given prior to stimulating nursing procedures.

Other methods of assessing neurologic changes include serial computed tomographic (CT) scans, electroencephalography and evoked potentials, and ultrasonography in the infant with open fontanelles.

Specific Considerations

Head Trauma

Head trauma is a leading cause of pediatric mortality. The primary event cannot be reversed, but secondary damage can be prevented or minimized by prompt action. Pediatric outcomes are better than those for adults who present with the same neurologic state. Children respond to head trauma with intracranial hypertension and increased cerebral blood flow, this hyperemia causing diffuse cerebral edema and petechial subarachnoid hemorrhages. A surgically drainable lesion is less common than in adults but must be suspected if focal neurologic signs develop. Although not as specific as in adults, the Glasgow Coma Scale allows repeated neurologic assessments to be compared along with changes in pupil size, pulse rate, respiratory rate, and blood pressure. Unless the patient is rapidly awakening, an aggressive regimen is necessary to optimize outcome.

If the child is comatose or semicomatose, institute the following measures:

1. Check the airway. Is it patent, unobstructed by soft tissues (e.g., tongue), blood, mucus, or vomit? Is the patient protecting the airway?
2. Check breathing. Is the patient breathing adequately? Has aspiration occurred? Is the patient hypoxic? Give supplemental oxygen.
3. Check circulation. Assess capillary refill and palpate the peripheral pulses. An absent radial, ulnar, dorsalis pedis, or posterior tibial pulse indicates a 5% loss of blood volume; an absent brachial artery pulse suggests a 10% blood volume loss; and absent femoral or axillary pulses

mean a loss in excess of 15% of the blood volume.
4. Assess the neurologic state using the Glasgow Coma Scale, examination of the cranial nerves, and lateralizing or localizing signs.
5. Look for coincident injuries (see Table 13-5).

Intubate before proceeding to further diagnostic work-up (e.g., CT scan). To avoid the ICP rise associated with an awake intubation, a rapid-sequence induction is performed with full precautions for a full stomach (food or swallowed blood) as follows:

1. Establish venous access.
2. Preoxygenate.
3. Apply cricoid pressure.
4. Give lidocaine (1.5 mg/kg IV) to obtund the pressor effect of laryngoscopy. Give atropine (10 μg/kg IV) to prevent succinylcholine-induced bradycardias.
5. Give pentothal in an adequate dose (depending on circulatory status), rapidly followed by succinylcholine (1 mg/kg).
6. Intubate orally, check bilateral breath sounds prior to removing cricoid pressure. Do not intubate nasally because of the risk of a basal skull fracture.
7. Use pancuronium, atracurium, or vecuronium by intermittent dosing or infusion for maintenance of neuromuscular blockade. Hyperventilate as required to reduce ICP. Consider using diuretics (furosemide or mannitol) to reduce the intracranial volume. Sedate with fentanyl and remember that hypertension may be due to a rising ICP or an "awake" patient. Persistent hypotension suggests bleeding from an extracranial source.
8. Reassess the circulatory and neurologic status, and establish further monitors as required (e.g., arterial catheter).
9. Once the patient is stable, perform diagnostic tests or proceed to the

Table 13-5 Common Coincident Injuries with Head Trauma

Injuries to Suspect	Signs/Management
Skeletal Injuries	
Cervical spine	If in doubt, assume a fracture until proved otherwise
	Intubate with an assistant holding the head to prevent flexion or extension
Ribs	Check for pneumo- or hemothorax
	Look for paradoxical movement
Pelvis, long bones	Cause considerable blood loss
Abdominal soft tissue trauma	If suspected, do paracentesis and lavage for free blood
Lung	Usually a delayed deterioration in function

operating room for intracranial bolt or craniotomy. Maintenance anesthesia for a CT scan can be provided with fentanyl and thiopental increments or short-acting benzodiazepines. Avoid nitrous oxide until air in the cranial cavity has been excluded. In 50% of cases, the CT scan shows slit-like ventricles, indicating diffuse cerebral edema. An ICP monitoring device and direct arterial and central venous pressure monitoring enable prompt action to be taken to keep CPP within acceptable limits.

Intracranial Tumors

Posterior fossa tumors are more common than supratentorial neoplasms in the pediatric population. Considerations for both include the following:

1. Give no sedative premedication if raised ICP is suspected. For antisialagogue purposes, intramuscular or oral glycopyrrolate may be given.
2. Gastric emptying may be delayed if ICP is increased; therefore, allow adequate preoperative fasting and use a modified rapid-sequence induction if the airway is normal. This consists of the following steps:
   a. Establish intravenous access, and apply monitoring as tolerated.
   b. Preoxygenate if possible.
   c. Induce anesthesia with thiopental, fentanyl, and a nondepolarizing muscle relaxant, while an assistant applies cricoid pressure.
   d. Immediately institute hyperventilation with a bag and mask using high gas flows to attain hypocarbia.
   e. When complete neuromuscular relaxation has occurred, intubate, check bilateral ventilation, release cricoid pressure, and hyperventilate to an end-tidal CO_2 of 25 to 30 mm Hg. Add small increments of isoflurane to control blood pressure.
   f. Establish further monitoring as required, depending on the magnitude of the operation and expected blood loss.
   g. Position the patient as previously described.
3. In addition, for posterior fossa tumors, consider the following:
   a. Position the patient in sitting or prone position. Watch for endotracheal tube kinking, and ensure secure tube fixation. In the prone position, ensure that the abdomen hangs free and that ventilation and venous return is uncompromised.
   b. Establish monitoring to detect air embolism, and consider using a "no nitrous" technique consisting of air, oxygen, isoflurane, and narcotics.
   c. Watch for brady- or tachyarrhythmias, nodal rhythm, and ectopic beats during surgical manipulation in the region of the fourth ventricle. Cessation of surgical stimulation or atropine is usually the only required treatment.
   d. At the end of surgery in the vicinity of the fourth ventricle, assess the protective airway reflexes and the respiratory drive carefully before extubation.

Neural Tube Defects

Neural tube defects result from failure of the neural tube to close and may affect the spine (meningomyelocele, incidence 1 to 4 per 1,000 births) or the cranium encephalocele, incidence 1 per 5,000 births). The measurement of maternal serum alpha-fetoprotein early in pregnancy detects severe neural tube defects. Eighty percent of meningomyeloceles occur in the lumbosacral region. Neurologic function below the lesion is usually compromised. The covering sac may rupture at birth with a subsequent high risk of infection. The defect is often closed within 24 to 36 hours of birth to reduce the risk of infection.

Anesthetic Considerations in the Neonate. Clotting and heat loss are the primary considerations in the neonate. To avoid clotting, check that vitamin K has been given. To minimize heat loss, warm the operating room and the anesthetic gases, lay the baby on a warming pad, and use an overhead radiant heater during induction. When the baby is turned prone for surgery, place the chest supports under the heating pad to ensure the largest patient-pad interface. Warm all fluids to be given.

Anesthetic Considerations of the Lesion. Ensure that the lesion remains covered with sterile dressings. Intubate the baby awake, either positioned supine with the lesion lying protected in a head ring, or lying in a left lateral position if the lesion is too large. The baby is preoxygenated and given atropine; an assistant holds the shoulders back with the heels of both hands and with the fingertips holds the head forward to prevent the baby extending the head. Once the airway is secure, induction of anesthesia is aided with a small dose of thiopental; ventilation is controlled; and nitrous oxide, oxygen, and a volatile agent are used to maintain anesthesia. Muscle relaxants are avoided if the surgeon proposes using a nerve stimulator to locate nerve roots.

Anesthetic Considerations of the Operation. Since the patient is positioned prone, the eyes must be protected. The endotracheal tube is checked for position and security and the abdomen allowed to hang freely. Blood loss may be considerable as the surgeon raises skin flaps to cover the defect. Therefore, good venous access and available cross-matched blood are essential.

Other Anesthetic Considerations. An encephalocele usually arises in the occipital region. The anesthetic considerations are those listed above. Special care must be taken to avoid compression of the lesion. The patient often has an associated abnormality such as Klippel-Feil syndrome (short webbed neck and fused cervical vertebrae), micrognathia, or cleft palate, all of which make intubation more difficult. Air embolism is a risk as the suboccipital venous plexuses are broached. Encephaloceles arising in the parietal, frontal, or nasal region usually present no specific anesthetic problem, although the latter may cause upper airway obstruction in the obligate nose breather, which can be relieved with an oral airway.

Eighty percent of these children develop hydrocephalus with the Arnold-Chiari malformation (downward displacement of the pons, medulla, and cerebellar vermis through the foramen magnum) and aqueductal stenosis. Stridor or laryngeal incompetence and aspiration may occur as a result of vagus nerve entrapment and traction. This necessitates prompt intubation and a relieving shunt operation or in some cases an occipital craniectomy to decompress the brain stem.

Hydrocephalus

Shunt insertion for hydrocephalus is the most common neonatal neurosurgical procedure. Hydrocephalus results from an abnormal accumulation of cerebrospinal fluid (CSF) and is caused by an excessive production or decreased uptake of CSF (communicating hydrocephalus), or most commonly, a blocked fluid pathway proximal to the subarachnoid space (noncommunicating hydrocephalus), as is seen in aqueductal stenosis (the aqueduct runs from the third to the fourth ventricle) and Arnold-Chiari malformation.

The incidence of hydrocephalus is 3 per 1,000 births and is usually secondary to meningomyelocele. The excess CSF causes ventricular dilatation, pressure destruction of surrounding neural tissue, and progressive enlargement of the cranium. Early signs include apnea, bradycardia, vomiting, and increasing head circumference. Late signs include bulging fontanelle, "setting sun" eyes (sixth cranial nerve palsy), and limb spasticity. A CT scan will confirm the diagnosis.

Current surgical treatment for noncommunicating hydrocephalus consists of the insertion of a ventriculoperitoneal shunt incorporating a low-pressure Spitz-Holter type valve. The CSF is reabsorbed through the peritoneum. Ventriculoatrial and ventriculopleural shunts are less popular because of the risk of infection and microemboli in the former and hydrothorax in the latter. For communicating hydrocephalus, a lumboperitoneal shunt can be established between the lumbar subarachnoid space and the peritoneal space.

Anesthetic considerations include raised ICP and a possible full stomach. A rapid, smooth induction avoiding hypoventilation, hypoxia, and hypertension is required. No premedication is given. A modified rapid-sequence intravenous induction consisting of atropine, thiopental, a nondepolarizing muscle relaxant, and cricoid pressure allows the immediate instigation of hyperventilation with a mask using high gas flows, while protecting against possible regurgitation. Once the airway is secure, hyperventilation is continued until the ventricles are decompressed.

Maintenance consists of nitrous oxide in oxygen and increments of pentothal if required until the ICP is reduced, at which stage isoflurane can be added. Sudden removal of a large volume of CSF may cause bradycardia and hypotension; rapid replacement with saline and a gradual release of fluid will prevent this. Heat loss can be considerable because of the wide surgical exposure needed from cranium to abdomen. Narcotic agents are avoided to enable rapid neurologic assessment on awakening. Intramuscular codeine phosphate provides adequate analgesia.

Patients who present with blocked shunts requiring revision require the same management as indicated above. If the blockage is distal to the shunt reservoir, this can be tapped preoperatively to reduce ICP. Shunts need to be revised several times during childhood to allow for growth.

Craniosynostosis

Craniosynostosis encompasses a spectrum of conditions ranging from premature fusion of a single suture (usually the sagittal) that is divided for cosmetic reasons to premature fusion of multiple suture lines. The latter are frequently associated with other congenital malformations (Apert's, Chotzen's, Crouzon's, and Noack's syndromes), but with the exception of Apert's syndrome, mental function may be normal.

Although the surgical procedure is extradural, blood loss is often large and difficult to estimate. For a single-suture synostosis, a single strip craniectomy is performed at about 3 months of age or when the child first presents. Since the ICP is not raised, the patient can be premedicated with a sedative premedicant and anesthesia induced by intravenous, inhalational, rectal, or intramuscular means. Good venous access must be secured and blood available, and blood pressure may be measured noninvasively. A light general anesthetic is usually sufficient, and the patient is extubated at the end of the procedure. Blood loss often continues in the postoperative period.

The anesthetic implications of multiple-suture synostoses or cranial reconstruction are far greater. These patients need careful preoperative assessment to detect raised ICP and airway abnormalities and thus a possible difficult intubation.

If ICP is raised, the induction of choice is an intravenous induction followed by assessment of ventilation using a bag and mask. If ventilation is easy, a nondepolarizing muscle relaxant can be given, hyperventilation performed by mask, and anesthesia deepened prior to intubation. If the airway is difficult to maintain, an inhalation induction is employed, and laryngoscopy is performed with deep halothane or isoflurane. Isoflurane is the preferred agent since it causes a smaller rise in ICP, but its pungent odor necessitates a slow induction and gradual deepening of anesthesia to avoid breathholding and coughing.

After initial orotracheal intubation, it is wise to change to an armored nasotracheal tube that can be sutured in place and provide a patent airway despite extremes of head movement. An additional venous line, an arterial catheter for direct reading of blood pressure and measurement of blood gases and hematocrit, a central venous pressure line (consider a femoral insertion if ICP is raised) to follow central blood volume changes, a urinary catheter, a temperature probe, precordial Doppler, and end-tidal CO_2 monitor complete the anesthetic preparation. A tarsorrhaphy is often necessary to protect the eyes. The patient is positioned prone and the usual post-positioning checks performed.

The surgical procedure consists of either multiple strip craniectomies or cranial vault removal and remodeling. Blood loss is usually considerable but rarely precipitates, and attempting to stay 10% ahead of the estimated blood loss allows for a margin of error. A head-up tilt and moderate hypotension helps reduce blood loss, but predisposes to venous air embolism. Normovolemic hemodilution techniques have been used to limit the total volume of blood infused and require careful frequent measurement of hematocrit, blood gases, and urine output to ensure that the oxygenation remains adequate. A mixed venous blood gas determination indicates the overall adequacy of oxygenation but does not indicate regional hypoperfusion. At the end of surgery the hematocrit is transfused up to 25%, and diuretics are given to aid excretion of excess crystalloid. These patients are electively ventilated postoperatively for 24 to 48 hours to allow fluid shifts to normalize, ICP to be controlled, and upper airway edema to resolve.

Intracranial Vascular Malformations

Infants may present with high-output cardiac failure secondary to an aneurysmal dilation of the vein of Galen. Initial therapy is aimed at controlling the cardiac failure. Surgical intervention consists of ligating or clipping the aberrant pathways. Blood loss may be sudden and catastrophic, so good venous access and full invasive monitoring is necessary. Cardiac failure may suddenly worsen on ligation of the feeding arteries.

Arteriovenous malformations may present in older children with an intracranial bleed. Because of the high incidence of rebleeding, arteriovenous malformations are resected if possible. Cerebral aneurysms may also present with bleeding in the older child. Anesthetic management for both these conditions is the same as for adults: a heavy sedative premedication, smooth induction of anesthesia with intubation when deep, full invasive monitoring, and hypotensive techniques as required.

Spinal Procedures

As in adults, spinal cord tumors can present at any site. A tethered cord presents with bladder or bowel dysfunction or lower limb weakness. A CT scan usually confirms the diagnosis. Anesthetic considerations are those of the prone position and include the avoidance of muscle relaxants if the surgeon is using a nerve stimulator.

Case History

Patient History, Physical Examination, Routine Laboratory Evaluation

A term baby, delivered by cesarean section after failure to progress in labor, was found on initial examination to have a 5-cm diameter lumbar meningomyelocele with intact sac. The Apgar scores were 7 and 9 at 1 and 5 minutes. The baby weighed 3.4 kg.

Neurologic testing was performed by observing the response to pinprick over the lower limbs: an intact neural pathway produces limb movement and central arousal and crying. Movement without arousal may be due to spinal reflexes. Denervated limbs are flaccid. Spontaneous voiding of reasonable volumes of urine suggests intact bladder innervation, whereas dribbling is indicative of denervation. Some normal infants do not pass urine in the first 12 hours. A non-patulous anus with an intact anal reflex indicates innervation. Formal testing revealed a low lesion, and a decision was made to close the defect to prevent further neurologic damage and infection.

The family history was unremarkable for anesthetic problems, serious medical illnesses, or allergies. Antenatal check-ups were poorly attended (neural tube defects can be detected by raised maternal serum alpha-fetoprotein levels or seen on ultrasound scan). The mother was well following the cesarean section and willing to donate a unit of fresh blood for the infant.

Examination revealed an awake, nonirritable term infant lying prone with a lumbar meningomyelocele. The intact sac was permeable to CSF, but fluid loss was decreasing as the membrane dried. The skin turgor was normal, the capillary refill brisk, the radial pulse easily palpable, and the anterior fontanelle neither bulging nor slack. Examination of the cardiovascular and respiratory systems was unremarkable.

A blood sample had been taken for determination of hematocrit (54%) and blood glucose level and for cross-match. The baby was currently receiving no medication, but vitamin K (1 mg IM) was given at birth. A 22-gauge cannula was sited on the dorsum of the hand, and 10% dextrose running at 2 ml/kg/hr was administered to maintain blood glucose and hydration. No premedication was ordered.

Anesthetic Management

The basic anesthetic principles for a neonate apply; therefore, the operating room is warmed to 78°F (25.5°C), a warming mattress placed on the operating table, and an overhead radiant heater obtained. The anesthetic machine, equipment, and drugs are checked and readied. The breathing circuit (with incorporated heater-humidifier) with which the anesthesiologist is most proficient is chosen. The Ayre's T-piece with Jackson-Rees modification or the semiclosed circle system with pediatric tubing are suitable, as breathing will be controlled. A neonatal straight-bladed (Miller) laryngoscope is most suitable for intubation. An awake intubation is being planned in order to secure the airway before the start of anesthesia and to avoid any problems with a difficult airway. Cardiovascular studies (albeit imperfect) on neonates suggest that a profound hypertensive response to awake intubation is not present in the first few days of life, but is a reality at 4 weeks of age. Experienced pediatric anesthesiologists may proceed with an inhalational or intravenous induction after careful evaluation of the airway to ensure that respiration can be controlled manually with a mask.

When preparations are complete, the baby is placed in the left lateral position on the operating table, and a precordial stethoscope, ECG, oximeter probe, and noninvasive blood pressure measuring device applied. If the defect is small enough, the baby can be placed supine with the sac protected by a foam ring. Intravenous access is secured or, if already present, checked for patency, and atropine (10 μg/kg IV) is given.

While the infant is preoxygenated, an assistant facing the head of the table grasps the shoulders in the palms of the hands and, with fingers applied to both sides of the head, flexes the cervical spine and extends the head at the atlanto-occipital joint. To obtain the best conditions for intubation it is important to prevent the baby from extending the cervical spine during laryngoscopy. Following 2 minutes of preoxygenation, laryngoscopy is performed in the usual fashion, the epiglottis being picked up if it is long or else the laryngoscope tip placed in the vallecula if it is short. The vocal cords will be seen to move with respiration, and intubation is timed to coincide with inspiration and abduction of the cords. Failure to wait for inspiration may cause vocal cord trauma. A small amount of cricoid pressure by a second assistant may improve the view at laryngoscopy by moving the larynx more posteriorly.

Once the patient is intubated, bilateral breath sounds are auscultated for in both axillae, and anesthesia induced with nitrous oxide, oxygen, and isoflurane, administered with assisted ventilation. The endotracheal tube is then secured, an esophageal stethoscope is passed, and once anesthetized, the baby is turned prone for surgery, with breath sounds rechecked when the patient is finally positioned.

Anesthesia is maintained with nitrous oxide, oxygen, and isoflurane. If the surgeon wishes to use a nerve stimulator to locate nerves, muscle relaxants are contraindicated; otherwise, atracurium (0.3 mg/kg) can be given and its effect monitored with a nerve stimulator. The use of a muscle relaxant will allow a reduced concentration of volatile agent and hence a lighter, more rapidly reversible anesthesia.

Maintenance fluid consisting of 10% dextrose is continued at 2 ml/kg/hr. Fluid loss secondary to the operation is given as lactated Ringer's solution and run at between 2 and 10 ml/kg/hr depending on the size of the surgical incision and consequent fluid loss.

The surgical raising of skin flaps to cover the defect may involve a relatively large blood loss. The weighing of swabs and the use of microburettes in the suction bottles give a conservative indication of blood loss. Clinically, the blood pressure and capillary refill time indicate blood loss fairly accurately. For this neonate with an estimated blood volume (EBV) of 90 ml/kg $\times$ 3.4 kg = 306 ml, we have a maximum acceptable blood loss (ABL) of:

$$ABL = \frac{(\text{Initial hct} - \text{Minimum hct}) \times EBV}{\text{Initial hct}}$$
$$= \frac{(54 - 40) \times 306}{54}$$
$$= 79 \text{ ml}$$

At one-third of this loss, colloid should be considered as the replacement fluid. Beyond this amount, blood, either maternal or freshly cross-matched, is given to replace losses.

At the conclusion of surgery, anesthesia is discontinued, muscle relaxants are antagonized, and the trachea is extubated when the patient is awake and breathing well in the left lateral position.

Postoperative Management

Postoperatively, the hematocrit, electrolytes, and blood glucose are measured and corrected if necessary. The patient is initially nursed in the prone position to reduce the risk of dural leak. Head circumference is measured daily, with a rapid increase in size suggesting the development of hydrocephalus (80% of these patients develop hydrocephaly). A CT scan will confirm the diagnosis. Lethargy, irritability, bradycardia, stridor, and "setting sun" eyes all indicate advanced raised ICP.

Surgical management of raised ICP usually consists of the insertion of a ventriculoperitoneal shunt. The anesthetic management is now that of a 10-day-old baby with raised ICP. Once again the patient is assessed preoperatively, attention especially being paid to signs of raised ICP, to the state of hydration, and to the respiratory system for signs of aspiration secondary to pharyngeal-laryngeal incoordination. The previous anesthetic chart is read and the patient's postoperative progress noted. The hematocrit, electrolytes, and blood glucose are checked; no premedication is ordered; and a preoperative fasting period of 3 hours is allowed if the baby has been well enough to take oral feeds.

The operating room and anesthetic equipment are prepared as before, heat-conserving measures again being important in view of the large surgical exposure needed from head to abdomen. An intravenous technique has been selected to provide a smooth induction of anesthesia, with rapid control of ventilation to produce hypocapnia and reduce ICP. The baby is placed on the warmed operating table and comforted to prevent crying, routine monitoring is begun, and intravenous access secured. Induction then follows with intravenous thiopental (2 to 4 mg/kg) and atracurium (0.5 mg/kg). If bradycardia is a problem, atropine (20 μg/kg IV) is given.

Hyperventilation is begun immediately with a mask and bag, using oxygen and small increments of isoflurane. Once relaxation has occurred, the patient is intubated, bilateral breath sounds confirmed, nitrous oxide/oxygen/isoflurane anesthesia commenced, and the endotracheal tube securely fixed, because the head will be extended and rotated by the surgeon. Ventilation is controlled to an end-tidal P_{CO_2} of 30 mm Hg. Rapid removal of CSF may cause a bradycardia or arrhythmia secondary to upward brainstem movement. Treatment is symptomatic, with reinfusion of CSF or saline and its subsequent slow removal. Once surgery is complete, anesthesia is reversed and the trachea again extubated with the child awake.

Suggested Reading

Cucchiara RF, et al. Air embolism in children undergoing suboccipital craniotomy. Anesthesiology 1982; 57:338.

McLeod ME, et al. Anaesthetic management of arteriovenous malformations of the vein of Galen. Can Anaesth Soc J 1982; 29:307.

McLeod ME, et al. Anaesthesia for cerebral arteriovenous malformations in children. Can Anaesth Soc J 1982; 29:299.

Single RC. Special techniques: deliberate hypertension, hypothermia and acute normovolemic hemodilution. In: Gregory GA, ed. Pediatric anesthesia. New York: Churchill Livingstone, 1983:553.

Swedlow MD. Anesthesia for surgical procedures. In: Gregory GA, ed. Pediatric anesthesia. New York: Churchill Livingstone, 1983:679.

Hilary A. Noble, B.M., F.F.A.R.C.S.

Anesthesia for Neuroradiology and Specialized Procedures 14

Radiology has played an important part in the diagnosis of neurologic and neurosurgical conditions since its introduction in the 19th century:

1918—Dandy injected air into the lateral ventricles of the brain to visualize their shape, size, and communications (ventriculography).

1919—Dandy injected air into the spinal subarachnoid space (pneumoencephalography).

1922—Sicard and Forestier injected a radiopaque substance into the spinal subarachnoid space (myelography).

1927—Moniz injected sodium iodide directly into the carotid artery to display the cerebral vasculature (angiography).

1973—First computed tomographic (CT) brain scanning units were introduced in the United States.

1980—Nuclear magnetic resonance units (NMR or MRI) were introduced.

1980—Digital subtraction angiography (DSA) was developed.

1986—Gamma knife was introduced.

All of these techniques are used today, and over the years improvements in apparatus and contrast media have produced better and safer results.

Anesthesia

General Considerations

1. X-ray rooms may be small, dark and unfamiliar; it is therefore necessary to have some means of checking the patient's color for cyanosis and to monitor vital signs such as respiratory rate, pulse rate, and blood pressure. Pulse oximetry is very valuable and should be available. Anesthetic machine flow meters should have luminous backdrops and be easy to read in the dark; vaporizers and cylinders should be checked and full at the beginning of the procedure with spares immediately available (often these rooms have no piped oxygen). Alarms should be checked and made use of in these conditions.

2. Often x-ray rooms were constructed before anesthesia became commonly used during these procedures; because of this, the anesthesiologist may find an unfamiliar environment where space is limited, bulky equipment is present, and personnel are unused to anesthetic demands. Always check the room for essential requirements, e.g., oxygen and suction, and make certain you have all the necessary equipment and drugs you may require for monitoring and resuscitation before commencing anesthesia. These should be equivalent to those present in a standard operating room and include electrocardiograph (ECG), automatic blood pressure machine, pulse oximeter, and capnograph. A defibrillator should be close at hand. Be prepared to instruct someone to assist you as required during the anesthetic administration.

3. X-ray rooms are often not well ventilated, and therefore anesthetic gases may accumulate with long procedures. Ensure that proper scavenging devices are available.

4. Access to the patient may be difficult during the investigation if the patient has to be moved or "disappears" into a machine. The airway must always be protected and monitoring used during these procedures, and both must be secured carefully to prevent detachment during the investigation.

5. Both patient and anesthesiologist must be protected from excessive radiation. Any anesthesiologist spending considerable time in the x-ray suite should be carefully monitored for overexposure.

6. Finally, many of these procedures may be long and repetitive. Care should be taken to remain vigilant and alert.

Remember, perfect x-ray films are useful only if the patient is still available to appreciate them.

Patient Considerations

1. All patients should undergo a full preanesthetic assessment to determine their fitness and the type of anesthetic required for the procedure. This should consist of a full history and examination with the appropriate laboratory investigations.

2. Certain neurologic patients will be unable to give a history, e.g., those with head injuries, those suffering from dementia or cerebral edema. The suspected diagnosis, level of consciousness, and any neurologic deficit should be noted together with signs or symptoms of raised intracranial pressure (ICP), e.g., papilledema, headache, or vomiting.

3. Hyperkalemia in response to succinylcholine has been noted in patients with neurologic conditions, e.g., motor neuron disease, multiple sclerosis, and some muscular dystrophies.

4. Check cardiovascular status. Systemic vascular disease may be related to cerebral vascular disease. Hypertension and ECG changes may be related to subarachnoid hemorrhage.

5. Check fluid balance. Depressed levels of consciousness, hemiplegia, or head injuries may result in hypovolemia due to poor hydration, producing hypotension during anesthesia. Electrolytes should be checked in these conditions.

6. Know the patient's drug history. Steroids are often used in various neurologic conditions, and additional doses will be required. Hypertensive patients should continue on their medication and be well controlled before their investigation. Antidepressant drugs may interact with various anesthetic agents.

7. Remember also the association of acute neurologic injuries with cervical spine injuries, multiple other organ injuries, and the risk of a "full stomach."

Anesthetic Management

Although most neurodiagnostic procedures are invasive and may produce considerable discomfort, none are so unpleasant as to make general anesthesia mandatory. However, these procedures do require immobility and therefore the cooperation of the patient. Certain groups of patients, such as young children, severely ill patients, and patients with neurologic conditions producing tremor or other uncontrollable movements, may require assistance to obtain suitable conditions to produce good x-ray films and diagnostic results. Other groups of patients in whom the airway may not be adequately protected or in whom there is cardiovascular instability may require anesthetic intervention.

Neuroradiologic procedures may be performed under local anesthesia, with or without sedation, or under general anesthesia. There is no "best" method, but each patient should be assessed separately with regard to their medical needs, age, and procedure required.

Computed Tomography

The introduction of CT in the 1970s has proved a major advance in the radiologic diagnosis of intracranial lesions. Although conventional radiographs can often provide important information in many clinical situations, they suffer the disadvantage that a three-dimensional structure is being portrayed by a two-dimensional image. Therefore, structures lying above and below the focused plane cause shadowing. Linear tomography overcomes this problem by holding the tomographic section under review in focus while surrounding structures are blurred by the relative motion of the x-ray source and film receptor. However, this method allows the patient to be exposed to a high radiation dose.

Computed tomography reduces this hazard and produces a clearer image. Using computers, the data obtained from the x-ray source is formed into tomographic "slices" of the head in which the brain tissue, the ventricular system, and any intracranial pathology can be easily visualized. When tumors are suspected, intravenous contrast medium (see below) may be injected. This diffuses more readily into the vascular tumor than into normal tissue, producing identification of the lesion. Because the procedure is noninvasive, rapid, and provides high-quality images, the need for other more invasive procedures has been greatly reduced, resulting in up to a 25% decrease in angiography and a 75% decrease in air-contrast studies in many centers.

Procedure

The patient lies on a table during the procedure with the head immobilized by a Velcro belt in a rotating gantry (previously the head was surrounded by a water jacket to eliminate computer artifact). One rotation of the gantry produces one axial slice, taking 2 to 4 seconds (in early scanners each "cut" took 4 to 5 minutes). A series of slices are made with a complete examination of the head consisting of about 6 slices. The whole procedure is then repeated after the infusion of contrast media if enhancement is indicated.

To obtain a successful radiologic scan the patient must lie absolutely still throughout the whole examination. Anesthesia may be needed for (1) cooperative patients with movement disorders; (2) patients who are confused or uncooperative, such as those with head trauma; and (3) pediatric patients.

Anesthesia for outpatient scanning is also becoming more routine because, due to its noninvasive nature, CT is being used more frequently for early detection of intracranial pathology.

Complications

Because CT scanning is noninvasive, there are no complications with its performance. However, when intravenous dye is injected as part of the examination, the problems of anaphylactoid reactions occur. (For details, see later in this chapter.) Examination of the posterior fossa may require extreme flexion of the head, which may obstruct the airway or kink an endotracheal tube. This position may also compromise blood flow to the brain or cause brainstem compression. Therefore, body scanners, which can tilt on their axis, are better used to carry out this part of the examination.

Clinical Uses

Since its introduction, a vast amount has been written testifying to the accuracy of CT scanning. It is reported to be 96% accurate in the diagnosis and detection of cerebral tumors. It has also proved useful in the investigation of cerebral trauma, cerebral ischemia, intracranial hemorrhage, and infection.

Anesthetic Considerations

Most adults and older children require no medication for CT scanning. However, certain adults (see above) and up to one-half of all children requiring a CT scan need anesthetic assistance. This may consist of either sedation or general anesthesia.

Sedation

Virtually all sedative techniques may be used, but it must be remembered that on occasions any technique may be inadequate to produce an acceptable examination. Also, with all techniques there have been reports of respiratory depression and cardiac arrest. Therefore, monitoring is essential even with sedation. Young children respond well to either oral or intramuscular sedation. However, it must be remembered that intravenous access is often required for the injection of contrast medium. Suggested regimens and routes of administration are given in Table 14–1. Caution must also be applied in the administration of sedatives to the patient who has head injuries or suspected raised ICP. Perhaps here there is a good argument to carry out a full general anesthetic.

General Anesthesia

In both children and adults, general anesthesia is the most effective way to produce a motionless patient with a protected airway. It is used when (1) sedation is either hazardous or ineffective, (2) patients have potential airway problems, and (3) control of ICP is critical. Induction may be performed either by the intravenous route or an inhalation technique.

For the intravenous route, use thiopental 4 to 5 mg/kg or propofol 1 to 2 mg/kg, the latter if the patient is to be discharged the same day.

Table 14–1 Suggested Regimens for Children and Adults Who Require Sedation for CT Scanning*

Route of Administration	Agent	Dosage
Children		
Oral	Chloral hydrate	40–75 mg/kg
Rectal	Methohexital	20–25 mg/kg
Intramuscular	Mixture of Meperidine hydrochloride 25 mg Chlorpromazine 6.25 mg Promethazine hydrochloride 6.25 mg in each ml	1 ml/10–12 kg Maximum dosage 200 mg given 20–30 min before the examination
	Ketamine†	5–10 mg/kg
Intravenous	Ketamine†	1–2 mg/kg
Adults	Same as for children, plus:	
Intravenous	Diazepam or midazolam	Incremental doses of 2.5 mg ± small doses of a short-acting narcotic (e.g., fentanyl 25 µg/dose)
	Thiopental	1–2 mg/kg with further small increments of 25 mg as required
	Propofol	1 mg/kg as required

* Remember: All of the sedation agents listed may cause respiratory depression with a rise in CO_2, a fall in oxygen saturation, and the loss of both airway and associated reflexes, all of which may be disastrous for a patient with even mild neurologic damage.
† The use of ketamine may be associated with an unacceptable incidence of patient movement.

When using the inhalation technique, since the head is inaccessible, an endotracheal tube should be placed, preferably via the oral route, and strapped securely to prevent movement or disconnection. Care should be taken to avoid kinking of the tube during the examination. This can be carried out either by using succinylcholine 1.5 mg/kg after pretreatment with tubocurarine 3 mg or either of the newer intermediate-duration, nondepolarizing muscle relaxants, e.g., vecuronium 1 mg/kg or atracurium 0.5 mg/kg.

The decision to employ either controlled or spontaneous respiration will depend on the condition of the patient, since the sole requirements are that the patient lie still and tolerate the endotracheal tube. If spontaneous ventilation is used, the vocal cords should be sprayed with topical anesthesia, e.g., lidocaine 4%, to improve tolerance of the tube. Although any volatile anesthetic may be used, isoflurane has several advantages over the other agents. It has no epileptogenic activity, has less effect on ICP than other anesthetics, and may be repeated without hepatic toxicity (important because follow-up scans are often performed within short periods of time).

When ICP is increased, controlled hyperventilation should be used. Nitrous oxide and oxygen with a nondepolarizing muscle relaxant and small dose of a short-acting narcotic, such as fentanyl, with or without a volatile agent, e.g., isoflurane, may be used with the aim of providing rapid postoperative recovery, so that early assessment of neurologic status may be performed. Ketamine increases cerebral blood flow and ICP and is not advocated in this situation.

Monitoring for this examination should be as for any neurosurgical procedure, consisting of ECG, automated blood pressure measurement, capnography, and pulse oximetry.

It is important to remember that the room in which the scanner functions must be kept cold (approximately 65°F) to avoid artifacts and damage to the machine's circuits. Therefore, young children and babies will rapidly lose heat. Standard techniques to avoid heat loss—warming lamps, warm fluids, and blankets—should be employed.

Caution should also be employed in relation to the hypertonic iodinated contrast media used, since it may precipitate fluid overload and therefore pulmonary edema, as well as an unrecognized full bladder. Contrast media may cause renal shutdown in dehydrated patients.

Angiography

Angiography consists of the percutaneous injection of contrast medium into an artery to demonstrate the position and state of the associated vasculature. With the increased use of computerized tomography, the incidence of angiography in the diagnosis of neuropathology has decreased. However, it is still used to picture the vasculature of the brain and spinal cord and is still carried out for investigation of intracerebral hemorrhages and intracranial vascular lesions, especially aneurysms, arteriovenous malformations, and arteriosclerotic cerebrovascular disease. It is also of value in determining the position of space-occupying lesions, such as tumors, abscesses, or hematomas.

Spinal Angiography

Spinal angiography was pioneered by Djindjian in France and is often used on patients who have already sustained damage to their spinal cords. The possibility of further damage to the cord is significant. The procedure almost always uses selective studies and subtraction techniques and therefore tends to be prolonged and uncomfortable. However, it is usually performed without general anesthesia so that the patient's neurologic status can be assessed after each injection of contrast. Paroxysmal contractions of the lower limbs may occur and will respond to the injection of 5 mg of diazepam through the angiography catheter.

Spinal angiography visualizes the circulation to the posterior fossa and occipital lobes.

Cerebral Angiography

Cerebral angiography is performed by the percutaneous puncture of the common carotid or vertebral arteries or by the retrograde catheterization of the subclavian, brachial, or femoral arteries, the femoral technique being the least disturbing to the patient and producing the fewest complications.

Injection into the internal carotid artery displays the distribution of the anterior and middle cerebral arteries and the venous distribution on the same side of the brain.

Complications

Site

Arterial puncture may cause hematoma, arterial spasm, or embolism of atherosclerotic plaques. Damage to the vessel wall may cause occlusion or subintimal dissection.

Contrast Medium

Reactions to intravascular contrast media are not uncommon. Of the millions of studies performed in the United States each year, some signs of adverse systemic reaction occur in approximately 5%, one-third of these being severe enough to require immediate medical treatment. It was estimated in 1984 that 500 fatalities per year followed examinations using intravascular contrast media.

Reactions occur frequently in young healthy patients, most often in those with a history of allergy or asthma. Patients with a history of allergy to seafoods have a 15% incidence of reaction, and a history of a previous reaction increases the incidence to 17 to 35%. Anaphylactoid reactions have been described in all age groups including infants; however, younger patients tend to have milder reactions than older groups. Patients with cardiac disease have a four to five times greater risk of having a systemic reaction, which if it occurs will also be more dangerous. Dose is also important; the lower the dose of contrast medium, the lower the incidence of reactions.

Owing to the properties of the iodinated contrast media, certain reactions occur in all patients injected: decreased hematocrit, increased osmolarity, and an osmotic diuresis are seen, the clinical significance of these being related to the cardiac status of the patient and the quantity of dye used.

Some patients, however, show other idiosyncratic reactions to the dye involving vasomotor, vasovagal, dermal, osmotic, or anaphylactic manifestations. These can be seen either individually or in a variety of combinations.

Nausea and vomiting occur, often within a few minutes of injection, in 20% of all anaphylactoid and fatal reactions. Other classic signs and symptoms consist of urticaria due to histamine release (often made worse by the patient's own anxiety), fever and facial flushing due to increased cutaneous blood flow, and changes in mental status shown by anxiety, restlessness, and individual reports of "feeling strange." These symptoms may remain of nuisance value only or may progress to more serious reactions. As many examinations occur in darkened rooms with sedated patients, care must be taken to note these prodromal signs. If general anesthesia is used, these symptoms may be missed or hidden by the normal clinical changes seen under anesthesia.

Anaphylactoid shock usually presents immediately and is probably the result of the nonimmunologic release of histamine and other vasoactive substances. Clinically the patient may present with dyspnea, wheezing, syncope, and cardiovascular collapse. Unfortunately there are no accepted predictive tests, intradermal tests having been shown to be unreliable.

Patients who either are allergic or have a history of reaction may be given steroids and antihistamines prior to being investigated; however, this is still controversial. Since stress may increase the severity of a reaction, a benzodiazepine may also be used before the examination.

Treatment. Rashes or mild reactions require only reassurance and an intravenous antihistamine such as diphenhydramine. The most severe reaction including bronchospasm, laryngeal edema, and severe hypotension needs to be treated with epinephrine 1:1,000 subcutaneously or intravenously (3 to 5 μg/kg boluses), which will improve both the bronchospasm and the hypotension. Rapid infusion of intravenous fluids will also be necessary, and arrhythmias should be controlled with antiarrhythmic drugs, cardioversion, or both. Corticosteroids may have a place in treatment, and aminophylline and nebulized isoproterenol may also be used to treat the bronchospasm. Endotracheal intubation with positive pressure ventilation may become necessary to ensure adequate oxygenation, and cardiopulmonary resuscitation must be commenced should cardiac arrest occur.

All emergency equipment and drugs necessary to deal with these situations should be readily available in all x-ray units.

Late Complications

At the end of the procedure, pressure should be applied to the puncture site until there is no sign of hematoma formation. This is especially important when the neck is used as the puncture site, where neglect may allow the formation of a massive hematoma with associated respiratory distress. Similarly, care should be taken at the femoral site, since femoral arterial spasm may occur.

Anesthesia for Angiography

Using the femoral site, either local or general anesthesia may be used. However, if the direct approach (into the carotid or vertebral artery) is used, general anesthesia is preferable.

Local Anesthesia

Although the patient may suffer slight discomfort, provided he or she is able to cooperate, less risk is involved using local anesthesia plus sedation. However, if the patient becomes confused or unconscious or develops hypoxia or hypercarbia, with or without raised ICP, the benefits of local anesthesia will be lost. The patient's neurologic state and general condition can be closely observed under local anesthesia, and the procedure can be abandoned at the first sign of neurologic problems.

Benzodiazepines such as midazolam and diazepam may be used both preoperatively and during the procedure. Doses of fentanyl (25 to 50 μg) may be given incrementally with or without the addition of droperidol (1.25 to 2.5 mg). Close observation of both the patient's circulatory and respiratory status must be maintained throughout the procedure, since these may be altered not only by the drugs used but also by manipulation of the carotid vessels in the neck.

General Anesthesia

General anesthesia is required for the semicomatose patient, who may move in response to painful stimuli or the injection of contrast medium, and for children or confused patients.

Advantages include increased patient comfort and immobility during x-ray procedures as well as the removal of emotional stress. The sternomastoid muscles are relaxed so that accurate puncture of the carotid artery may be obtained. However, hypotension produced by isoflurane may make arterial puncture more difficult.

A standard anesthetic technique consists of an intravenous induction with thiopental, followed by intubation and then either an inhalation technique with isoflurane and spontaneous respiration or a nitrous/narcotic/relaxant technique with controlled ventilation. The latter technique is more popular because of its rapid reversibility, allowing early neurologic assessment, and the advantages of hyperventilation when raised ICP is present, since it allows the control of arterial CO_2. Hypocarbia slows the cerebral circulation, therefore allowing greater concentration of contrast medium, and by constricting cerebral vessels improves the quality of the angiogram. This is particularly important in children with increased cerebral blood flow, in whom good angiograms are hard to obtain (however, with new rapid filming techniques this is becoming less of a problem), and in patients with brain tumors, in whom provoking an intracerebral steal (hypocarbia does not constrict tumor vasculature) will delineate the tumor sharply.

Controlled ventilation should, however, be used with care in patients with suspected ruptured aneurysms, as the spasm and impaired cerebral circulation may be worsened by further hypocarbic vasoconstriction. Normocarbic anesthesia is probably the most appropriate anesthetic here. However, this question is becoming more and more academic as neurosurgeons become increasingly reluctant to perform these procedures in the early posthemorrhagic state, relying instead on CT scanning. Whichever technique is used, continuous monitoring of blood pressure, pulse, and respiration is necessary. Mild hypotension may occur owing to baroreceptor discharge, usually transient. However, more severe falls may occur in patients with cerebrovascular disease or subarachnoid aneurysms. Serious neurologic complications may occur after angiography, caused by thrombosis, embolism, or an increase in vascular spasm. The development of new noninvasive techniques should, however, supplant the need for angiography and is to be welcomed.

Digital Subtraction Angiography

Digital subtraction angiography (DSA) involves computer processing of a fluoroscopically acquired analog image into a digital image, which can then be manipulated by computer to obtain maximum information. In the most usual configuration, the information from an image intensifier is converted to digital form and introduced into the computer as an array of numbers according to the density of each point on the image. The image obtained just before the injection of the contrast and the image just after the injection are stored by the computer, and the second image is then subtracted from the first so that only the vessels containing the contrast medium are visualized on the resulting third image. Advantages include greater sensitivity than standard x-ray films, immediate availability of the image, and cheaper storage on magnetic tape. Also, because the sensitivity is so great, images may be obtained after intravenous injection as opposed to intra-arterial injection, thus removing the need for intra-arterial cannulation. Image contrast is under computer control, so that exposures are not critical and small changes in the patient's position are not as important as in conventional angiography. Disadvantages include the poor imaging of some structures, such as the base of the skull, where bone interferes with visualization of the structures and vasculature present.

Anesthesia for Digital Subtraction Angiography

Anesthesia for DSA is essentially the same as for angiography, as these procedures are often performed sequentially. If, however, only intravenous contrast is used, very little discomfort is felt and often only sedation is employed. However, the same considerations regarding patient cooperation in lying still apply in deciding between local and general anesthetic techniques. DSA studies may also require a technique involving the control of respiration during injection sequences, necessitating general anesthesia with controlled ventilation. Monitoring is the same as for angiography, since the same problems with contrast medium may occur.

Therapeutic Embolization

Using the skills obtained during selective angiography, it is now possible to cannulate specific cranial vessels and obliterate them. This technique is used to eliminate such vessels as those arteries feeding arteriovenous malformations, to decrease the vascularity of tumors, or to close carotid cavernous sinus fistulas. Glue, gelatin sponge, or balloons may be used.

Complications

Injury to a vessel wall may occur, causing hemorrhage; the wrong vessel may be accidentally obliterated; and, as always, the usual complications involving contrast medium may occur.

Anesthesia for Therapeutic Embolization

Since it is important to recognize neurologic complications early, it is usually preferable to carry out these procedures under sedation. However, because they are often long and painful, the anesthesiologist may be involved to ensure the patient's comfort, improve conditions, and provide constant monitoring of both cardiovascular and neurologic conditions. If signs of impaired neurologic function occur, the procedure should be halted immediately with measures employed to maintain cerebral blood flow, such as administration of low-weight dextrans and preservation of normal blood pressure. Small doses of fentanyl (25 to 50 μg) with droperidol (1.25 to 2.5 mg), with or without small doses of a short-acting benzodiazepine such as midazolam (1 to 2 mg), may be used and repeated throughout the procedure.

General anesthesia may be necessary to prevent movement in small children; therefore, any technique producing normocapnia and an early return to consciousness may be used. Nitrous oxide and oxygen with a muscle relaxant and controlled ventilation may be used after an induction of choice.

Magnetic Resonance Imaging

Nuclear magnetic resonance (NMR), now termed magnetic resonance imaging (MRI), is a new concept representing a radically different technique for imaging body structures, not relying on ionizing radiation but instead using magnetic fields and radiofrequency pulses for the production of images. The introduction of MRI into clinical practice has been dependent on the production of suitable magnet systems and the reconstructive algorithms developed for CT scanning. The existence of nuclear spins is essential to the concept of MRI, which depends on the responses of atomic nuclei in a magnetic field.

Only certain nuclei occur in sufficient abundance in biologic tissue to yield an MRI signal, hydrogen nuclei being one of these. When these nuclei are placed in a strong magnetic field, they align themselves in the direction of the field.

The equilibrium of these nuclei may then be perturbed by the application of a second field perpendicular to the first, energy being absorbed in this process. Thus, for the hydrogen atom, if radiofrequency is applied in pulses of sufficient power, the axis of nuclear spin is deflected by 90 to 180 degrees. When this magnetic field is switched off, the nuclei return to their original position, the absorbed energy being emitted as radiofrequency radiation. This is detected as an MRI signal by the same coils used to transmit the radiofrequency signal.

Physical Forces and Their Ramifications

There are three physical forces involved in this equipment with which the anesthesiologist must be familiar: magnetic attraction, induced currents, and radiofrequency.

Magnetic Attraction

A strong magnetic field is produced by the large magnetic instruments. This is most powerful at the center of the machine and fades as the distance from the magnet increases. The strength of this field is such that metal objects may become lethal projectiles as they approach the magnet. This prevents the use of ferromagnetic materials such as cobalt, nickel, and some types of stainless steel in the same room. Metallic implants in patients will also be subjected to these forces with potentially serious consequences. Ferromagnetic aneurysm clips may be dislocated from blood vessels, and cardiac pacemakers may change from demand mode to continuous mode under the influence of these fields. The induced voltages produced in the pacemaker leads can also mimic cardiac function and lead to pacing failure. Pacemakers with ferromagnetic coverings may be rotated or displaced within the chest wall. Therefore, such patients are at present excluded from these investigations. Analog wristwatches, credit cards, and other magnetic encoded media are also at risk from these force fields.

Magnetic fields, however, cause no known injury to living organisms, and thus the anesthesiologist may remain close to the patient at all times without risk, obviously not the case with conventional radiation. There is a strong pull by the magnet on conventional anesthesia machines (especially on the gas cylinders); therefore the machine must be kept away from the magnet and a long breathing system such as an elongated Bain (Mapleson D) system used to administer the gases. The expiratory port should be made of aluminum. A "zone of risk" can be established, inside which there should be no loose objects. The anesthesia machine and other ancillary equipment will distort the magnetic field produced by the magnet; thus, when a suitable position is found, adjustments to the field can be made to compensate for this. Anesthetic gases are best supplied by pipeline, but spare cylinders should be available and stored outside the room.

Other anesthetic equipment can be altered to cope with these fields. A brass precordial or a plastic esophageal stethoscope, both with plastic tubing, can be used safely. Oscillatory blood pressure cuffs can be used by adding long, wide-bore tubing to the cuff and replacing the adapter junctions with plastic. The ideal ventilator should be of low mass, of the fluidic type, and have few ferromagnetic components, e.g., the Penlon. Cathode ray tubes used in many monitors can distort the field if placed too close.

Induced Currents

When a conductor moves in a magnetic field, a voltage is induced. If the conductor forms a circuit, a current will flow. This may occur in the patient. A current of 1 to 10 A/m^2 induces fibrillation in the heart, and 30 A/m^2 can induce a nerve action potential. During MRI the current density produced is about 10 mA/m^2, and as yet there have been no reports of fibrillation or epileptiform movement.

Radiofrequency

Most of the radiofrequency power used to excite the nuclei is dissipated as heat, and the levels reached currently with the MRI are unlikely to cause adverse effects. However, the radiofrequency signals do cause background noise and will interfere with the electrocardiogram. This noise will also interfere with the heart sounds heard through the precordial stethoscope; however, a discerning ear will still be able to distinguish the patient's actual heart sounds. The conducting wires for monitoring electrical signals will likewise degrade the radiofrequency signal. Elimination of this by either telemetry or fiberoptic transmission has been somewhat successful. The pulse oximeter can be used in the initial stages of adjustment; however, during the actual scanning when the radiofrequency signal is on (5- to 8-minute periods) the signal from the oximeter will interfere with the imaging.

Magnet Failure

These systems work at extremely low temperatures. Should the cooling system fail, heat will be produced, causing the helium and nitrogen components to boil off. Although these gases are nontoxic, they may be produced in large enough volumes to reduce oxygen levels and cause asphyxiation.

Anesthesia for Magnetic Resonance Imaging

At present the number of patients requiring anesthesia for MRI procedures is small, because it is a noninvasive, nonpainful procedure. However, the same concerns exist as with the CT scanner, and the patient must be willing to cooperate and lie still. As mentioned, monitoring does present difficulties, and during the procedure the head (and sometimes the body) disappears into the machine, further complicating monitoring.

The principal problems associated with anesthesia are therefore (1) airway management, (2) patient inaccessibility, (3) the effects of magnetism on the anesthetic equipment, and (4) the effects of the equipment on the magnets.

Oral sedation may be safely used, especially with children. Chloral hydrate (40 to 75 mg/kg) is acceptable, as is rectal methohexital (20 to 25 mg/kg).

If a general anesthetic is required, it is safest to anesthetize the patient at a distance from the magnet, where standard monitoring can be used, and move the patient to the magnet when stabilized. Since airway access is limited, endotracheal intubation is often the method of choice, using plastic connectors. The choice of either spontaneous or controlled ventilation, as with CT, depends on the condition of the patient.

As with all other imaging procedures, when anesthesia is administered, full resuscitation equipment must be available. However, in the event of a cardiac arrest, it must be remembered that portable ECGs, defibrillators, and other equipment will malfunction in close proximity to the magnet. Intubation with a laryngoscope will also be difficult, as the highly ferromagnetic batteries will make it very unwieldy; thus, the safest practice is to remove the patient from the magnet.

Contrast Agents

Little is known about contrast agents used with MRI. They rely on intrinsic paramagnetic properties to produce local magnetic field effects. Iron, manganese, and chromium have all been found effective, but their free ions are toxic. Further research is needed before the substances are fully assessed and their clinical usefulness determined.

Pneumoencephalography

Pneumoencephalography is today rarely performed, its use decreasing with the advent of the CT scanner, and it will almost certainly be totally eliminated when MRI techniques are readily available. However, it still plays an important role in the diagnosis of small mass lesions in the sellar and cerebellopontine angle regions, as well as being helpful in the investigation of epilepsy and cerebral atrophy.

The procedure involves the injection of air into the lumbar subarachnoid space, after which the patient is maneuvered into various positions to move the gas intracranially. With the patient erect, the air arrives in the ventricular system via the cisterna magna, outlining its shape, size, and symmetry. Air also passes over the hemispheres, outlining the brain sulci. Radiographs are therefore taken with the patient in the erect, supine, and prone positions.

Complications

The investigation is not without risk. Air embolism or brainstem herniation may occur, both resulting in acute respiratory and cardiovascular insufficiency and often cardiac arrest. However, diagnosis is often difficult to make. If the symptoms just described occur directly after lumbar puncture, herniation is likely, especially if the injection has been rapid. If air has just been injected, air embolism is likely. Anesthetic-induced circulatory collapse must also be considered.

Treatment of all three complications consists of rapid return to the supine position with full cardiopulmonary resuscitation. If air embolism is suspected, the left lateral position may be beneficial, whereas if brainstem herniation is confirmed, reinjection of fluid into the lumbar subarachnoid space may help.

Pneumoencephalography is absolutely contraindicated in any patient with signs or symptoms of raised ICP. Minor complications may occur, including headache, nausea, vomiting, tachycardia, bradycardia, extrasystoles, hypotension, and hypertension, making this one of the most uncomfortable and unpleasant examinations a patient may undergo.

Anesthesia for Pneumoencephalography

General anesthesia or local anesthesia with sedation may be used. Because of the unpleasantness of the procedure, its prolonged duration, extreme position changes, and airway inaccessibility, many centers prefer general anesthetic techniques, especially in children. However, some still prefer to use local anesthesia, partly because the serious complications described above are more easily recognized in a conscious patient, and partly to reduce the complications that arise when extreme changes in position are associated with general anesthesia.

Sedation

Intermittent benzodiazepines, e.g., diazepam in 2.5-mg increments, plus a short-acting narcotic, e.g., fentanyl in 25-μg increments IV, have been used successfully. Hypotension and bradycardia in response to position changes should be treated aggressively, e.g., ephedrine in 5-mg boluses. Nausea and vomiting respond well to droperidol (1.25 to 2.5 mg IV), while the headaches usually respond to further narcotic. Care must, however, be taken in using the latter, since excess may produce hypoventilation and changes in the patient's level of consciousness.

General Anesthesia

Any anesthetic may impair normal cardiovascular responses to positional change. Nitrous oxide should not be used as part of the anesthetic technique when air is used as the gaseous medium, as N_2O, being more soluble in blood than nitrogen, will be displaced into the ventricles, causing distention and an increase in ICP, contraindicated in this examination. The anesthetic technique chosen should avoid excessive responses to position changes and alterations in ICP by preventing hypercapnia, coughing, and straining. Therefore, it should involve a smooth induction in a relaxed patient. Thiopental, muscle relaxant, and controlled ventilation with small doses of narcotic or a volatile agent such as isoflurane have been found satisfactory. Ketamine was at one time thought of as a useful drug for this procedure, maintaining cardiovascular and respiratory reflexes; however, its effect on ICP makes it unsuitable.

After the procedure the patient should lie flat for 24 hours to prevent the low-pressure spinal headache which may occur.

Gamma Knife

Closed stereotactic procedures or radiosurgery using a single high dose of focused radiation energy instead of electrodes to affect or destroy intracranial tissue was first introduced by Leksell. Following much experimental and clinical research, a stereotactic gamma unit was constructed as a clinical tool for radiosurgery. This is as yet a relatively new technique used only in a few centers.

Although the actual procedure of radiosurgery may only take minutes, the entire investigation may take several hours. The patient first has a stereotactic frame placed under local anesthesia and then a series of normal investigations, usually including CT scanning and angiography, are carried out. The patient then proceeds to the gamma room for treatment. Often it may take up to 1 hour to calculate and compute the isotope configurations and treatment times for the radiosurgery after angiography but before the actual therapy can commence. The treatment or surgery itself usually lasts about 20 minutes.

At present, most adults are treated without any form of anesthesia since the therapy is not painful and the patient's cooperation is needed throughout. However, occasionally small amounts of intravenous sedation (e.g., diazepam or midazolam) may be used. The patient is in the sitting position for the frame to be placed and the rest of the procedure is carried out in the semi-erect position. Occasionally, vasovagal reactions requiring intravenous atropine occur while the patient is in the sitting position.

The patient is monitored as for any neuroradiologic procedure, using both ECG and arterial blood pressure, and the investigator continuously communicates with the patient to assess consciousness. During irradiation all personnel must be outside the room containing the knife; thus all monitoring equipment must have consoles outside, while cameras continuously monitor the patient inside. In the event of a problem the radiation can be terminated and the room entered relatively quickly.

The anesthesiologist becomes more important when children are involved. Here, cooperation is more difficult to obtain and so the child is anesthetized for the frame to be placed and angiography performed. The patient must then be moved to the gamma knife room, involving all the complications of transportation. The patient is then placed in the correct position, but during the short bursts of radiation the anesthesiologist has to leave the room and monitor the child using the outside cameras and monitors. The technique of intubation with either spontaneous or controlled ventilation has been used safely in various centers.

As yet we have little knowledge of the exact role and all the problems to be encountered by the anesthesiologist during this procedure.

Summary

The anesthesiologist today plays an important role in the management of patients requiring neuroradiologic investigations not only by helping ensure their comfort and cooperation during these procedures and in the treatment of any problems that may arise in their course, but also by ensuring the production of the best radiographic results and conditions to aid in successful diagnosis and treatment. As further advances in this field occur, the role of the anesthesiologist will also expand to provide assistance to both the patient and the neuroradiologist in an ever-widening range of challenging situations.

Suggested Reading

Aidinis S, et al. Anesthesia for brain computer tomography. Anesthesiology 1976; 44:420.

Andrews C. Anesthesia management for neuroradiologic diagnostic procedures. In: Frost EAM, ed, Clinical anesthesia in neurosurgery. Stoneham, Mass: Butterworth, 1984.

Campkin TV. General anaesthesia for neuroradiology. Br J Anaesth 1976; 48:783.

Goldberg M. Systemic reactions to intravascular contrast media. A guide for the anesthesiologist. Anesthesiology 1984; 60:46.

Hirsch NP, et al. Advances in clinical imaging. In: Jewkes DA, ed, Bailliere's clinical anaesthesiology—anaesthesia for neurosurgery. London: Bailliere Tindall, 1987.

Wolfson B, et al. Anesthesia for neuroradiologic procedures. In: Cottrell J, et al, eds, Anesthesia and neurosurgery. 2nd ed. St. Louis: CV Mosby, 1986.

Cary S. Sternick, M.D., and Joseph A. Stirt, M.D.

Anesthesia for the Patient with Neurologic Disease   15

This chapter focuses on the patient whose ongoing neurologic disease represents a distinct risk in terms of perioperative and anesthetic management. The following diseases are considered: amyotrophic lateral sclerosis (ALS), myotonic dystrophy, Duchenne muscular dystrophy, myasthenia gravis, multiple sclerosis, Parkinson's syndrome, seizure disorders, Alzheimer's disease, and migraine headaches.

Amyotrophic Lateral Sclerosis

Amyotrophic lateral sclerosis (ALS) may affect a person of any age, but generally involves males and females between the ages of 30 and 60. Ten percent of ALS cases are hereditary, but the vast majority are not. Clinically, the manifestations of ALS include both upper motor neuron and lower motor neuron symptoms and signs. Thus, in addition to weakness and atrophy of the upper extremities, lower extremities, and bulbar muscles, there may also be spasticity and rigidity of those same muscles.

In most cases the initial signs are asymmetrical, and over the course of 2 to 3 years of progressive involvement, profound weakness of all extremities, the bulbar musculature, and finally significant respiratory insufficiency secondary to muscle wasting are seen. Aspiration secondary to weakness of the pharyngeal musculature is a common complication.

Although there are exceptions, the average patient succumbs with respiratory insufficiency within 3 to 4 years after the onset of the disease. The etiology of ALS is unknown, and currently, despite a multitude of research trials, no medication has been shown to alleviate or arrest the progression of this disease.

Anesthetic Considerations

In the ALS patient there is no evidence of cardiac involvement. The respiratory system is the focus in the anesthetic management of a patient with ALS. Intercostal muscle weakness causes respiratory insufficiency and alveolar hypoventilation, and this must be addressed by the anesthesiologist. Neuromuscular blocking drugs employed should be exclusively of the nondepolarizing variety, with dose directly titrated to clinical effect with the use of a nerve stimulator. Similarly, antagonism of neuromuscular blockade must be carefully assessed prior to extubation of the trachea in order to minimize the risks of aspiration.

Any surgical procedure on a patient with moderate to advanced ALS must be considered carefully as to its absolute necessity, since weaning patients from the ventilator after surgery and general anesthesia can be very difficult. We have personally cared for a number of patients who could not be weaned from the respirator after a surgical procedure under general anesthesia.

Myotonic Dystrophy

Myotonic dystrophy is a multisystem degenerative disease inherited in an autosomal dominant pattern. The diagnosis of myotonic dystrophy is easily made clinically by a combination of myotonia (a failure of relaxation of muscles), distal muscle weakness, ptosis, and bitemporal muscle atrophy. Common findings include cataracts, testicular atrophy, mental retardation, and cardiac abnormalities. To confirm the diagnosis, electromyography is performed. Electromyographic testing of numerous muscles reveals the classic "dive bomber" phenomenon pathognomonic for myotonia. The average age at clinical onset is between 20 and 25 years. The etiology of myotonic dystrophy is unclear, but it appears that muscle membrane hypersensitivity and abnormalities of membrane conduction are involved.

Anesthetic Considerations

The anesthetic considerations are twofold. Cardiac involvement is perhaps the most significant factor that the anesthesiologist must consider. Although the patient may be asymptomatic and have no cardiac complaints, almost all patients with myotonic dystrophy are found to have cardiac abnormalities when extensive testing is performed. The conduction system appears to be involved frequently. First-degree heart block is perhaps the most common abnormality. Atrial arrhythmias and flutter are often reported. Sudden death is known to occur in myotonic dystrophy.

The second important consideration in the patient with myotonic dystrophy is respiratory insufficiency secondary to weak intercostal muscles. Atrophy and wasting of the muscles of the airway and swallowing mechanism put these patients at increased risk for aspiration. Thus, similar considerations in the use of muscle relaxants to those noted above for ALS apply. Respiratory response to carbon dioxide is diminished in some patients, which must be taken into account during anesthesia, especially in the postoperative period.

Patients must also be questioned carefully regarding medications used to reduce their underlying myotonia. Phenytoin (Dilantin), quinine sulfate, procainamide, and tocainide are medications currently in widespread use. Dilantin use increases the requirement for nondepolarizing muscle relaxants. Quinine sulfate and procainamide are less than optimal choices for chronic use because of their increased tendency to depress cardiac conduction, which is already a significant problem. Because interaction of these drugs with general inhalation anesthetics may lead to cardiac depression, caution is advised.

Duchenne Muscular Dystrophy

Duchenne muscular dystrophy is the most common of all the muscular dystrophies. It is inherited through an X-linked recessive pattern and occurs in 1 in 4,000 births. Clinically, it is characterized by the onset of an abnormal waddling gait, usually before the age of 4 years; hypertrophy of the calves; progressive muscle weakness, proximal more than distal; and loss of the ability to walk between the ages of 7 and 15 years. Death usually occurs before the age of 20 as a result of myocardial insufficiency. The diagnosis is made by reviewing the family history. In addition, a finding of high levels of muscle enzymes is the rule. A muscle biopsy shows idiopathic changes with fatty replacement of muscle fibers. There is no treatment. Although males are overwhelmingly affected, some female carriers have mild to moderate symptoms.

Anesthetic Considerations

Patients with Duchenne muscular dystrophy take no particular medications. Cardiac and respiratory problems, however, are typical. Electrocardiographic (ECG) findings include tall R waves in the right precordial leads and deep Q waves in the left precordial and limb leads. T-wave inversion over the precordial leads is also common. Persistent tachycardia and sudden death from cardiac failure have frequently been reported. The ECG may be absolutely normal, yet the patient may have significant cardiac disease. The anesthesiologist must be aware of this potential danger.

Because of weakness of the intercostal muscles, respiratory insufficiency is common, and considerations in the use of muscle relaxants are similar to those noted above for ALS. Choice of anesthetic is made on the basis of individual pathology, with no one regimen currently being considered superior to any other. These patients are very sensitive to sedatives and narcotics, and caution is advised when using such drugs. In addition, patients with Duchenne muscular dystrophy have an increased propensity for malignant hyperpyrexia.

Myasthenia Gravis

Myasthenia gravis is a neuromuscular disease that can be divided into three types:

1. Acquired—myasthenia acquired after birth.
2. Congenital—myasthenia present at birth.
3. Neonatal—transient myasthenia noted in approximately 10% of the children of myasthenic mothers.

Myasthenia is frequently a disease of young women and old men, but there are no absolute rules. Myasthenia gravis usually begins with weakness and fatigue, most often in the extraocular muscles and eyelids, making double vision and ptosis the most common initial symptoms. Weakness and fatigue of extremities, respiratory muscles, and bulbar muscles are not unusual. The course of the disease is unpredictable, and there are both nonprogressive and acute fulminating forms. A small percentage of patients with myasthenia have a complete remission, which can be permanent.

Myasthenia is an autoimmune disease in which there is a loss of acetylcholine receptors at the postsynaptic membrane secondary to antibody attack. The diagnosis of myasthenia requires a careful clinical evaluation in addition to nerve conduction studies to determine whether the classic decremental response is present on repetitive nerve stimulation. A positive acetylcholine receptor antibody blood test is helpful.

The treatment of myasthenia gravis is aimed at increasing the amount of acetylcholine available to the diminished number of receptors and/or reducing the antibody activity. In order to increase the amount of acetylcholine available, anticholinesterases, which reduce the amount of acetylcholine breakdown, can be employed. Steroids, plasmapheresis, and immunosuppressive drugs are all used to decrease the antibody response.

Thymectomies are frequently performed, and statistics claim that two-thirds of myasthenia patients improve after undergoing this procedure. The exact relationship of the thymus gland to the production of myasthenia is unclear, but there does seem to be a definite relationship between the thymus gland and the autoimmune component of the disease.

Anesthetic Considerations

Myasthenia does not cause cardiac difficulties, but can cause respiratory insufficiency (secondary to weakness), which must be given careful consideration. Great controversy exists regarding the two major issues involved in the anesthetic management of myasthenia patients. The first concerns the use of muscle relaxants. Suffice it to say that in most cases, anesthesia and surgery may be performed safely without employing muscle relaxants, which also obviate considerations involved in the use of nondepolarizing relaxant antagonists. If relaxant use is required, succinylcholine should be avoided. These patients appear to respond normally to atracurium. If any other nondepolarizing agent is employed, markedly reduced doses (i.e., 1 to 3 mg of *d*-tubocurarine) may be sufficient. The duration of relaxation may be far longer than normally seen.

The second source of controversy involves maintenance of anticholinesterase therapy in the perioperative period. Again, simplicity provides the safest course. Continuation of the preoperative medication regimen, following consultation with the patient's internist or neurologist, in most cases will produce little problem for the anesthesiologist, especially if muscle relaxants have been eschewed. Should the patient be unable to resume oral medications soon, neostigmine, 0.5 mg IV every 4 to 6 hours, will provide adequate coverage.

Multiple Sclerosis

Multiple sclerosis produces its multitude of neurologic signs by damaging the myelin that surrounds the axons in the central nervous system. This damage occurs randomly throughout the central nervous system and can involve a very large or small portion of the brain and spinal cord. A variety of signs can occur because of the numerous different nerve tracts involved in the disease process. Multiple sclerosis is most common in the 20- to 40-year age group, although people as young as 5 and as old as 65 can present with the disease. Although it is more common in patients who have spent their formative years in a northern latitude, there is certainly no absolute rule.

The exact etiology of the production of the damaged myelin (plaques) is unknown, but most researchers think a combination of viral and immunologic interacaction is likely. The plaque formation causes a slowing and/or block of conduction in the axon itself and thus abnormal or no function through the damaged nerves.

The course of multiple sclerosis is unpredictable. Exacerbations and remissions of neurologic symptoms are the general rule, except in the later-onset type, which generally shows a gradually progressive course. The patient with multiple sclerosis can never be sure when an exacerbation or a remission will occur. In addition, the patient cannot predict the duration of either an exacerbation or remission.

Anesthetic Considerations

Studies to determine the effects of anesthesia on the course of a patient's multiple sclerosis have been extremely difficult to interpret because of the random exacerbations and remissions of the disease. In addition, it is hard to separate the effects of surgery on the disease course from the effects of the anesthetic. However, certain patterns have emerged from the numerous studies performed to date:

1. Most surgical procedures in and of themselves do not appear to have any effect on multiple sclerosis, with the exception of genitourinary surgery, which does increase the likelihood of an exacerbation.
2. General anesthesia does not increase progression of the disease nor the risk of an exacerbation.
3. There is a slightly increased risk of causing exacerbation by performing spinal anesthesia in an affected patient.
4. Local nerve blocks do not increase the chance of exacerbation.
5. Elevated body temperature should be avoided, since increased temperature raises the likelihood of further nerve slowing or conduction block and can exacerbate the disease. Postoperative infection and fever should be treated aggressively.

Multiple sclerosis usually does not affect the patient's cardiopulmonary status and therefore is not a major consideration in performing anesthesia. Most patients with multiple sclerosis are not taking any medication for the disease itself, and thus concurrent drug therapy is rarely an issue. Baclofen (Lioresal) is sometimes used for neurogenic bladder but should not pose a risk of interaction with the anesthetic. Patients with increased spasticity may take dantrolene. In such patients, the use of a non-depolarizing neuromuscular blocking drug titrated to effect with the use of a nerve stimulator is acceptable. Succinylcholine should be avoided because of the unpredictable potential for a hyperkalemic response.

Parkinson's Syndrome

Parkinson's syndrome is a disease of unknown etiology occurring generally between the sixth and eighth decade of life, equally frequently in males and females. The disease is characterized by a slow-resting tremor (generally of the pill-rolling type), bradykinesia, rigidity, a slow festinating gait, and expressionless facies. It may present with a unilateral tremor or rigidity. Even with treatment the disease is relentless, causing disability secondary to rigidity and bradykinesia in addition to tremendous ambulatory difficulty. There is no hereditary component identified. The etiology is unknown, but pathologically there is a loss of dopamine cell bodies in the substantia nigra in the brain. The dopamine deficiency causes the clinical symptoms and signs. Treatment is designed to increase the activity of the remaining dopaminergic cells in the substantia nigra. This is accomplished in three ways:

1. Oral administration of a dopamine precursor (L-dopa) such that there is an increased concentration of dopamine in the substantia nigra.
2. Oral administration of a medication such as bromocriptine, which increases the dopamine receptor activity in the substantia nigra. Other such medications used occasionally are trihexyphenidyl hydrochloride (Artane) and amantadine, but these are less effective.
3. Oral administration of a newer drug, Deprenyl (Selegiline), which works by inhibiting the enzymes that break down dopamine in the substantia nigra.

Anesthetic Considerations

Parkinson's syndrome does not affect respiratory or cardiac function. Patients receiving L-dopa, which sensitizes the cardiovascular system, have an increased risk or perioperative arrthythmias. Nevertheless, medication should be continued throughout the perioperative period. Patients receiving long-term L-dopa therapy have a tendency to autonomic instability and blood pressure fluctuations, and special attention should be directed to monitoring venous and arterial pressures, sometimes necessitating use of invasive techniques. Phenothiazines and butyrophenones should be avoided in these patients, since their dopamine blocking properties may exacerbate parkinsonism.

Transplantation therapy for Parkinson's syndrome remains highly experimental, but the tantalizing successes reported to date appear to herald an entirely new era in the treatment of this disorder.

Seizure Disorders

Seizures, which affect approximately 1% of the population in the United States, exist in numerous forms. The most commonly appreciated are generalized tonic-clonic seizures consisting of rhythmic jerking of all four extremities with occasional associated tongue biting and urinary incontinence. Absence seizures (petit mal) are also generalized seizures involving seconds of brief staring. Other common seizures, such as complex partial seizures, cause their abnormal effects on the basis of where the focus of aberrant electric discharge is located in the brain. Since a seizure results from an abnormal electrical discharge in the brain, the different seizure types can be distinguished clinically in many instances by determining exactly what the abnormal paroxysmal activity is. Most generalized seizures are idiopathic, but many partial seizures are secondary to an irritative phenomenon in the brain, such as a tumor, stroke, or previous trauma.

Anesthetic Considerations

Patients with seizure disorders have no particular cardiopulmonary dysfunction. The anesthesiologist need not be concerned about a seizure if the patient is under general anesthesia. General anesthesia is, in fact, an uncommonly employed treatment for status epilepticus. A patient with a seizure disorder has no increased risk of having a seizure under regional anesthesia.

The main concern of an anesthesiologist caring for a patient with seizures is knowledge of the anticonvulsive medications being used, their possible effect on the patient's cardiopulmonary status, and the potential for interaction with the anesthetic employed. Dilantin, phenobarbital, primidone, carbamazepine (Tegretol), valproic acid, and ethosuximide (Zarontin) are the anticonvulsants most frequently used today. Apart from Dilantin, use of which by rapid injection has resulted in respiratory arrest, hypotension, and death both in and out of the operating room, it is unlikely any of the other agents will be administered during general anesthesia. Patients receiving Dilantin or Tegretol have an increased requirement for nondepolarizing relaxants, and titration with the aid of a nerve stimulator is advised.

Alzheimer's Disease

Alzheimer's disease is a neurodegenerative affliction that causes a gradual decline in cognitive functioning. Clinically it has become a diagnosis of exclusion; however, with a characteristic history, a normal spinal fluid examination, and no evidence of toxic-metabolic cause, the diagnosis can probably be made accurately 95% of the time. A short-term memory dysfunction is the usual initial clinical complaint, but variations do exist, with language dysfunction occasionally the sentinel event. The clinical examination of a patient with Alzheimer's disease is generally normal, with the exception of abnormal frontal-lobe release signs such as grasp, sucking, and snout reflexes.

The course of the disease is progressive dementia without remission or improvement. No medications or treatments have been effective in either treating the disease or stopping its progress. Pathologically, abnormal proteins are seen in the form of plaques and neurofibrillary tangles. Most commonly these are seen first in the hippocampal area (accounting for memory loss), but with evolution of the disease these tangles and plaques are found diffusely in the gray matter throughout the brain. The etiology of Alzheimer's disease is unknown, although a deficiency in acetylcholine and enzymes involved in its production have been reported.

Anesthetic Considerations

Alzheimer's disease does not affect the cardiac or pulmonary systems. No medicines are used at present to treat Alzheimer's disease. Regardless of the surgical procedure or the anesthetic used, it is common to have a cognitive deterioration after surgery. Patients with Alzheimer's disease frequently decompensate with any systemic insult. Frequently, in hospitalized patients, an acute deterioration in mental status is seen in conjunction with a urinary tract infection or mild bronchitis. Therefore, it is expected that after administration of any anesthetic, whether general or regional, decompensation may occur, and this must be discussed candidly and frankly with the patient's family.

Migraine Headaches

Although statistics vary, approximately 20% of the population of the United States have a migraine headache sometime during their lives. For simplicity, migraine headaches are frequently divided into two types: classic and common.

Classic migraines usually start with an aura, most commonly scintillating scotomata (lightning-like flashing lights in the eyes), numbness or tingling in an arm or leg, or a general feeling of being unwell. The headache thereafter is no different in classic migraines from that in common migraines. The headaches are frequently unilateral but may be bilateral, bifrontal, holocephalic, or occipital. The hoary adage that a migraine is unilateral is no longer considered valid. Associated with the headache, which generally lasts from 2 to 6 hours but can last as long as 24 hours, are photophobia, phonophobia, nausea, and occasional vomiting. Diarrhea is seen in approximately 10% of patients.

A family history is common in migraines, and approximately 35% of patients have a first-degree relative with the same affliction. In children, migraines are found equally in males and females, but after puberty, migraines are significantly more common in women. Menstrual migraines are a common phenomenon and are extremely difficult to control medically. Usually as patients approach their 40s and 50s the frequency, duration, and severity of their migraines diminish. The pathophysiology of migraines is unknown. Multiple theories exist as to the involvement of serotonin receptors, increased release of substance P, extrinsic neuromuscular system causation, and the like, but thus far no exact mechanism has been elucidated.

Anesthetic Considerations

Migraines do not cause any cardiac or pulmonary dysfunction. The major consideration in providing anesthesia to a migraine patient is to determine whether that patient is taking any medications for migraines. Migraines are treated medically in three separate ways: general analgesics at the time of the headache; ergotamines at the onset of the headache to prevent pain; and prophylactic drugs that are taken daily to prevent the episodic migraine. The former two types of medicines are not an important consideration for the anesthesiologist, but the latter is.

Propranolol (Inderal) is the most common prophylactic medicine employed. It is a beta-blocker and the presumed mechanism in migraine is as a serotonin receptor antagonist. Calcium-channel antagonists such as verapamil are rapidly becoming a staple in the prophylactic treatment of migraines. It is not known whether their action in blocking calcium entry into cells or their action in inhibiting platelet release or some other mechanism produces their effect on migraines. In any event, the anesthesiologist should continue the preoperative prophylactic drug regimen throughout the perioperative period.

Suggested Reading

Hyman SA, et al. Perioperative management for transplant of autologous adrenal medulla to the brain for Parkinsonism. Anesthesiology 1988; 69:618.

Jones RM. Anaesthesia and demyelinating disease. Anaesthesia 1980; 35:879.

Leventhal SR, et al. Prediction of the need for postoperative mechanical ventilation in myasthenia gravis. Anesthesiology 1980; 53:26.

Ngai SH. Levodopa treatment and anesthesia for patients with Parkinsonism. Anesthesiology 1972; 37:344.

Richards WC. Anaesthesia and serum creatinine phosphokinase levels in patients with Duchenne pseudohypertrophic muscular dystrophy. Anaesth Intens Care 1972; 1:150.

Rosenbaum KJ, et al. Sensitivity to nondepolarizing muscle relaxants in amyotrophic lateral sclerosis: report of two cases. Anesthesiology 1971; 35:638.

Stirt JA, et al. Atracurium in a child with myotonic dystrophy. Anesth Analg 1985; 64:369.

C. Morgan Cooper, M.D., and David J. Stone, M.D.

Anesthesia for Head Trauma   16

Overview

Incidence

One of every 12 deaths in the United States results directly from head trauma. Approximately 50% of these are the result of motor vehicle accidents, and roughly two-thirds of those involved are alcohol-impaired. More than 50% of all patients with motor vehicle–associated head trauma die before arriving in the emergency room. Males are involved 2.5 times more often than females, and the peak incidence is during the late teens and early twenties. Falls, firearm assaults, and sports-related injuries also commonly contribute to head trauma, with an overall prehospital mortality of approximately 15%.

Outcome

Outcome studies of head-injured patients have been extremely difficult to analyze given the many variables involved, such as type of injury, associated injuries, and type of therapy administered. Patient outcome has been categorized into five groups by Jennett and Bond:

> Group 1: good recovery
> Group 2: moderate disability
> Group 3: severe disability
> Group 4: persistent vegetative state
> Group 5: death

Classification of head trauma patients in the emergency room based on the Glasgow Coma Scale (Table 16-1) is shown in Table 16-2. Of the roughly 400,000 annual hospital admissions for head trauma, 80% are mild, 10% moderate, and 10% severe (Table 16-2). In one series, all patients with mild head injuries were discharged alive; 93% of the moderate group and 42% of the severe group were also discharged alive. The in-hospital mortality rate for severe head trauma approximates 40%, secondary complications being the major cause of death. Although there is evidence that a vigorous approach in the

Table 16-1 The Glasgow Coma Scale

Activity	Qualification	Response	Score
Eyes	Open	Spontaneously	4
		To verbal command	3
		To pain	2
	No response		1
Best motor response	To verbal command	Obeys	6
	To painful stimulus	Localizes pain	5
		Flexion-withdrawal	4
		Flexion-abnormal (Decorticate rigidity)	3
		Extension (Decerebrate rigidity)	2
		No response	1
Best verbal response		Oriented and converses	5
		Disoriented and converses	4
		Inappropriate words	3
		Incomprehensible sounds	2
		No response	1

From Teasdale G, Jennett B. Assessment of coma and impaired consciousness. Lancet 1974;2:81. Reproduced with permission.

Table 16-2 Classification and Incidence of Head Trauma

Classification	Glasgow Coma Scale Score	Incidence (%)
Mild	13-15	80
Moderate	8-12	10
Severe	0-7	10

treatment of head-injured patients can influence recovery, the major improvement in the morbidity and mortality due to head injuries has come not from improved medical care, but from mandatory seat-belt and helmet legislation.

The Glasgow Coma Scale (GCS) is a valuable, reproducible tool in quantifying and predicting outcome in head-injured patients, especially those with scores of 8 to 15 and 0 to 4. An overview of several studies suggests a 95% confidence level of favorable outcome when the GCS score is greater than 8, and 95% confidence level of an unfavorable outcome when the score is less than 5. The predictive value of the GCS is less accurate in the middle scores. Other variables such as pupillary reactivity, brainstem function, vital signs, hematocrit, age, and type of injury can be used as a basis for predicting outcome. Comparative analysis of clinical signs, CT scanning, evoked potentials, and intracranial pressure monitoring suggests that the clinical examination remains the strongest basis for prognosticating outcome in severe head injury. Prognostication for the individual patient remains uncertain, however.

Initial Assessment

Two major factors associated with the majority of severe head injuries are hypoxia and hypovolemia (shock). These complications are most often associated with a bad outcome and should be initially addressed in the field.

Hypoxemia is defined as a PaO_2 less than 60 mm Hg. Patients with altered states of consciousness have difficulty maintaining and protecting their airway. Respiratory obstruction is the primary cause of death in 15% of these patients. Hypoxemia may be worsened by airway obstruction, aspiration, pneumo- and/or hemothorax, lung contusion, or neurogenic pulmonary edema associated with head trauma.

Shock is defined as a systolic blood pressure of less than 90 mm Hg. Decreased blood pressure in the face of increased intracranial pressure (ICP) and hypoxia results in a significant reduction in the delivery of oxygen to the brain cells (because cerebral perfusion pressure [CPP] equals mean arterial pressure [MAP] minus ICP). Systemic hypotension is rarely due to brain injury alone, except as a terminal event. The normal CPP is around 80 to 90 mm Hg. When CPP falls below 40 mm Hg, ischemia may develop.

Primary Versus Secondary Injury

The primary injury to the brain occurs at the time of injury. Damage results from the direct disruption of structures within the cranium, such as arteries, veins, and white and gray matter. Closed-head injuries usually involve the shearing of white matter with injury to the axons and dendrites.

Secondary injury probably begins at the time of the initial insult, although its impact is not immediately apparent. The factors contributing to secondary injury include tissue hypoxia, lactic acidosis, hypercapnea, and elevation of ICP with possible herniation.

Four mechanisms appear to contribute to brain damage in the head-injured patient: (1) mechanical injury, (2) hemorrhage, (3) edema, and (4) ischemia. It is the last two that are of concern to the anesthesiologist. Ischemia is the final common pathway resulting in injury. Most ischemia is the result of compression from an extra- or intracerebral hematoma, or from diffuse brain swelling, resulting in elevation of ICP. Recent studies of elevations in ICP suggest that there is a point at which brain swelling becomes irreversible (around 60 mm Hg) and that the ability to control brain edema physiologically and pharmacologically correlates with this initial opening pressure. The loss of vasomotor regulatory mechanisms probably accounts for this finding.

Neurologic Assessment

History

During the initial evaluation, information about time, location, and mechanism of injury should be gathered. Occasionally the underlying cause of the trauma may be missed, such as a stroke, seizure, arrhythmia, or drug-related loss of consciousness prior to the accident. The patient's level of consciousness is the single most important clinical sign in the assessment of the severity of head injury, and this should be noted at the scene immediately following the accident.

Glasgow Coma Scale Score and Intracranial Hypertension

As previously mentioned, the GCS score correlates well with the severity of injury and outcome. Of the three components of the score, the motor response is the most sensitive. The accuracy of the GCS score is affected by intoxication, hypoxia, a postictal state, other drugs, and most important, shock. Signs or symptoms of intracranial hypertension are of special importance to the anesthesiologist. These include papilledema, asymmetric pupils, nausea, vomiting, headache, tinnitus, and visual symptoms.

Head Examination

Obvious injuries to the scalp, lacerations, and palpable depressed skull fractures with a "fall off" sign may be noted. Hemotympanum, ecchymosis over the mastoid area (Battle's sign), and periorbital edema are highly suggestive of a basilar skull fracture. Drainage of cerebrospinal fluid (CSF) from the nares should be suspected. This can be investigated by using a paper test-strip for glucose or the classic "double ring" sign on a piece of blotter paper. The glucose test is of little value because it may give a positive reaction with as little as 5 mg/dl glucose concentration and is positive in 75% of patients with normal nasal secretions.

Neck Examination

In most severe head injuries resulting from motor vehicle accidents there is associated neck injury. Almost 20% of persons killed in vehicular accidents had isolated upper cervical spine injuries. Fractures of the cervical spine usually occur at the C1-C2 or C5-C6 vertebrae. All suspected cervical spine injuries should be carefully immobilized, preventing extension, rotation, or flexion until a thorough physical and radiologic examination has occurred. Spinal trauma may not become apparent until the patient's cerebral insult begins to clear.

Types of Injuries

Injuries to the Brain Coverings

Any depressed skull fracture under a laceration should be considered an open fracture and treated appropriately. For the anesthesiologist this is significant, because it is important that any bony fragments not be manipulated except in the operating room. Any fragment, like any penetrating foreign body, could well be serving to tamponade a ruptured artery or vein. Therefore, great care must be taken when managing the airway or placing an endotracheal tube.

Signs of a basilar skull fracture are important to the anesthesiologist. Look for hemotympanum, otorrhea, ecchymosis over the mastoid area (Battle's sign), and ecchymosis around the eyes without extension beyond the orbit (raccoon eyes). Nasal intubation in patients suspected of having a basilar skull fracture is relatively contraindicated because of the significantly increased likelihood of seeding the CSF with bacteria, which causes infection, and because of the risk of inadvertently placing the tip of the endotracheal tube into the cranium. If the patient cannot be intubated orally, the clinician must make a judgment as to whether nasal intubation has more or less risk than cricothyroidotomy or tracheostomy.

Penetrating Brain Injury and Traumatic Intracranial Hematoma

Epidural Hematoma

Epidural hematomas are most often caused by disruption of the middle meningeal artery or its branches because of fracturing of the temporal bone. Traumatic epidural hematoma occurs in about 1 to 2% of head injuries and is usually associated with automobile accidents. Ninety percent of epidural hematomas are associated with skull fractures discovered at the time of surgery. It is not until adulthood that the middle meningeal artery becomes secured in its bony groove, and this is probably why epidural hematomas are infrequent in children.

Another cause of epidural hematoma is disruption of a venous sinus. In this case, epidural hematoma is more slowly progressive, usually becoming apparent a few days after the original injury.

The classic textbook description of a patient with an epidural hematoma is a transient loss of consciousness, followed by a return to a lucid interval and a normal neurologic examination. This then proceeds to complaints of increasing headache, decreasing consciousness, and finally the sequelae resulting from intracranial hypertension and impending herniation, including signs of dilatation of the ipsilateral pupil from third-nerve palsy and contralateral extremity weakness and decerebration. Often these patients are functionally hypovolemic from being NPO, having had an osmotic load from a dye study, mannitol, or both. Some patients with elevations in ICP may develop a rise in systolic blood pressure (Cushing's response). Induction of anesthesia may add insult to injury with hypertension or hypotension and resultant ischemia.

Subdural Hematoma

Subdural hematomas (SDH) are usually classified as acute, subacute, and chronic.

Acute Subdural Hematoma. The most common cause of SDH is trauma. The collection of blood between the dura and subarachnoid membranes is considered acute when it becomes clinically significant within 72 hours from the time of initial injury. Acute SDH is the most common intracranial hematoma to require surgical removal. The classic presentation of an acute SDH is that of unconsciousness without a lucid period and associated signs of a mass lesion that causes intracranial hypertension. A simple SDH is usually the result of a rupture of the bridging veins to the sagittal sinus following an acceleration-deceleration injury. Complicated SDH is associated with an underlying cerebral contusion or lacerations, and this type is far more serious. The mortality rate is more than 50% when SDH is bilateral or when multiple lacerations are present. The subdural space allows for a larger spread of hematoma, and although it may appear less significant on CT scan, it can occupy a volume that reduces intracranial compliance. Early evacuation of the mass is advocated, because half of the patients will experience significant intracranial hypertension. Most patients should have ICP monitoring and receive appropriate medical therapy.

Subacute Subdural Hematoma. Subacute SDH is one that manifests clinically between 3 and 15 days after the initial injury.

Chronic Subdural Hematoma. Defined as a hematoma of greater than 2 weeks duration, a chronic SDH is usually seen in alcoholics, epileptics, and the elderly. The mechanism is thought to be leakage from disrupted capillary endothelium or rehemorrhage of the thin-walled vessels of the subdural membrane. A history of head trauma is often absent. The clinical presentation varies from a mild organic brain dysfunction to focal signs. Diagnosis is made by CT scan. Treatment can be as simple as a needle aspiration under local anesthesia or as complex as craniotomy for removal of a solid clot. Surgical intervention may not be required.

Intracerebral Hematoma

This relatively uncommon form of bleeding is seen with coup and contrecoup injuries. Gunshot wounds to the head often cause this type of bleeding. The associated tissue damage from the high pressure wave generated upon impact may be devastating, and ICP may climb transiently to 2,000 to 3,000 mm Hg. Large hematomas and delayed intracerebral hematomas should be removed surgically; however, small, multiple hematomas are not amenable to surgical evacuation. The presence of intracerebral hematomas can be detected with ICP monitoring, since the rise in ICP usually precedes neurologic changes seen on examination.

Associated Injuries

Between 35 and 50% of patients with severe head injuries have associated life-threatening multisystem trauma. A scalp laceration alone may bleed enough to produce hypovolemia, especially in children. Since the majority of cases of severe head trauma are associated with motor vehicle accidents, injuries may include cervical spine injury from the head hitting the windshield or dashboard; pulmonary or cardiac contusions; pneumothorax; hemothorax; aortic disruption and cardiac tamponade from impact upon the steering column; and lumbar spine injury, splenic injury, and retroperitoneal bleeding from seat-belt impaction. Aspiration of vomitus and blood is also common. These are discussed in detail in Chapter 18.

Early Management

Initial care of the head-injured patient involves addressing any associated life-threatening injuries such as those mentioned above. The patient must be stabilized prior to undertaking diagnostic studies such as CT scan, radiography, arteriography. Laboratory tests to be completed prior to surgery include hemoglobin, hematocrit, blood chemistry, arterial blood gas, coagulation profile with platelets, and a toxicology screen. Cross-matched blood should be in the operating room ready for use if needed.

Airway

Providing an airway is one of the most important functions served by the anesthesiologist. The tongue is the most frequent cause of obstruction. This may be the result of relaxation of the intrinsic muscular structures of the oropharynx or secondary to a bimandibular fracture with loss of support and posterior displacement. Inability to open the mouth may be caused by muscle spasm associated with focal trauma or by temporomandibular joint (TMJ) dislocation. Spasm will disappear with neuromuscular blockade but if the TMJ is involved, awake intubation is required. If the patient is combative, uncooperative, anxious, or incoherent, hypoxia should be the first concern. Simple maneuvers including jaw thrust, placement of a nasopharyngeal airway, or the simple removal of vomitus or other debris may be enough to provide a patent airway. Of special concern to the anesthesiologist is an associated cervical spine injury. The seventh cervical vertebrae must be seen on the cross-table x-ray film in order to ensure completeness in evaluating plain films. Cervical spine injuries should be assumed in any patient who is unconscious or has fallen from a height of 10 feet or greater. Airway management of the spinal-cord-injured patient is discussed in Chapter 12.

Any patient who is apneic, unconscious, or with signs of deterioration should be intubated. Almost 75% of seriously head-injured patients are hypoxic. Hypoxia is prevented by the administration of oxygen (50 to 100%), and hypercarbia is avoided by hyperventilation. These requirements are facilitated by the placement of an endotracheal tube, which also allows for protection of the airway and reduces the chance of aspiration. Although there will be a rise in ICP with laryngoscopy and intubation, this concern forms a lower priority than treatment of hypoxia and hypercapnea. Much of the secondary injury to the brain is caused by poor ventilation. When the PaO_2 is lower than 50 mm Hg, or when the $PaCO_2$ is greater than 50 mm Hg, there are increases in cerebral blood flow (CBF), cerebral blood volume (CBV), and ICP. Intubation of the patient with head injury should be performed with the patient properly anesthetized, if possible. The inexperienced trainee should solicit more senior back-up for such intubations outside the operating room. The details of anesthetic induction and intubation are found in the section on induction of anesthesia later in this chapter.

Many patients with head trauma spontaneously hyperventilate, because of the presence of elevated catecholamines, hypoxic drive, and the central effect caused by intracerebral acidosis, which is created by the brain lesion itself. It has been reported that small changes in the pH of CSF of 0.1 are enough to cause apnea or hyperventilation, depending on the direction of the change. This fact alone leads many practitioners to intubate their patients electively so that the airway and ventilation can be controlled during potentially compromising situations, such as CT scan of the head. For these reasons, some clinicians maintain that all patients with a GCS score less than 8 should be intubated. Additional criteria for intubation (when available) are listed below:

1. Irregular respirations
2. Respiration rate < 10 or >40 per minute
3. V_T (tidal volume) <3.5 ml/kg
4. VC (vital capacity) <15 ml/kg
5. PaO_2 <70 mm Hg
6. $PaCO_2$ >50 mm Hg

The lowering of $PaCO_2$ by controlled hyperventilation is the fastest way to raise CSF pH. This is because CO_2 diffuses rapidly across the blood-brain barrier and is then trapped in its ionized form. The ICP-reducing effects of hyperventilation are discussed in Chapter 2. Local "inverse steal" induced by hyperventilation in head-injured patients, resulting in increased blood flow to injured areas, remains a controversial area requiring more study. In neural tissue in which autoregulation is preserved, the extracellular alkalosis caused by hypocapnea directly affects vascular smooth muscle, causing constriction of cerebral resistance arterioles. Normalization of CSF pH occurs after several hours, although the release of acid metabolites from damaged tissue continues as long as focal ischemia and tissue hypoxia are present. Moderate hyperventilation to a $PaCO_2$ of 25 to 30 mm Hg is the standard of care in most cases.

Once the airway has been controlled, small doses of fentanyl (50 to 100 μg) may be used to attenuate the hypercatecholamine, central hyperventilatory state.

Positive end-expiratory pressure may be used judiciously with the patient in a 15- to 30-degree head-up position as long as ICP is being monitored. Improving oxygenation may result in a lowering of ICP.

Cardiovascular Volume Status

Prehospital shock occurs in one-third of patients sustaining severe head trauma. Acute hypotension must be treated with volume replacement. Lactated Ringer's or a balanced isotonic salt solution may be used to correct hypovolemia. The administration of free water should be avoided in order to minimize cerebral edema associated with hyponatremia. Military antishock trousers (MAST) can be used to support the circulation without increasing ICP and will support the patient until more definitive therapy is initiated at the hospital. The use of the head-down Trendelenburg position to maintain blood pressure is to be avoided, since this will cause an unacceptable amount of cerebral edema and an elevation of ICP.

Osmotherapy

It is now generally accepted that increases in intracranial hypertension are associated with increased mortality. For this reason, individuals with an increase in ICP above 20 mm Hg or severely head-injured patients who are unconscious require osmotherapy. Some authors feel that diuretics should not be used unless ICP monitoring is in place. In the United States, mannitol and furosemide are the mainstays of therapy. Along with hyperventilation, osmotherapy gives the neurosurgeon time to perform essential diagnostic studies. One caveat in the use of mannitol is with children. Often, the lesion in a head-injured child is not amenable to surgical correction and is caused by a swollen, hyperemic brain. Therefore, many centers advise against the use of mannitol unless the presence of an epidural hematoma is suspected. The dosing and mechanisms of action of mannitol and furosemide are discussed later in this chapter.

Indications for Monitoring Intracranial Pressure

Monitoring of ICP should be applied in all patients who have a GCS score of 7 or less after resuscitation. ICP should be monitored as soon as possible after the injury, especially in adult patients with no eye opening, no verbal response, and nonpurposeful motor movements. The presence of compressed ventricles on CT scan also suggests intracranial hypertension. All patients who undergo surgery for head injury and show signs of swelling and edema should be monitored postoperatively. It is important to note that in the unconscious patient, early changes in ICP may not be reflected in the physical examination, and an elevation in ICP may occur with or without a surgical lesion. ICP monitoring is also important in order to verify the results of other therapies, such as barbiturates or muscle relaxation, since traditional findings in the physical examination may be lacking.

Diagnostic Studies

X-ray Studies

Plain skull films are of limited value in any patient with a GCS score less than 8. In a patient who has a lucid interval followed by deterioration, the finding of a linear skull fracture on plain film may suggest an ipsilateral epidural hematoma. When deterioration occurs, this line can be used as the site to define the location of surgical craniotomy. There is a 17 to 20% incidence of cervical spine fractures in the severely injured group; therefore, cervical spine films from C1 to the top of T1 should be completed before any manipulation of the neck is attempted. A chest film should also be completed preoperatively to screen for significant injury to structures within the thorax and the possibility of hemo- and/or pneumothorax.

Computed Tomography

The CT scan is the most important diagnostic test that can be performed on the head-injured patient. It is the initial procedure of choice in evaluating intracranial mass lesions, and its use has greatly helped in differentiating surgical from nonsurgical lesions. Patient care must be assigned and responsibility shifted appropriately so that the patient is not placed in the radiology department without proper attention.

Arteriography

When a CT scanner is not available, the next diagnostic method of choice is arteriography, which helps to delineate the vascular pathology. Some clinicians have stated that any patient in a deep coma or with signs of clinical deterioration and a focal neurologic finding should have arteriography performed in addition to a CT scan.

Magnetic Resonance Imaging

Magnetic resonance imaging (MRI) appears to be more sensitive than CT in the diagnosis of contusions and residual parenchymal shearing-type injuries after head trauma. There have been practical problems with the use of metallic instruments and monitors placed in a strong magnetic field and the interference these devices may cause in distorting the image. Because of the excessive amount of time required to complete an MRI study, CT scanning is still the radiographic method of greatest value in the initial evaluation for the head-injured patient.

Anesthetic Management

Premedication

The head-injured patient generally needs no premedication for the purpose of sedation. The effect of increasing $PaCO_2$ is undesirable, and controlled ventilation is required if respiratory depressants are given.

Glycopyrrolate (0.2 mg IV) may be given for its effect on drying secretions. It is preferred over atropine for its longer duration of action and minimal cardiac effects. Metoclopramide (10 mg IV) can also be administered to help gastrointestinal motility, although its effects are diminished when used in the presence of an anticholinergic. If the patient is cooperative and has intact protective airway reflexes, a standard Bicitra or Shohl's solution should be given PO in order to reduce the risks of pulmonary complications, should aspiration occur. An H_2-blocker such as ranitidine (50 mg IV drip) may also be helpful if surgery might be delayed because of diagnostic testing. H_2-blocking drugs have no effect on the preexisting acidic contents of the stomach, and therefore their protective benefits may not be realized at the time of induction.

Monitoring

Routine monitors should be used. This includes electrocardiography, pulse oximetry, precordial or esophageal stethoscope, temperature monitor, urinary catheter, and blood pressure cuff. In addition, direct arterial blood pressure monitoring and measurement of end-tidal CO_2 are recommended. The arterial line is placed prior to induction, and blood pressure is transduced at the level of the external auditory meatus in order to track CPP. Central venous pressure (CVP) or pulmonary artery catheters may be used if there is a question about fluid or cardiovascular status. A long-arm CVP can often be placed rapidly, although exact positioning may be difficult. Special catheters are available for treatment of air embolism when it is a potential problem. We do not use them routinely for head-trauma patients unless a venous sinus has been disrupted or the operative site is significantly above the level of the heart (i.e., surgery is performed in the sitting position). If a trauma patient is to be operated on in the seated position, a precordial Doppler is also used. Blood samples are taken frequently from the arterial line to verify the reading of the end-tidal CO_2 monitor and to follow electrolyte and osmolarity shifts resulting from diuretic therapy. ICP monitoring may be used preoperatively, although in our institution, ICP monitors are usually placed at the end of the operative procedure to monitor pressures postoperatively.

Anesthesia Induction

The ideal induction of anesthesia should avoid swings in blood pressure or elevation of ICP. The cerebral effects of anesthetic and neuromuscular blocking agents are described in Chapter 3.

In preparation for anesthesia induction, painful maneuvers should be minimized (e.g., suctioning of the endotracheal tube, manipulation of traumatized areas). Coughing, bucking, and straining are undesirable, since they may aggravate an already hypersympathetic state and cause an elevation in blood pressure, brain bulk, ICP and increase the risk for catastrophic herniation.

Positioning of the head in a neutral supine position and avoidance of any position that limits venous return (e.g., extreme flexion or rotation of the head) help prevent decreases in CPP, since the effect of raising or lowering the head is unpredictable.

After the application of all appropriate monitors the patient is preoxygenated to 100% saturation and, if able, is directed to hyperventilate. In most circumstances, thiopental is the induction agent of choice, given its ability to reduce CBF and ICP secondary to its rapid vasoconstrictive effect. Small repeated doses may be carefully administered, while cricoid pressure is maintained, remembering that the head-injured patient is likely to be hypovolemic.

Etomidate, an imidazole derivative, appears to be a suitable alternative to thiopental. An induction dose of 0.2 to 0.4 mg/kg IV provides rapid onset of action while providing cardiovascular stability and the absence of histamine release. CBF, $CMRO_2$, and ICP are all lowered while CPP is maintained. Because etomidate lacks analgesic properties, the concomitant use of a narcotic such as fentanyl is indicated.

Lidocaine (1.5 mg/kg) may be given 1 to 3 minutes before intubation in order to blunt changes in blood pressure and ICP.

Narcotics may be used to help smooth induction; given with thiopental in reduced amounts, cardiovascular stability is maintained. Fentanyl (1 to 4 μg/kg) given 3 to 4 minutes prior to laryngoscopy may accomplish this. If intracranial hypertension is present, morphine, sufentanil, and alfentanyl are less desirable than fentanyl because of possible cerebrovasodilation.

Ketamine is relatively contraindicated because of its tendency to increase CBF and ICP and inability to lower $CMRO_2$.

A rapid-sequence induction using lidocaine, a low dose of fentanyl and a carefully chosen dose of thiopental are probably optimal in most patients unless there is severe cardiovascular compromise.

Vecuronium may be the relaxant of choice because of its cardiovascular stability and minimal effects on ICP. The combination of vecuronium and fentanyl may result in bradycardia. Historically, pancuronium has been used because of its ability to maintain CPP, offsetting the depressant effects of thiopental. However, in patients with intracranial pathology and defective autoregulation, large increases in CBF and ICP might be expected to follow pancuronium-induced hypertension. Agents releasing histamine, such as curare, metocurine, and extremely large doses of atracurium, should be avoided if possible. Atracurium also yields a metabolite, laudanosine, which readily crosses the blood-brain barrier and can cause seizures in animals. Its clinical relevance in humans remains unproven.

The use of succinylcholine has been controversial. It has been shown that succinylcholine causes an increase in muscle spindle activity resulting in increased cerebral afferent input. Increases in CBF, ICP, and $PaCO_2$ as well as electroencephalographic arousal may then occur. A defasciculating dose of metocurine (0.03 mg/kg) has been shown to block this effect completely in humans, yet the use of pancuronium in animals has had no effect. There have also been case reports of hyperkalemia associated with the use of succinylcholine in the head-injured patient. One could argue that the benefits of adequate relaxation for a rapid-sequence intubation in a patient with a full stomach outweigh these reported risks. The use of succinylcholine in the acutely injured patient remains a matter of balancing risks.

Maintenance

The ideal anesthetic technique for the patient with multisystem trauma should be one that has the least effect on cerebral autoregulation and CO_2 responsiveness, while maintaining cardiovascular stability. It should also lower ICP, thereby increasing CPP. Often after head injury, the cerebral autoregulatory mechanisms are disrupted. This renders the patient vulnerable to cerebral edema and hyperemia as a result of increases in mean arterial pressure from surgical stimulation. One of the primary goals of anesthesia is to minimize this response. At our institution, an intravenous technique has generally been used. Narcotics, barbiturates, and benzodiazepines all have the effect of lowering CBF, $CMRO_2$, and ICP. A residual narcotic effect may be beneficial in the postoperative management of the severely injured patient requiring continued hyperventilation.

Anesthetic technique may depend on the type of injury. For example, hyperventilating a patient with elevated ICP, who also has areas of focal cerebral ischemia secondary to vasoconstriction, may be unwise. Titration of ventilation may be enhanced by measuring the difference between arterial and jugular venous bulb oxygen content ($AJDO_2$) as follows:

$$AJDO_2 = \frac{CMRO_2}{CBF}$$

This measurement reflects the balance between supply and demand. The normal oxygen content of venous blood returning from the brain is approximately 13 to 14 vol% compared with the arterial value of 20 vol%. The normal oxygen gradient is therefore 6 to 7 vol%. A narrow $AJDO_2$ gradient ($<$10 vol%) suggests that blood flow to the brain is adequate and the use of barbiturates and hyperventilation to control ICP is appropriate. In the patient with blunt trauma and a wide $AJDO_2$ ($>$10 vol%), brain ischemia may be better served with drugs that improve blood flow and help to reduce $CMRO_2$. Isoflurane, in a dose below 1 MAC, may be added to help improve brain ischemia by enhancing blood flow.

Jugular oxygen content is measured through a small catheter placed in the jugular venous bulb connected to a pressurized, heparinized flush system. Intermittent sampling of jugular venous blood allows for the above calculations. This monitoring technique is not current standard practice at most trauma centers and its use is yet not fully defined.

The use of nitrous oxide remains controversial. Past practice has accepted adding a mixture of N_2O after hyperventilation had been initiated and the $PaCO_2$ lowered to 25 to 30 mm Hg. Nitrous oxide administered after doses of thiopental and narcotic usually has minimal deleterious effects on ICP. The cerebrovascular-dilating effects of N_2O appear to be blunted by the vasomotor tone previously generated by the intravenous agents and by hyperventilation. Concerns of tension pneumocephalus and elevations in ICP from direct vasodilation have led some centers to avoid any use of N_2O, an approach that is gaining wide acceptance.

All volatile agents abolish cerebral autoregulation to some extent in a dose-dependent manner. Halothane is a potent cerebrovasodilator. The head-injured patient usually has high levels of circulating catecholamines and may have sustained injury to the vagus nerve. Halothane's arrhythmogenic side effects may make it a poor anesthetic choice. Enflurane, also a cerebrovasodilator, has the additional problem of generating seizure-like activity in the hyperventilated patient. Isoflurane appears to be the most suitable volatile agent for the patient who sustains blunt head trauma. It does not have the problems listed above, is effective in helping to reduce $CMRO_2$, and may be beneficial in the setting of intraoperative hypertension. Cerebral vascular responsiveness to CO_2 is maintained to some degree with isoflurane so that hyperventilation will constrict vessels in uninjured areas of brain while injured areas may receive an increase in blood flow. If the injured areas are ischemic, as may occur in closed head injury, this increase in flow will be beneficial. If edema (rather than vasoconstriction) is limiting flow, vasodilation may increase the edema, limit local blood flow, and actually worsen the situation. Our current state of understanding and monitoring does not allow for such precise administration of the "right" anesthetic. However, empiric observations in patients imply that in blunt and penetrating head injury nitrous oxide has an adverse effect on outcome. In blunt head injury, the dilating effect of isoflurane may have a beneficial effect on outcome.

Patients who sustain penetrating trauma are likely to do better with the use of fentanyl and barbiturates. These patients may sustain intracranial pressures of 2,000 to 3,000 mm Hg at the time of impact, and require maintenance of cerebral vasoconstriction. A continuous narcotic infusion (e.g., fentanyl at 1 to 4 $\mu g/kg/hr$) may be used to help maintain anesthesia. It should be discontinued near the end of surgery if immediate postoperative emergence is desired. Thiopental (1 to 6 mg/min) or lidocaine (1 to 4 mg/min) may also be given by continuous infusion.

Emergence

Generally, if the patient was awake and breathing spontaneously at the beginning of a case, he should be in the same condition postoperatively. Extubation, performed in the operating room, unless mitigating circumstances dictate otherwise, requires close communication between the anesthesiologist and the surgeon. With the release of a mass lesion, consciousness should return postoperatively. Associated chest injury, facial fractures, cervical spine injury, or postoperative brain tissue swelling secondary to traumatic injury may indicate a need for continued endotracheal intubation in the intensive care unit for continued hyperventilation, airway maintenance, and airway protection. Continued hyperventilation and sedation may obscure early signs of rebleeding and other serious postoperative complications. A significant percentage of patients with severe brain injury (GCS score <8) will go on to eventually have a tracheostomy for airway management.

If continued intubation is required for transport to the intensive care unit, a small dose of narcotic and/or thiopental will help the patient tolerate the endotracheal tube. Coughing and bucking on the tube is to be avoided, and lidocaine (1.5 mg/kg) can also be used to help smooth emergence. The patient should be transported with the head of the bed flat or slightly elevated (0 to 15 degrees) and with the appropriate monitors and oxygen en route.

Adjuvant Therapy

Anticonvulsants

It has been estimated that 5% of patients with blunt head injuries and 40 to 60% of those with missile injuries suffer a seizure, and 75% of these will continue to have seizures. The incidence of epilepsy after 1 week in those suffering a depressed skull fracture may be as high as 10% and is related to post-traumatic amnesia and dural tear. Seizures within the first week after injury may also be caused by hypoxemia, electrolyte abnormalities, or bleeding. Seizures can contribute to increases in ICP and further tissue ischemia by increasing $CMRO_2$ and CBF. Prophylactic phenytoin (Dilantin), 10 to 15 mg/kg IV, may be given slowly (50 mg/min) as a loading dose and then dosed according to blood levels. Phenytoin has the added effect of reducing cerebral blood volume and may afford some degree of metabolic brain protection.

Steroids

In some centers, children with a GCS score of less than 6 and adults with scores less than 8 receive high-dose dexamethasone (1 to 1.5 mg/kg), which is then tapered after a short course. Other prospective studies have shown no benefit from steroids and describe the inherent complications associated with steroid use, with hyperglycemia the most frequent problem. Given the lack of strong evidence of improvement in head-injured patients receiving steroids, many centers have stopped this practice, and we do not use them in the head-injured patient.

Fluid Management

In the operating room, intravenous solutions of lactated Ringer's solution, normal saline, or Plasmalyte are used. No free water is given to minimize or retard the degree of cerebral edema. Sugar-containing solutions are avoided, given studies suggesting poorer outcomes when brain ischemia and high blood glucose (>150 mg/dl) conditions exist conjointly. The theoretical concern is that high glucose levels will result in increased CSF lactate production by anaerobic metabolism. The subsequent acidosis is damaging to neurons.

Initially, the patient may be hypovolemic secondary to blood loss, and this should be corrected. Once fluid resuscitation is adequate, the patient is kept slightly dehydrated, with serum sodium in the high-normal range and serum osmolality in the 295 to 315 mOsm/L range. This may result from mild fluid restriction with administration of 20 to 30 ml/kg/day. Electrolytes and serum osmolality should be monitored throughout the perioperative period.

Any significant blood loss should be replaced with blood products to avoid anemia and ischemia. The hematocrit should remain above 30%. In head-injured animal studies, a replacement of one-half blood volume with NaCl 0.9% or 5% dextrose will elevate ICP 90% and 150%, respectively. Hetastarch 6% appears to have little effect on ICP. Hetastarch has colloidal properties similar to that of human albumin. It may interfere with platelet function and may transiently prolong clotting times when doses above 30 ml/kg are given. Albumin has been used in an attempt to prevent increases in brain edema and ICP. Generally, it is excluded from the brain extravascular space unless there has been a disruption of the blood-brain barrier. When a disruption occurs, osmotic pressure gradients tend to be lost, and fluid movement into the brain becomes a function of hydrostatic pressure. A more complete discussion can be found in Chapter 6.

The insertion of a central line or pulmonary artery catheter is indicated when fluid status is in doubt. In order to avoid the risks of pneumothorax with the subclavian approach and possible disruption of carotid blood flow with an internal jugular approach, a basilic vein approach is preferred. The associated use of a head-down, Trendelenburg position to facilitate line placement is absolutely contraindicated in the head-injured patient.

Diuretics and Osmotherapy

Mannitol

Mannitol is a 6-carbon sugar that is filtered through the kidney without reabsorption in the tubules. The molecule is large enough to be unable to pass through the intact blood-brain barrier. It does not undergo metabolism and does not enter cells. In addition to increasing serum sodium by generating a large amount of hypotonic urine, administration of mannitol also increases plasma osmolarity, drawing fluid from intracellular to extracellular spaces. There is concern that in the contused brain any disruption of the blood-brain barrier will allow mannitol to leak into the brain tissue, causing localized edema and increased ICP. The effects of mannitol include a possible initial increase in CBF and CBV, decreased viscosity, and a free radical scavenger capability. ICP usually falls within 10 to 20 minutes after administration of mannitol if pressure autoregulation is intact. The typical dose is 0.5 g/kg given over 10 to 20 minutes. Repeated doses are given every 3 to 6 hours as needed.

A special consideration exists with the hyperemic post-traumatic state seen in children. In this case, the increase in ICP is primarily caused by increased blood volume, not brain edema as is seen typically in adults. Therefore mannitol may not be indicated in this specific situation.

Furosemide

Furosemide is a loop diuretic that works on the distal tubule in the kidney to inhibit sodium reabsorption. It also inhibits carbonic anhydrase, thereby reducing the rate of production of CSF. Generally, 0.5 to 1.0 mg/kg is given IV, and this may be administered before mannitol in order to prevent the rebound of increased ICP and CBV seen with that drug. Titration of the drug to keep serum osmolality approximately 30 mOsm above normal can be accomplished while monitoring potassium levels. A rise of 10 mOsm is adequate to initiate dehydration of brain tissues.

Barbiturates

The use of barbiturates in the management of intracranial hypertension in the intensive care setting, specifically barbiturate coma, is discussed in Chapter 18.

In the operating room it should be remembered that thiopental may cause severe hypotension in the presence of hypovolemia, a state which may or may not be corrected prior to surgery. The major effects of barbiturates are anesthesia, scavenging of free radicals, increasing cerebral vascular resistance thereby reducing CBF, CBV, and ICP, and reduction of $CMRO_2$. Although all of these may be of benefit to the head-injured patient, attention should also be focused on cerebral perfusion pressure, since drastic reductions in mean arterial pressure with thiopental will occur in the face of hypovolemia. If there are refractory elevations in ICP after conventional, conservative measures have been tried, reduction of ICP in 75% of patients occurs when high-dose barbiturates are added to the therapeutic regimen. Unfortunately, there remains doubt as to the improvement in outcome in randomized clinical trials.

Intraoperative Complications

Cardiovascular Complications

The most common cardiovascular responses to head injury are characterized by sympathetic hyperactivity. This results in elevated blood pressure, both systolic and diastolic, and increases in cardiac output, oxygen consumption, systemic vascular resistance, intrapulmonary shunt, and $\dot{V}/\dot{Q}$ mismatch.

Almost every arrhythmia and change in waveform morphology has been described in the setting of intracranial pathology. Most of these appear to be mediated by a central hyperadrenergic discharge, although metabolic and cardiac causes need to be considered in the differential. A loading dose of lidocaine (1 to 1.5 mg/kg IV) and titration of a lidocaine drip (1 to 4 mg/min) may be beneficial.

Intraoperatively, treatment of hypertension may be accomplished with IV hydralazine, nitroprusside, or nitroglycerin. Although these agents are effective in lowering systemic blood pressure, they are also potent cerebrovasodilators, which make them undesirable for use in the patient with head trauma. Beta-blockers such as esmolol, propranolol, or labetalol (also an alpha-blocker) are preferred.

These should be titrated to effect, and systolic blood pressure should be close to the patient's "normal" baseline pressure, or in the 160 mm Hg range (systolic). This helps to maximize CPP until the dura is opened.

Neurogenic Pulmonary Edema

Neurogenic pulmonary edema includes an increase in pulmonary venous pressure as well as a component of increased capillary permeability. The permeability of the alveolar capillary endothelium is affected by hypothalamic autonomic neural outflow to the lung. These leaky capillaries cause interstitial edema resulting in shunting, decreased compliance, and loss of lung volumes. The onset of neurogenic pulmonary edema may be rapid and is usually associated with a significantly abrupt increase in ICP.

Signs and symptoms of neurogenic pulmonary edema include dyspnea, cyanosis, pallor, sweating, and a weak, rapid pulse. The typical pink, frothy sputum of pulmonary edema is also apparent.

Treatment consists of surgically decompressing or removing the compressive intracranial lesion (hematoma) and pharmacologically instituting measures to reduce ICP. Additionally, antiadrenergics may be of value. Treatment of pulmonary edema consists of dehydration, increasing FiO_2 to maintain PaO_2 of 70 to 80 mm Hg, achieving "optimal" positive end-expiratory pressure (minimal increase in ICP with minimal decrease in cardiac output), and maintaining a $PaCO_2$ of 25 to 30 mm Hg. Patient positioning may help control ICP in light of necessary therapeutic measures.

Fat Embolism

Because one of the major signs of fat embolism is decreased consciousness, fat embolism is difficult to diagnose in the head-injured patient. The etiology of this process is mechanical or biochemical release of lipid-rich bone marrow into the circulation from disruption of the long bones of the extremities or pelvis. These globules become lodged in the lung where free fatty acids are released, causing increased pulmonary capillary leakage. Fluffy infiltrates are seen on chest films in association with hypoxemia and pulmonary edema. The complications of cerebral edema and disseminated intravascular coagulation may also become apparent, usually at least 12 to 24 hours after the initial injury.

Treatment is supportive, and steroids may be of some benefit, although high morbidity and mortality remain associated with this complication.

Air Embolism

Venous air embolism is a common occurrence when there is disruption of a venous sinus or when bony sinusoids are exposed to air. The risk is increased any time the operative site is elevated above the level of the heart, allowing entrainment of air down a pressure gradient to the right atrium.

The most sensitive indicators of venous air embolism include transesophageal-precordial Doppler changes and end-tidal nitrogen, followed by an increase in pulmonary artery pressures, a fall in end-tidal CO_2, a rise in CVP, and finally a drop in mean arterial pressure and PaO_2. A classic "mill-wheel" murmur may eventually be heard through the esophageal stethoscope. Diagnosis starts with a high index of suspicion. Treatment of air embolism involves notifying the surgeon of the problem, placing the patient's head down, immediately flooding the operative site with normal saline, discontinuing N_2O, and providing ventilation with 100% oxygen. Aspiration of entrained air through a multiorificed central line placed at the superior vena cava-right atrial junction may be tried. Turning the patient left-side down may also keep air from progressing into the pulmonary outflow tract. Cardiovascular support may be enhanced by the use of pressors or inotropes.

Case History

An 18-year-old male, brought to the emergency room by the county rescue squad, had been the driver in a motor vehicle accident involving a two-car collision. At the scene he had been thrown from his car, was unresponsive to verbal stimuli, and withdrew to pain. His vital signs were blood pressure 100/60, pulse 110, respiration rate 36. Pupils were 2 mm, equal and sluggish. There was a large 12-cm laceration exposing bone over the left frontotemporal area. No other injuries were apparent on initial examination in the field. Two large-bore intravenous lines were started; the patient was given oxygen by a 100% nonrebreathing mask and was brought to the emergency room in stable but critical condition. He was secured on a backboard with cervical spine stabilization using sandbags and a cervical collar. No other history or review of systems was available.

In the emergency room the patient was noted to have irregular respirations at a rate of 12/min, stable blood pressure, and full pulses. His pupils were 3 mm and equal bilaterally, although they remained sluggish to light. He withdrew from painful stimuli but did not localize. He opened his eyes with stimuli and muttered incomprehensible sounds. Laboratory studies were drawn and the patient was scheduled for a computed tomographic (CT) scan emergently.

Suggested Reading

Adams RW, et al. Isoflurane and cerebrospinal fluid pressure in neurosurgical patients. Anesthesiology 1981; 54:97.

Adams RW, et al. Halothane, hypocapnia and cerebrospinal fluid pressure in neurosurgery. Anesthesiology 1972; 37:510.

Artru AA, et al. Anoxic cerebral potassium accumulation reduced by phenytoin: Mechanism of cerebral protection? Anesth Analg 1981; 60:41.

Becker DP, et al. The outcome from severe head injury with early diagnosis and intensive management. J Neurosurg 1977; 47:491.

Bedford RF, et al. Lidocaine or thiopental for rapid control of intracranial hypertension? Anesth Analg 1980; 59:435.

Bruce DA, et al. Outcome following severe head injury in children. J Neurosurg 1978; 48:679.

Campkin TV, et al. Neurosurgical anaesthesia and intensive care. 2nd ed. London: Butterworths, 1986.

Cooper PR. Head injury. 2nd ed. Baltimore: Williams & Wilkins, 1987.

Cooper PR, et al. Pulmonary complications associated with head injury. Respir Care 1984; 29:263.

Cottrell JE, et al. Intracranial and hemodynamic changes after succinylcholine anesthesia in rats. Anesth Analg 1983; 62:1006.

Darby JM, et al. Local "inverse steal" induced by hyperventilation in head injury. Neurosurgery 1988; 23:1.

Donegan MF, et al. Intravenously administered lidocaine prevents intracranial hypertension during endotracheal suctioning. Anesthesiology 1980; 52:516.

Eisenberg HM, et al. High-dose barbiturate control of elevated intracranial pressure in patients with severe head injury. J Neurosurg 1985; 69:15.

Faupel G, et al. Double-blind study on the effect of steroids on severe closed head injury. In: Pappius HM, Feindel W, eds. Dynamics of brain edema. New York: Springer-Verlag, 1976:337.

Frankville DD, et al. Hyperkalemia after succinylcholine administration in a patient with closed head injury without paresis. Anesthesiology 1987; 67:264.

Frost EAM. Anesthesia and outcome in severe head injury. Br J Anaesth 1981; 53:310.

Giannotta SL, et al. High dose glucocorticoids in the management of severe head injury. Neurosurgery 1984; 15:497.

Gobiet W, et al. Treatment of acute cerebral edema with high-dose dexamethasone. In: Beks JWF et al, eds., Intracranial pressure III. New York: Springer-Verlag, 1976:231.

Gordon E. The management of acute head injuries. In: A basis and practice of neuroanesthesia. New York: Elsevier, 1981.

Hamill JF, et al. Lidocaine before endotracheal intubation: intravenous or laryngotracheal? Anesthesiology 1981; 55:587.

Horton JM. The anesthetist's contribution to the care of head injured patients. Br J Anaesth 1976; 48:767.

Jamieson KG. Surgically treated hematomas. J Neurosurg 1972; 37:137

Jennett B, et al. Assessment of outcome after severe brain damage. A practical scale. Lancet 1972; 1:734.

Langfitt TW. Measuring the outcome from head injuries. J Neurosurg 1978; 48:673.

Langfitt TW, et al. Can the outcome from head injury be improved? J Neurosurg 1982; 56:19.

Marshall LF, et al. Mannitol dose requirements in brain-injured patients. J Neurosurg 1978; 48:169.

Matjasko J, et al. Controversies in severe head injury management. In: Clinical controversies in neuroanesthesia and neurosurgery. Orlando: Grune and Stratton, 1986.

Minton MD, et al. Serum potassium following succinylcholine in patients with brain tumors. Can Anaesth Soc J 1986; 33:328.

Molofsky WJ. Steroids and head trauma. Neurosurgery 1984; 15:424.

Piatt JM, et al. High dose barbiturate therapy in neurosurgery and intensive care. Neurosurgery 1984; 15:427.

Pollay M, et al. Effect of mannitol and furosemide on blood-brain osmotic gradient and intracranial pressure. J Neurosurg 1983; 59:945.

Raphaely RC. Central nervous system trauma in children. In: Rogers M, ed. Current practice of anesthesiology. Toronto: BC Decker, 1988.

Rose J, et al. Avoidable factors contributing to death after head injury. Br Med J 1977; 2:618.

Stevenson PM, et al. Succinylcholine-induced hyperkalemia in a patient with a closed head injury. Anesthesiology 1979; 51:89.

Willatts SM, et al. Anesthesia and intensive care for the neurosurgical patient. Oxford: Blackwell, 1986.

David J. Stone, M.D.

Recovery Room Care   17

Careful recovery room management is essential to maintain the high standards of patient care necessary for successful neuroanesthesia. This chapter first addresses the general principles of recovery room care and then focuses on the problems of specific types of surgery.

Recovery Room Report

The report given to the recovery nurse is a complete summary of all information on the patient's prior medical history as well as the anesthetic care that may have a bearing on the recovery period. In addition to the patient's routine drugs, drugs given preoperatively and drugs (including dosage) used intraoperatively are listed. The surgery is described, as well as the names of the surgeons responsible for the surgical aspects of recovery care (position, drains, neurosurgical complications such as bleeding or cerebral edema). The status of the airway, neuromuscular blockade, and intravascular cannulas are described as well as fluids lost and administered. Any special aspects of the patient's situation are noted (dementia, underlying neurologic deficits such as quadriplegia, psychosis, drug addiction). The anesthetist assists with recovery room care, if necessary, until the patient is acceptably stable or the anesthetist is relieved by an appropriately trained and informed clinician.

Problems in Management of the Respiratory System

Airway Maintenance and Bronchospasm

After most neurosurgical procedures the patient is awake and able to maintain his airway. However, obstruction may occur because of residual anesthesia or brainstem or cranial nerve edema or injury. After cervical spine surgery, it is especially important not to extubate the trachea until the patient is fully awake, because neck extension is contraindicated and reintubation may be difficult. In patients with normal cervical spines, the neck can be extended and the jaw lifted or thrust forward to open the airway. Positioning the patient on the side and insertion of a nasal or oral airway may help relieve the obstruction. After transsphenoidal surgery, the airway should be examined for remnants of surgical packing if obstruction occurs. Oxygen should be administered; occasionally reintubation and rarely cricothyroidotomy are required to reestablish the airway.

In addition to cervical spine surgery, the patient should remain intubated if the airway or intubation was difficult, reversal of neuromuscular blockade is inadequate, or the patient has inadequate blood gases or hemodynamic instability. The latter statement is modified in that the hypertensive neurosurgical patient may require extubation to relieve the stimulus that is causing the hypertension. This is a judgment call, and it may be more prudent to resedate the patient with narcotic (fentanyl 1 to 4 μg/kg), thiopental (1 to 2 mg/kg), and/or lidocaine (1 to 1.5 mg/kg) if the wisdom of extubation is in doubt.

After surgery that may impair the patient's ability to protect the airway, intubation should be continued until the patient demonstrates a cough or gag response to the endotracheal tube. These situations include posterior fossa surgery with brainstem manipulation or any intracranial procedure that has been unduly compli-cated. If the patient began surgery unable to protect the airway because of neurologic disease, he should remain intubated postoperatively. The patient with a "full stomach" also should not be extubated until there is some evidence of airway responsiveness and the patient is awake. Patients with elevated intracranial pressure (ICP) should remain intubated until airway protection and hyperventilation are no longer necessary. Although cranial nerves may be damaged after carotid endarterectomy, a conservative approach is usually not necessary and deep extubation is acceptable.

Laryngospasm and airway swelling (glottic, subglottic edema) are discussed in the pediatric section of this chapter. In the extubated patient, upper airway obstruction may be mistaken for bronchospasm. Upper airway obstruction produces inspiratory wheezing when the trachea is auscultated, because extrathoracic obstruction is exacerbated when the negative pressure of inspiration tends to bring laryngeal surfaces closer together. Congestive heart failure can mimic bronchospasm in the extubated or intubated patient because small airways are mechanically compressed by peribronchial edema. In the patient who remains intubated, what sounds like bronchospasm may be caused by obstruction of the endotracheal tube (biting by patient; kink, clot, foreign body, or mucus in the tube; bevel against tracheal wall; overinflated cuff; tension pneumothorax; or endobronchial intubation). The presence of the tube itself results in some degree of reflex bronchospasm, which may be severe in those already predisposed to bronchospasm. After mechanical problems have been ruled out (cuff deflation, turning tube 90 degrees, passing a small catheter through tube, possibly chest film), bronchospasm can be approached pharmacologically. Treatment includes humidified oxygen plus the following drugs as necessary:

1. Inhaled beta-2-agonists—nebulized metaproterenol (0.2 to 0.3 ml in 2 ml normal saline) or isoetharine (0.5 ml in 2 ml normal saline) or salbutamol (2 puffs by metered inhaler)
2. Anticholinergics—glycopyrrolate 0.5 to 1 mg IV or nebulized glycopyrrolate (0.5 to 1 mg in 2 ml normal saline) or atropine (1 to 2 mg in 2 ml normal saline). These will also reduce secretion volume without increasing viscosity.
3. Corticosteroids—hydrocortisone 3 to 4 mg/kg IV or equivalent dose of other preparation (prednisolone 0.5 to 1 mg/kg) or dexamethasone (0.2 mg/kg IV)

4. If the patient is intubated, lidocaine (1 to 1.5 mg/kg IV) or fentanyl (1 to 2 μg/kg IV) decreases reactivity to the endotracheal tube. Deeper anesthesia and even muscle relaxants with mechanical ventilation may be necessary if bronchospasm is severe.

5. Parenteral beta-2-agonists—Terbutaline 0.25 mg SQ with careful monitoring for arrhythmias.

6. Aminophylline—5 to 6 mg/kg IV over 20 minutes and then infusion of 0.6 mg/kg/min (normal adults); 0.3 mg/kg/min (elderly patients, adults with liver or heart failure) or 0.9 mg/kg/min (children, healthy adult smokers). Aminophylline may produce tachyarrhythmias as well as nausea but has the possible advantage of improving respiratory muscle strength.

7. Intravenous beta-2-agonists—isoproterenol or epinephrine (start 0.25 μg/min and titrate)—both may produce tachyarrhythmias and myocardial ischemia and should be used only for severe bronchospasm.

8. Other measures—Severe refractory bronchospasm has been treated with deep inhalational anesthesia. The three potent agents are about equally potent bronchodilators, and the choice of drug should be made for other considerations. Chest physical therapy may help loosen secretions plugging up airways. While positive end-expiratory pressure is thought by some to be contraindicated in this situation, I have found it to be useful when hypoxemia is still present in the patient on 100% oxygen. It may act by stenting open airways that would otherwise close during expiration in the bronchospastic patient. It is also advisable to obtain a chest film and to consider the possible presence of a foreign body in the airway.

Hypoxemia

After general anesthesia, lung volumes may be reduced by about half for approximately 4 hours. After surgery, that does not involve the thorax or abdomen, such as intracranial surgery, endarterectomy, or cervical or lumbar laminectomy, abnormalities in lung volumes should not persist to a significant degree. After extensive and painful spinal procedures such as Harrington rodding, abnormalities probably continue past this early postoperative period.

Unlikely causes of hypoxemia postoperatively include low inspired-oxygen concentration or diffusion hypoxia. Upper airway obstruction and bronchospasm have been addressed. Hypoventilation with hypercarbia may result in hypoxemia unless the inspired concentration of oxygen is increased. If hypoventilation results in actual atelectasis, hypoxemia may be caused by the resultant $\dot{V}/\dot{Q}$ abnormalities. Increased oxygen consumption (fever, sepsis, seizures, shivering) or decreased cardiac output may cause hypoxemia by decreasing the oxygen saturation of mixed venous blood and subsequently, PaO_2. Pneumothorax is uncommon after neurosurgery unless central lines have been placed via subclavian or internal jugular veins or spinal surgery was performed in the area of the thorax. Pulmonary thromboembolism is another possible cause of postoperative hypoxemia that is difficult to diagnose (atelectasis affecting nuclear scan results) and treat (anticoagulation contraindicated) postoperatively.

Pulmonary edema may occur on a cardiogenic (high pulmonary venous pressures) or noncardiogenic (increased permeability) basis. Unless there is underlying cardiac dysfunction, cardiogenic pulmonary edema is uncommon postoperatively. This should be especially so in the neurosurgical patient in whom fluids are meticulously managed. Special causes of noncardiogenic pulmonary edema in the neurosurgical patient include neurogenic pulmonary edema and edema as a sequela of venous air embolus. Neurogenic pulmonary edema actually may have a component of high pulmonary venous pressures as well. It is associated with sudden increases of ICP, such as seizures, and may be difficult to differentiate from aspiration acutely. However, neurogenic pulmonary edema will usually resolve more quickly with the measures discussed below. Other causes of noncardiogenic pulmonary edema include allergic reactions to drugs or the white blood cell components of blood transfusion, sepsis as a sequela of upper airway obstruction, and the above mentioned aspiration.

As previously noted, residual anesthesia may cause $\dot{V}/\dot{Q}$ mismatching for some time into the postoperative period. This is exacerbated by underlying pulmonary disease, obesity, and old age. Atelectasis may or may not be apparent on the chest film. After specific etiologies are dealt with, hypoxemia should be treated with an increase in FiO_2 via nasal prongs, mask, or endotracheal tube; encouragement of deep breathing and cough in the awake patient (this must be done with caution if ICP is a concern, since cough will cause an ICP spike); and use of positive end-expiratory airway pressure, which is PEEP in the ventilated patient or continuous positive airway pressure (CPAP) in the spontaneously breathing patient. In the patient who is not intubated, mask CPAP can be used (5 to 15 cm H_2O for 15 to 30 minutes every 2 hours) if the patient is awake. These airway pressure modalities must be used with caution since they may increase ICP. However, a neurosurgical patient who develops postoperative pneumonia has a very serious problem, as well. Careful suctioning is also an important part of care with attention to the influence of suctioning on ICP. Spikes in ICP with suctioning can be prevented with lidocaine 1 to 1.5 mg/kg IV.

Hypercarbia

Hypercarbia results when pulmonary ventilation is not adequate to expel the CO_2 produced during metabolism. In general, $PaCO_2$ is proportional to CO_2 production and inversely proportional to ventilation. Hypercarbia will occur for one (or more) of the following four reasons:

1. *Increased CO_2 production.* Normal CO_2 production (Vco_2) is about 150 to 200 ml/min in the adult. Shivering, seizures, fever, sepsis (especially with shaking chills), emergence excitement, central hyperthermia, malignant hyperthermia, or the neurolept malignant syndrome all increase Vco_2.

2. *Decreased central drive to breathe may occur after neurosurgical injury to the central respiratory centers.* Even in neurosurgical patients, drugs are a more likely cause of diminished central drive to breathe. Potent inhalational anesthetics, narcotics, benzodiazepines and barbiturates all can contribute. Naloxone given in 40-μg increments will reverse narcotic-induced respiratory depression, but care must be taken that the naloxone effect does not wear off before the narcotic effect. Naloxone can also cause hypertension, dysrhythmias, and even pulmonary edema. Physostigmine in 1-mg increments up to 4 mg will act as a central cholinesterase inhibitor, which may cause a general arousal reaction. I give 0.2 mg glycopyrrolate with physostigmine to prevent peripheral cholinergic side effects.

3. *Dysfunction of nerve, neuromuscular junction, and/or respiratory muscles.* After anesthesia, residual neuromuscular blockade is the most likely cause of this problem. If relaxants have been fully reversed pharmacologically and reversal is inadequate, the patient should be mechanically ventilated (and respiratory acidosis

avoided) until there is evidence of adequate reversal (ability to lift head or stick out tongue for 5 seconds; sustained tetanus; train-of-four fourth stimulus height more than 70% of first stimulus). Underlying myopathy (e.g., muscular dystrophy) may contribute to weakness. Extreme sensitivity to relaxants suggests the possibility of underlying myasthenia gravis.

4. *Intrinsic lung dysfunction with baseline increased dead space areas of lung and resting hypercarbia.* This results in exacerbated postoperative hypercarbia, and is usually seen in patients with underlying chronic obstructive pulmonary disease. Any pulmonary process that increases dead space will make ventilation less efficient and potentially contribute to hypercarbia.

Cardiovascular Problems

Hypertension

The problem of hypertension is also addressed in the chapters on postoperative care of patients after intra- and extracranial vascular surgery (Chapters 9 and 10). Hypertension must be treated in patients with increased ICP to a degree that lowers ICP without contributing to further cerebral ischemia. Theoretically, drugs that are cerebrovasodilators (nitroprusside, nitroglycerin, hydralazine, calcium channel blockers) should be used with caution to avoid actually increasing cerebral blood flow, volume, and pressure. Hypoxemia, hypercarbia, bladder distention, or pain should be investigated as causes for hypertension.

Beta- and alpha-blockers reduce blood pressure with minimal increase in cerebral blood flow (CBF). Propranolol (in 0.5-mg increments) or metoprolol (in 5-mg increments) can be given intravenously with caution regarding heart rate, contractility, and bronchospasm. I have noticed that when beta-blockers cause undue bradycardia or a slow, irregular heart rhythm, there may be underlying brainstem compression or increased ICP. Labetalol is a combined alpha- and beta-blocker which has proved very useful in general neurosurgical and neurovascular patients. It is begun in 5-mg increments intravenously, and the doses can be doubled (10 mg to 20 mg to 40 mg) if there is no effect 5 minutes after a smaller dose.

The use of nitroprusside and nitroglycerin is discussed in the cerebrovascular sections. They are begun at 0.25 μg/kg/min IV and titrated to blood pressure. Nitroprusside is especially potent and should be used with an arterial line. Besides severe hypotension, nitroprusside may cause cyanide toxicity, and doses should be limited to less than 8 μg/kg/min. Toxicity may be manifested by tachyphylaxis, acidosis, hypotension, or an increase in mixed venous oxygen saturation. Treatment includes discontinuation of nitroprusside, thiosulfate (150 mg/kg IV) to accelerate conversion to thiocyanate, and correction of blood pressure and acid-base abnormalities. The main toxicity of nitroglycerin is hypotension, but the solvent of some preparations may be a myocardial depressant. Nitroglycerin is especially useful in patients with known or suspected coronary disease.

Hydralazine can be given in 5- to 20-mg IV boluses but takes about 15 to 20 minutes to work, is associated with reflex tachycardia, and its action cannot be rapidly terminated. Other treatments include nifedipine 10 to 20 mg sublingually, nitroglycerin paste (1 to 4 inches), phentolamine (an alpha-blocker) in 5-mg boluses, or trimethaphan, a ganglionic blocker as an infusion begun at 1 mg/min and titrated. Trimethaphan has the disadvantages of causing pupillary dilatation and possibly contributing to patchy cerebral ischemia during hypotension.

Dysrhythmias

Dysrhythmias are common postoperatively and may be due to hypoxemia, hypercarbia, acid-base disturbances, hypokalemia, and myocardial ischemia, among treatable causes that should be investigated. However, they may simply be due to surgical stress, pain, and hypothermia with a resultant high catecholamine state.

Premature Atrial Contractions

These are common and do not usually necessitate treatment. If conduction is aberrant, they may be difficult to differentiate from premature ventricular contractions.

Sinus Bradycardia

This may occur as a result of narcotization, beta-blockade, and administration of cholinesterase inhibitors. More worrisome is an association with high ICP (Cushing reflex) or brainstem compression. In these pathologic situations the rate may be irregular as well.

Sinus Tachycardia

This may be due to pain and stress but hypovolemia, congestive heart failure, hypoxemia, also should be investigated. In patients with coronary artery disease, heart rate may have to be empirically lowered with beta-blockers (while observing carefully for congestive heart failure or hypovolemia) to lessen the likelihood of ischemia.

Premature Ventricular Contractions

Again, these are common and may not represent underlying heart disease. The above-mentioned etiologies should be ruled out as causes. If pain is the cause, morphine may be the solution. Central venous catheters may cause dysrhythmias by irritating the endocardium. Cardiac ischemia should be sought and, if it is the cause, the dysrhythmia should be treated with lidocaine (1.5 mg/kg bolus IV) followed by an infusion of 1 to 4 mg/min. If the dysrhythmia is very frequent, multifocal, or causing hemodynamic problems, it should also be treated.

Atrial Fibrillation

This may occur because of the high catecholamine state or stretching of the atria from volume shifts. Treatment may include verapamil (2.5- to 5-mg IV boluses), digoxin (0.25- to 0.5-mg bolus) or propranolol (0.5-mg IV boluses). If hypotension is associated, cardioversion should be employed. Care must be taken to avoid hypotension, heart block, or bradycardia if drug combinations are employed.

Myocardial Ischemia

Myocardial ischemia is discussed in the extracranial vascular surgery section of this chapter, since it is mainly in this patient population that the problem arises.

Hypotension

After ruling out technical problems and artifact due to vascular stenosis, true hypotension can be treated by raising the legs, a fluid bolus (250 to 500 ml normal saline or lactated Ringer's solution) and, if necessary, a small dose of vasopressor such as ephedrine (5- to 15-mg IV bolus). The special problem of hypotension after carotid artery surgery is addressed in that section of this chapter.

Hypotension is frequently caused by hypovolemia in surgical patients. Neurosurgical patients generally do not have significant fluid shifts or major blood loss, but may have extensive diuresis from mannitol and inadequate fluid replacement. Hypotension may be caused by myocardial ischemia or residual anesthetic effect; cardiac tamponade or tension pneumothorax related to central venous catheter placement; anaphylaxis; sepsis; adrenal or thyroid deficiency; vasodilation secondary to drugs or rewarming; hypoxia; or bleeding.

On occasion, a central venous pressure or pulmonary artery catheter is required to sort out the etiology and guide the treatment of hypotension. Blood should be given to replace blood losses as indicated. Otherwise, a normotonic crystalloid (saline, Ringer's) or the colloid of choice (Plasmanate, hydroxyethyl starch) may be used to replace volume. Some clinicians may choose to avoid hydroxyethyl starch (Hetastarch) in neurosurgical patients because of the possible contribution to a coagulation disturbance.

Oliguria

Oliguria is listed under cardiovascular problems because it is frequently caused by hypovolemia in this setting. After ruling out mechanical problems (kinked Foley, urinary retention), intravascular volume should be optimized quickly to avoid actual acute tubular necrosis. Diuretics should not be given until intravascular volume is repleted and appropriate urine studies performed (U_{Na}^+, U_{OSM}, U_{CR}, specific gravity, urinalysis), is judged necessary.

Other Postoperative Problems

Hypothermia

Hypothermia is a common sequela of general anesthesia given without humidified, warmed gases and warmed fluids in a cold operating room. Although some degree of intraoperative hypothermia may provide some small degree of brain protection, a shivering hypothermic recovery room patient will raise $CMRO_2$ (cerebral oxygen consumption) and possibly ICP, become hypertensive, and generally awaken less smoothly. Carbon dioxide production will increase and may result in an undesirable increase in $PaCO_2$. Hypothermia can be treated with warm blankets, heating lamps, warming of intravenous fluids, and covering the head, especially in infants. In the intubated patient, it may be best to sedate the patient until rewarming is achieved more smoothly, but resedation is not generally desirable in neurosurgical patients. The goal should be to avoid hypothermia in the operating room except in the rare cases when it is employed as part of the neuroanesthetic.

Hyperthermia

Hyperthermia is somewhat uncommon in the recovery room. Although it may be due to simple atelectasis, aspiration or impending infections are worrisome causes. Malignant hyperthermia may first occur in the recovery room and can be evaluated with an arterial blood gas analysis, searching for combined respiratory and metabolic acidosis. The malignant neuroleptic syndrome may occur after the use of phenothiazines or buty-rophenones (such as droperidol), but is unlikely to occur as early as the recovery room period. Other pharmacologic causes of fever include anticholinergic toxicity with rash, delirium, and the absence of sweating (treat with physostigmine, 1 to 4 mg IV) or the interaction of monoamine oxidase inhibitors with meperidine. The latter may result in severe hyperpyrexia with seizures and death. Thyroid storm, adrenal insufficiency, and even pheochromocytoma are endocrinologic causes. Neurosurgery involving the hypothalamus may theoretically result in a central fever.

After the fever is noted, it should be treated in these patients to avoid increased CO_2 production, increased $CMRO_2$ and possibly increased ICP, and interference with evaluation of mental status. In adults, rectal acetaminophen can be used in 650–1,300 mg doses; in children, the dose is 10 mg/kg. Cooling blankets may help as well.

Nausea and Vomiting

Nausea and vomiting are particularly worrisome in neurosurgical patients because they may represent an intracranial problem, such as increased ICP, or they may themselves increase ICP. They are common sequelae of general anesthesia, and patients should be worked up for aspiration if vomiting occurred during a period of decreased consciousness.

Antiemetics do tend to cause slight sedation. Commonly used drugs include droperidol (Inapsine) 0.625 to 2.5 g IV, haloperidol (Haldol) 0.5 to 2.0 g IV, prochlorperazine (Compazine) 5 to 10 g IM or IV, or promethazine (Phenergan) 12.5 to 25 g IV or IM. All these drugs are dopamine antagonists and may cause dystonic reactions or exacerbation of Parkinson's disease. Dystonia can be treated with diphenhydramine (Benadryl) 25 to 100 mg IV or IM, or benztropine (Cogentin) 1 to 2 mg IV. Alternative treatments for nausea include benzquinamide (Emeticon) 25 mg IV or 50 mg IM, dexamethasone (10 mg IV), or metoclopramide (10 mg IV). Acute hydrocephalus or increased ICP should be considered if nausea is unusually severe or refractory to mild treatment.

Special Neuroanesthetic Concerns

Supratentorial Surgery

Anesthesia for neurosurgery is generally designed to allow prompt awakening in most circumstances. Head injury care is discussed in Chapter 16 as well as in Chapter 18. When awakening is unduly delayed or unexpected new focal neurologic findings are present, the following possibilities should be considered. Metabolic derangements are less likely to cause focal findings than they are to cause global dysfunction. However, the combination of differences in blood flow (i.e., underlying vascular stenoses) and metabolic abnormalities (especially hypoglycemia) may result in focal findings. Vital signs should be reviewed for gross derangements in cardiovascular or respiratory function. Stat laboratory evaluation of glucose, sodium, and arterial blood gases should be obtained to evaluate these possible etiologies for central nervous system dysfunction.

While the above work-up is proceeding, the responsible neurosurgeon should be contacted to inform him of a possible problem. The decision can then be made as to whether a CT scan is required for investigation of a structural cause of neurologic dysfunction. These problems include bleeding, edema, tension pneumocephalus, and hydrocephalus.

Postoperative intracranial hemorrhage is uncommon because neurosurgeons take great care to prevent it. It may be epidural, subdural, parenchymal, or intraventricular. The patient may or may not have a lucid interval after the anesthetic. The anesthetist may aid in its prevention by raising blood pressures to the normal range while the dura is closed after a procedure employing hypotensive anesthesia. This allows for detection of bleeding that might be masked by continued hypotension. The diagnosis is made by CT scan, and the neurosurgeon must decide whether the anatomic derangement justifies reoperation for drainage.

Brain edema is usually maximal from 24 to 72 hours postoperatively. Its occurrence in the immediate postoperative period may be anticipated when dural closure is "tight" even after a mass has been removed. It is more likely after meningioma than glioma removal, because the former are often quite large and prolonged and extensive brain retraction may be involved in their exposure and resection. The diagnosis may be made from the absence of blood or presence of hypodense areas with or without midline shift on CT scan. Treatment follows the principles previously given for increased intracranial pressure. Briefly, this includes hyperventilation to $PaCO_2$ 20 to 25, reduced fluid input, administration of mannitol (0.25 to 1 g/kg IV), head-up position, increased dose of steroids, and avoidance of drugs that might increase CBF (ketamine, vasodilators other than alpha-antagonists, inhaled anesthetics). If refractory, a pentothal drip may be begun with or without a lidocaine infusion. ICP monitoring may be indicated (see Chapter 4).

Tension pneumocephalus is discussed more extensively in the following section on infratentorial surgery because it is more common after using the seated position. It may occur occasionally after supratentorial operations. In absolute frequency, it is very unlikely to cause postoperative neurologic dysfunction.

Acute hydrocephalus is detected by CT scan and may be treated with ventricular shunting if the neurosurgeon judges that this is indicated.

Although most patients in this setting are receiving an anticonvulsant, seizures may occur at this time. It is critical to maintain the airway and oxygenation; seizures may be treated with increments of pentothal (25 to 100 mg) or diazepam (2 to 20 mg IV). The patient should be reintubated if necessary for maintenance of oxygenation, ventilation, and airway protection. Muscle relaxants will stop motor activity but not the deleterious increase in $CMRO_2$ and CBF caused by the seizure. Midazolam may be useful in this setting, but there is not yet much experience with this usage. The treatment of status epilepticus is outlined in the chapter on critical care. The patient should be loaded with phenytoin (15 mg/kg at 50 mg/min) if this was not previously done, and the patient already on phenytoin should receive an additional dose of 100 to 200 mg per the neurosurgeon.

Infratentorial Surgery

Bleeding and edema may also occur after infratentorial surgery. Since brainstem compression and ischemia result, the patient may present with irregular breathing or even respiratory arrest, hypertension, and changes in heart rate. In any case, the neurosurgeon must be quickly informed of this dangerous complication. Occasionally supratentorial epidural (and rarely intracerebral) clots will occur after surgery in the sitting position. They may occur at the site of a burr hole made for ventricular decompression but more commonly occur at a remote site, possibly due to tearing of bridging veins. They may be caused by sudden relaxation of the dura when intraventricular pressure is relieved. Hydrocephalus may occur because of obstruction in cerebrospinal fluid flow due to edema or clot. Postoperative hypertension should be treated to reduce the likelihood of bleeding or edema. Cerebral vasodilators are best avoided in attempting to decrease blood pressure. Labetalol, a combined beta- and alpha-blocker, in 5-mg increments is an excellent choice.

Cranial nerve dysfunction may involve cranial nerves IV through XII. Dangerous sequelae include loss of corneal sensation due to trigeminal injury, facial nerve injury, with impairment of eye closure, and injuries to nerves IX to XII, which may impair the ability to protect and maintain the airway as well as cause dysphagia. Damage to the respiratory centers may impair or result in absence of spontaneous ventilation.

The sitting position may result in several special complications. There may be ischemia at points of pressure and stretching of the sciatic nerve. Upper airway obstruction caused by head and tongue swelling has been reported and attributed to position-related venous obstruction. Quadriplegia has been reported in patients positioned with extreme neck flexion causing cord ischemia. If venous air embolism has occurred during the case, the patient may have postoperative noncardiogenic pulmonary edema. If paradoxical embolism has occurred, there may be dysfunction of the organs affected, especially heart and brain. Finally, if the sitting position resulted in marked hemodynamic instability, there may be ischemic injuries to the brain and myocardium.

The timing of extubation is a somewhat difficult problem in these patients. If the patient was wide awake preoperatively, there are no undue surgical problems, and breathing appears adequate, the patient may be extubated awake in the operating room. Some clinicians bring all of these patients to the recovery area with the endotracheal tube in place. In these cases, the patients can be extubated when they are awake, with adequate ventilation, oxygenation, and gag reflex, if there is no new head or neck edema. The inability to maintain the airway may only be realized when the tube is removed, and these patients must be carefully observed for airway obstruction, aspiration, and irregular breathing.

Tension pneumocephalus (TPC) occurs when an excessive amount of air accumulates in the subdural space and is trapped by dural closure. The amount of air is increased when the brain sinks down as a result of the sitting position, ventricular shunts, lumbar fluid drainage, and other attempts to collapse the brain to improve surgical exposure. Consequently, the brain swells to some extent postoperatively and pressure increases in the fixed cranial volume available to brain and air. Patients may then have global or focal neurologic signs due to the pressure. If suspected, the diagnosis can be made by plain skull films, but more often the diagnosis will be made when CT scanning is performed to check for bleeding and edema. A small burr hole placed with the patient under local anesthesia can be used by the neurosurgeon to vent the air under pressure if necessary. There has been some controversy of late whether N_2O should be turned off before dural closure to prevent TPC. TPC has been reported even when N_2O was discontinued 90 minutes prior to dural closure, so TPC may occur even when N_2O has no bearing on its formation. The percentage of N_2O in the gas trapped under the dura may be important. If it is low and N_2O is continued or begun, the space will expand. If it is high, not much more nitrous can enter and the outflow of N_2O at the end of the case will actually make the gas volume smaller. If N_2O has not been used during the case, it should not be turned on after dural closure because this will in fact cause an increase in pneumocephalus. The latter is not just a theoretical possibility, because some clinicians will avoid N_2O at times to lessen the impact of venous air embolism, to diminish the increase in sympathetic tone due to N_2O (which may counteract hypotensive measures), and to avoid the occasional marked increase in CBF due to N_2O.

Pituitary Surgery

If a cranial approach has been taken, the previously noted problems of supratentorial surgery apply. It is especially important to monitor visual activity and fields, as they may be affected by postoperative bleeding or migration of the fat or muscle plug used to seal up the sella.

After a transsphenoidal approach, the patient is unable to breathe through his nose. The patient is generally extubated awake because of this requirement as well as a propensity to vomit because of swallowed blood and secretions. Before extubation, any packing placed in the oropharynx to soak up blood should be removed. Nasal packing may cause gagging, coughing, and vomiting if it is displaced. Patients who have been operated on for acromegaly may have a difficult airway because of a large tongue, bony mandibular overgrowth, and glottic narrowing.

Hypertension is commonly observed in this patient population and hypoxemia and/or hypercarbia due to airway obstruction should be checked for as the hypertension is treated. Patients with preoperative Cushing's syndrome may have hyperglycemia and hypokalemia as well as the anesthetic complications of obesity. These include compromise of the airway, occasional marked sensitivity to sedation (in those with sleep apnea), and overloaded cardiovascular and respiratory systems, which have little reserve even at rest. Care should be taken to avoid oversedation and overhydration, and respiratory measures to prevent postoperative complications should be begun. These include coughing and deep breathing, chest physical therapy, and mask CPAP during the recovery room period.

Other patients may have adrenal insufficiency on the basis of pituitary disease and should be covered with steroids through the perioperative period (hydrocortisone 100 g IV, for 6 to 8 hours and taper). The combination of hypotension, nausea, hyponatremia, hyperkalemia, and fever should bring the diagnosis of adrenal insufficiency to mind. Hypothyroidism will not be a factor in the immediate postoperative period unless it was present and undetected before and during the operation. Rarely, severe hyperthermia due to central neurogenic (hypothalamic) pathology will occur and should be treated with sufficient intravascular volume, physical cooling measures, and steroid coverage. Malignant hyperthermia should be considered, since this can first appear in the postoperative period.

The most common postoperative endocrinologic problem is diabetes insipidus (DI) in which insufficient antidiuretic hormone is secreted so that the kidneys excrete large volumes of dilute urine. This usually begins 1 to 4 days postoperatively, but can begin in the recovery room or even in the operating room. It generally lasts less than a week because it is due to local edema that is reabsorbed, but it may be permanent if there is sufficient local structural damage. Osmotic diuresis caused by mannitol, glucose or simple fluid overload should be ruled out. In DI the urine is very dilute (specific gravity < 1.005; osmolality < 200 mOsm, frequently < 150 mOsm) and inappropriately so in the presence of increasingly hyperosmolar serum. The urine osmolality is less than the serum osmolality, and serum sodium concentrations are elevated as free water is excreted. In the past, small doses of vasopressin (Pitressin) have been used (5 to 20 IU per day) but at present desmopressin (DDAVP) is favored because of its ease of administration and lack of vasoactive properties in the doses required. DDAVP is given in 1- to 2-μg doses once or twice a day, so a 2-μg IV dose in the recovery room would be adequate to treat the problem during the patient's stay in the recovery room. These drugs cannot be given nasally for some time (up to 2 weeks) after transsphenoidal procedures.

Other postoperative problems include the sequelae of venous air embolism, which may occur during surgery. These include pulmonary edema, right ventricular overload due to pulmonary hypertension and infarcts of various organs, especially the heart and brain. The patient requiring hypophysectomy for metastatic cancer is frequently debilitated and requires postoperative ventilation as well as meticulous attention to intravascular volume, pain control, and other organs affected by the cancer (pericardial effusion, lung and cardiac metastases, pleural effusions).

Extracranial Vascular Surgery

The cardiovascular and cerebrovascular systems are the two keys in the postoperative management of this group of patients. These patients may be cared for in a recovery room or intensive care unit postoperatively.

Cerebral ischemia in this setting is most commonly due to intraoperative emboli resulting from manipulation of the diseased vessel. Other intraoperative causes of ischemia include carotid cross-clamping and marked hypotension. The patient may therefore arrive in the recovery room with a neurologic deficit present, and it is essential to document the status of the neurologic examination in the recovery room as soon as the patient is sufficiently awake to cooperate. Postoperative causes of neurologic deficit include new emboli, thrombosis of the vessel, severe hypotension, or intracerebral hemorrhage caused by hyperperfusion in the area supplied by the previously stenotic vessel. The latter is likely to be associated with hypertension. This is why the postoperative systemic blood pressure is kept at normal levels or slightly (about 10%) above normal.

The incidence of neurologic deficits after carotid endarterectomy ranges from 2 to 20% and depends on patient pathology as well as the skills of the surgeon and anesthesiologist in operative and postoperative care. The best monitor of a neurologic problem is repeated neurologic examinations to test for focal weakness that would be referable to a hemispheric deficit. The responsible surgeon should be notified and blood pressure adjusted to the desired range as discussed above. Thrombosis of a vessel may be amenable to emergency reoperation.

Myocardial ischemia is a common, serious problem in this population which has a high incidence of underlying coronary artery disease. Myocardial infarction reportedly occurs in about 2% of patients, but the incidence is higher in those who have had a recent myocardial infarction. Although postoperative cardiac ischemia may be caused by hemodynamic aberrations such as tachycardia, severe bradycardia, hypotension, or marked hypertension, it may occur in the absence of these factors. Esophageal echocardiography cannot be used in these awake patients, so the electrocardiogram (ECG) remains the diagnostic standard of perioperative ischemia or infarction. Thus it is essential to have the baseline ECG available for comparison. The ischemic ECG may reveal S-T depression or elevation; T-wave inversion, flattening or hyperacuity (increase in size); or Q waves as well as various dysrhythmias. After any operation the ECG may be nonspecifically altered by stress, drugs, temperature, and electrolyte shifts, resulting in a mildly changed but suspicious ECG.

After carotid artery surgery, T-wave changes that may not represent myocardial ischemia are especially common. It is possible that this is due to surgery in the area of the stellate ganglia that have autonomic input to the heart. If a preoperative two-dimensional echocardiogram is available, a postoperative echocardiogram may demonstrate diagnostic focal wall motion and wall thickening abnormalities that are more specific for ischemia than is the ECG. One approach is to observe minimal ECG changes (< 1 mm S-T shift, T-wave flattening) if the patient is asymptomatic and stable. More significant changes must be treated as presumptive myocardial ischemia with nitrates, beta-blockers, and calcium channel blockers as well as oxygen and pain relief.

Intravenous nitroglycerin (begin at 20 μg/min and titrated) can be employed and the ECG reexamined after blood pressure is reduced to 10% below baseline. If there is no change in the ECG, a clinical judgment must be made as to continuance of the drug. Nitroglycerin paste 1 to 4 inches may be used once the situation is stabilized. Sublingual nitroglycerin can be used until the intravenous drug is prepared. Intravenous beta-blockers (propranolol in 0.5-mg increments, labetalol in 2.5-mg increments, metoprolol in 2.5-mg increments) should be used to slow heart rate unless they are contraindicated. In addition Nifedipine can be given sublingually (10 mg). In general, a cardiologist should be consulted for help in postoperative care and because the newer means of managing myocardial infarction may require a specialist's input. In fact, the role of clot dissolution and/or angioplasty in the management of perioperative myocardial infarction is not clear at the present.

Hypotension occurs in about 15 to 20% of these patients postoperatively and is sometimes explained as the sudden exposure (after removal of plaque) of the carotid sinus to true arterial pressures resulting in reflex vasodilation and bradycardia. Adequate volume should be given. If blood pressure is still unacceptably low, phenylephrine can be given as an intravenous infusion started at 20 μg/min and titrated. Phenylephrine has the potential to contribute to myocardial ischemia via coronary vasoconstriction and should probably be given with nitroglycerin if used to treat hypotension in the setting of myocardial ischemia. Sometimes, the postoperative hypotension persists for several days and the clinician has difficulty weaning the patient from phenylephrine. If volume does not suffice to maintain the blood pressure, a low dose of norepinephrine (start 0.5 μg/min) may allow for weaning of the phenylephrine, after which the norepinephrine is easily weaned. This may occur because phenylephrine indirectly releases catecholamines as well as directly stimulating alpha receptors. If given for many hours or for days, catecholamines may become depleted and are repleted by the infusion of norepinephrine. Potent vasoconstrictors (norepinephrine, epinephrine) should be given through a central line in an elective setting, such as for weaning of phenylephrine.

Hypertension is more common than hypotension and occurs in more than half of postoperative patients. Many of these patients have baseline hypertension and should have their preoperative medication resumed as soon as possible. While they should not have an ileus, some of these patients have trouble swallowing pills in the early postoperative period and must be treated with parenteral or dermal preparations. Other patients may have hypertension due to edema or structural damage to the nerves supplying the carotid sinus so that the brainstem cardiovascular centers are not receiving the message that blood pressure is adequate and proceed to raise blood pressure to high levels. Hypertension may contribute to myocardial ischemia, bleeding at the wound site, and cerebral hemorrhage. Blood pressure should be kept within approximately 20% of normal mean pressure with drugs as required. While nitroprusside is effective and often recommended, it has the potential to produce severe hypotension and theoretically, some degree of coronary steal. It must be used slowly and cautiously with an arterial line in place. Since many of these patients have concomitant coronary artery disease, nitroglycerin is a good choice for hypertension, either intravenously or as paste. Beta-blockers, especially labetalol, and sublingual nifedipine are also useful. Hydralazine can be given as 2.5- to 10-mg IV boluses or as an infusion but takes about 15 to 20 minutes for onset and wears off over a prolonged period (unlike intravenous nitroglycerin or nitroprusside).

Cranial nerves, most commonly the hypoglossal, may be damaged during the surgical dissection. If bilateral (after being damaged after bilateral endarterectomies, for instance), hypoglossal dysfunction can result in airway obstruction. Injury to cranial nerves IX and X can produce various degrees of difficulty in swallowing, vocalization, and airway protection. After bilateral carotid endarterectomies, damage to both carotid bodies can result in diminished or absent hypoxic drive to breathe.

If there is excessive bleeding, a hematoma may form that can obstruct the airway. While the surgeons are called, reintubation is attempted but may be very difficult because of anatomical distortion. In a life-threatening situation, the wound may need to be opened and intubation performed. Pressure should be applied to the area until the surgeons arrive.

Intracranial Vascular Surgery

These patients are generally brought directly to an intensive care unit. Their care is discussed in detail in Chapter 18.

The immediate concerns in these patients are neurologic status and blood pressure control. The patient may be extubated awake at the end of the case, but if the patient was neurologically impaired preoperatively or if there were intraoperative problems (ruptured aneurysm, excessive retraction, or brainstem manipulation), the patient is likely to arrive in the recovery room still intubated and possibly requiring mechanical ventilation. The need for ventilation is determined by clinical observation (rate and depth of respirations), arterial blood gases, and bedside pulmonary function tests (tidal volume, vital capacity, inspiratory force), if available. In general, a minimal tidal volume of 5 ml/kg, vital capacity of 10 ml/kg, and inspiratory force of -20 cm H_2O are sought.

If a dose of narcotic has been used, it will likely smooth out the patient's tolerance of the endotracheal tube, but may delay emergence from a deep (for hypotension) isoflurane anesthetic. Doses of fentanyl greater than 12.5 μg/kg or of sufentanil greater than 2.5 μg/kg may saturate redistribution mechanisms and require metabolism (which is a slower process than redistribution) for their elimination. If the patient is fighting the endotracheal tube and becomes hypertensive, the clinician must decide whether extubation or resedation is appropriate. The latter can be accomplished with narcotic (fentanyl 1 to 2 μg/kg), thiopental 1 to 3 mg/kg, midazolam 1 to 5 mg or lidocaine 1.5 mg/kg. If in serious doubt, it is usually prudent to resedate the patient to allow for a smoother emergence.

There are several causes of neurologic problems postoperatively. Ischemia may occur as a result of vasospasm, surgical retraction, hypotension, or even a misplaced clip. Hemorrhage or hydrocephalus can also occur, and a CT scan will sort out these possibilities, if necessary. An angiogram provides definite evidence of vasospasm or misplaced clip, but is not often required in this setting.

Spinal Surgery

The postoperative care of these patients is discussed in Chapter 12, "Anesthesia for Spinal Cord Surgery." Special considerations include pressure on eyes, genitals, or nerves caused by the prone position; neurologic deficit secondary to hematoma; airway management after cervical surgery; blood pressure management in quadriplegia; and ventilatory management after scoliosis surgery.

Pediatrics and Neuroradiology

Complications after supratentorial or infratentorial surgery are similar to those in adults. The child must be carefully observed for postoperative neurologic deterioration, especially from bleeding. Although children are unlikely to have intracranial aneurysms, they may have intracranial vascular surgery for arteriovenous malformations, which have similar postoperative concerns, except that vasospasm is less likely. If a child has received a general anesthetic for a neuroradiologic procedure, he should receive the same level of recovery care given to a patient who has had a surgical procedure.

Children are more likely to develop laryngospasm after extubation than adults. This is prevented by extubating children while they are deeply anesthetized or wide awake. Intravenous lidocaine (1 to 1.5 mg/kg) given just before extubation may decrease the incidence of laryngospasm, possibly by making the airway less irritable. Laryngospasm is treated with 100% O_2, jaw extension, and gentle mask CPAP and eventually muscle relaxant and reintubation if necessary.

Another airway problem more common in children (especially age 1 to 4 years) is postintubation croup, which is due to edema of the glottic or subglottic (cricoid cartilage level) areas. Exacerbating factors include use of an endotracheal tube that is too large (inadequate leak), traumatic intubation, long operation, movement of head after intubation, and cough. There is inspiratory stridor, respiratory distress, and reduced air movement. Postintubation croup is treated with dexamethasone 0.5 mg/kg IV (up to 10 mg) and inhaled racemic epinephrine 0.25 to 0.5 ml in 2 ml of normal saline in a nebulizer. It can be repeated in 20 to 30 minutes if necessary, then every 2 to 6 hours as needed. On occasion, reintubation is necessary, especially if there is underlying laryngotracheal pathology (stenosis, malacia).

Temperature must be carefully monitored and hypothermia corrected, especially in small infants. In addition to adult techniques, heating lamps and blankets as well as covering of the head are helpful. If an infant has been brought to surgery from the neonatal intensive care unit (NICU), I generally maintain intubation and sedation until the infant is returned to the NICU where a controlled wake-up and extubation with careful regulation of temperature and fluids can be performed. Other considerations in this population are blood glucose and calcium, hematocrit, and the presence of previously undetected congenital anomalies.

Suggested Reading

Artru AA, et al. Cardiorespiratory and cranial-nerve sequelae of surgical procedures involving the posterior fossa. Anesthesiology 1980; 52:82.

Bedford RF. Perioperative air embolism. Semin Anesth 1987; 6:163.

Bedford RF, Durbin CG. Neurosurgical intensive care. In: Miller RD, ed. Anesthesiology. New York: Churchill-Livingstone, 1986.

Branson RD. PEEP without endotracheal intubation. Respir Care 1988; 33:598.

Breslow MJ, et al. Changes in T-wave morphology following anesthesia and surgery: A common recovery room phenomenon. Anesthesiology 1986; 64:398.

Colice GL. Neurogenic pulmonary edema. Clin Chest Med 1985; 6:473.

Craig DB. Postoperative recovery of pulmonary function. Anesth Analg 1981; 60:46.

Cully MD, et al. Hetastarch coagulopathy in a neurosurgical patient. Anesthesiology 1987; 66:706.

Donegan MF, Bedford RF. Intravenously administered lidocaine prevents intracranial hypertension during endotracheal suctioning. Anesthesiology 1980; 52:516.

Gal TJ. How does tracheal intubation alter respiratory mechanics? Problems in Anesthesia 1988; 2:191.

Guze BH, Baxter LR. Neuroleptic malignant syndrome. N Engl J Med 1985; 313:163.

Hess D. The use of PEEP in clinical settings other than acute lung injury. Respir Care 1988; 33:581.

Hitselberger WE, House WSA. Warning regarding the sitting position for acoustic tumor surgery. Arch Otolaryngol 1980; 106:69.

Horwitz NH, Rizzoli HV. Postoperative complications of intracranial neurological surgery. Baltimore: Williams & Wilkins, 1982.

Leslie JB, et al. Intravenous labetalol for treatment of postoperative hypertension. Anesthesiology 1987; 67:413.

Skahen S, et al. Nitrous oxide withdrawal reduces intracranial pressure in the presence of pneumocephalus. Anesthesiology 1986; 65:192.

Stone DJ. Recovery room. In: Firestone LL, ed. Clinical anesthesia procedures of the Massachusetts General Hospital. Boston: Little, Brown, 1988.

David L. Bogdonoff, M.D., and David J. Stone, M.D.

Neurosurgical Intensive Care   18

Satisfactory outcome for neurosurgical patients often requires that comprehensive management be available in an intensive care unit (ICU). Preexisting neurologic diseases or trauma, aggravated by operative interventions and residual anesthetic affects, require appropriate treatment to assure a functional recovery. A cornerstone of neurointensive care is clinical observation, although there is increasing use of sophisticated monitoring methods. An experienced ICU nurse is therefore invaluable. Several aspects of care of the neurosurgical patient are addressed in this chapter. These include the need for accurate assessment of neurologic changes, monitoring and treatment of increased intracranial pressure (ICP), cardiovascular and respiratory problems unique to neurosurgical patients, treatment of medical problems to which neurointensive care is clinical observation, although there is increasing use of sophisticated monitoring methods. An experienced ICU nurse is therefore invaluable.

Transport and Initial Assessment

During transfer to the ICU, intraoperative monitoring should be continued. Supplemental oxygen must be administered. Initial evaluation in the ICU includes the taking of basic vital signs, and the drawing of admission blood samples. Invasive monitoring should be continued, including on-line capnography if available. A careful neurologic assessment is extremely important at this time. Level of consciousness, degree of motor activity, and the size and reactivity of the pupils are important clinical signs. The Glasgow Coma Scale (see Table 16-1), initially developed as a prognostic indicator in head injury, is a useful scale in the assessment of postoperative neurologic status. Although level of consciousness is subject to variability between observers, measurement of motor activity and pupillary and respiratory signs are more objective. These latter signs are useful in the determination of intracranial integrity, particularly in the unconscious patient. Ipsilateral pupil dilatation, for example, is an excellent warning sign of uncal herniation. Midbrain compression may be diagnosed by constricted pupils. The development of localizing neurologic signs may suggest a developing intracranial catastrophe, such as hematoma formation, vasospasm, or regional edema formation. Focal muscle weakness is one of the best early signs of supratentorial lesions. In the future, the use of sophisticated monitoring of intracranial electrical activity by on-line encephalography (EEG) or by various manipulations of that data, may diminish our reliance on basic neurologic observations. For now, however, the neurologic examination remains the mainstay of assessment of neurologic integrity.

Intracranial Pressure

The monitoring and therapy of elevated ICP has been utilized in attempts to improve outcome in cases of head injury and Reye's syndrome. Its implementation may improve the outcome of other conditions associated with the risk of ICP elevation. The purpose of monitoring ICP is to detect situations of decreased cerebral perfusion pressure as well as to enhance early recognition of catastrophic intracranial events. Such early detection of conditions likely to lead to neurologic dysfunction facilitates successful intervention. Reliance on clinical examination alone may not reveal the true magnitude of the disturbance until such time as therapy will no longer be effective. Details of the pathophysiology of elevated ICP have been discussed in Chapter 2. Basically, three components affect ICP in the percentages shown: cerebral blood volume (10 percent), cerebrospinal fluid (CSF) (10 percent), and brain and interstitial tissue (80 percent). Reduction in the volume of any one of these will lead to a lowering of ICP. Decisions to be made include when and how to monitor ICP and when to treat ICP elevations. Therapeutic maneuvers affecting ICP are numerous and include respiratory manipulations, drug administration, blood and plasma volume adjustments, CSF drainage, and operative interventions.

Monitoring

Indications

Deciding when to initiate monitoring may be difficult. Candidates for monitoring may include those with a condition known to have a significant incidence of elevated ICP and in which it would be detrimental to neurologic function. When other forms of monitoring, i.e., neurologic examination, will be ineffective or unavailable, as during general anesthesia, ICP monitoring must be available. Specific guidelines for monitoring in individual situations are not universally agreed upon. Altered consciousness and/or Glasgow Coma Scale score of 7 or less are generally accepted indications for ICP monitoring in head trauma, Reye's syndrome, intracerebral hemorrhage, and persistent coma following neurosurgical procedures or cardiac arrest. Other situations that may warrant invasive pressure monitoring are those associated with diminished intracranial compliance, such as tumor, hydrocephalus, cerebral edema, and other causes of intracranial mass effect. Compliance ($\Delta V/\Delta P$), or its reciprocal, elastance ($\Delta P/\Delta V$), describes the interrelationship of changes in volume and pressure in the cranial vault. Conditions of reduced compliance place a patient at high risk from even small changes in any component of cerebral volume.

Techniques and Complications

There are three basic techniques for invasive ICP monitoring: intraventricular, subarachnoid, or subdural and epidural. The gold standard is the ventricular catheter, which yields the most accurate ICP readings. It allows access to CSF for purposes of therapeutic drainage. Measurements of pressure following aspiration or injection of fluid into the ventricle can yield valuable information about intracranial compliance or elastance. Disadvantages of the ventriculostomy include difficulty of placement into ventricles, which are small and slit-like, as well as a high incidence of infection (8% at 5 days to 40% at 12 days). Subarachnoid or subdural techniques involve the use of a "bolt" or a catheter to connect a pressure transducer to the intracranial compartments. More modern devices, such as the Camino monitor, make use of fiberoptic technology to transmit pressure information. Ease of insertion and lower infection rates offer advantages over ventriculostomy catheters. Questions of accuracy at high levels of ICP and an inability to routinely drain CSF or measure intracranial compliance limit the usefulness of subdural or subarachnoid techniques. Epidural sensing carries the lowest risk of infection and greatest ease of insertion. However, drainage of CSF is impossible. At present epidural sensing systems are complicated by questions of accuracy and zero baseline drift. With all systems, meticulous care and use of sterile technique is mandatory to prevent the devastating consequences of intracranial infection. In the future, implantable telemetric devices will be available for long-term monitoring without the risks of infection although their use for short-term problems with ICP will not be practical.

Caveats

Caveats for ICP monitoring include a possible lack of clinical relevance at times. Conditions such as posterior fossa or temporal lobe lesions may produce locally increased pressures and regional ischemia that are not detected by routine supratentorial ICP monitoring devices. In addition, knowledge of intracranial compliance is often not obtainable, making the true significance of a given absolute value of ICP unclear. One must be aware of the potential for occlusion of the devices and/or dampening of the signal and have a low threshold for correcting the problem. Devices may need to be replaced. The presence of a false-negative reading must be kept in mind, and one should not be lulled into a false sense of security by normal readings in the face of clinical deterioration.

Therapy

General Measures

Treatment of elevated ICP usually begins when a value of 20 to 25 mm Hg is reached in order to avoid the deterioration of neurologic function which occurs with ICPs of 40 to 50 mm Hg. However, the lack of knowledge of intracranial compliance and the inability to determine when the brain's compensatory mechanisms are exhausted precludes one from predicting when a rapid rise in ICP is imminent. Therapeutic maneuvers take time to have effects on ICP and should be started before rapid deterioration begins.

Treatment of elevated ICP requires two sets of interventions. Initiation of therapy is undertaken while a simultaneous search for the etiology is made. There are physiologic and structural causes of increased ICP. Elevated $Paco_2$, hyponatremia with brain swelling, hyperthermia, and bucking against the ventilator are physiologic causes that are easily diagnosed by clinical or laboratory observations. Their treatment is discussed elsewhere. Hydrocephalus, intracranial hematoma, and cerebral edema are structural lesions usually detected by computed tomographic (CT) scanning or other noninvasive diagnostic tests. Treatment is usually implemented in a series of steps that will be discussed.

General measures should be implemented prior to undertaking more specific interventions unless there is a rapidly progressing ICP elevation. Elevation of the head of the bed may be beneficial—15 to 30 degrees seems to be the optimal elevation. Individual variability does exist however. Occasional patients may be encountered who suffer elevations in ICP due to obstruction of CSF outflow through the foramen magnum when assuming an upright position. Therefore, one must measure cerebral perfusion pressure to ensure its preservation with position changes. Hyperthermia must be corrected because it leads to increased cerebral metabolism with accompanying cerebral vasodilatation. A cooling mattress is effective, but caution is necessary to prevent shivering. Should it occur, muscle relaxants may be necessary to eliminate shivering in the intubated and ventilated patient. Seizures lead to ICP elevation and need to be treated. Neurosurgical patients, even those in coma, are responsive to pain; sedatives and analgesics should be used as necessary. Especially when ventilation is being controlled, one should eliminate pain and anxiety if they are contributing to ICP elevations. Respiratory care interventions can lead to ICP changes; these are discussed elsewhere in this chapter. The presence of adequate alveolar ventilation must be guaranteed because elevated levels of $Paco_2$ lead to cerebral vasodilatation. Oxygen is administered to prevent hypoxia. Hypoxia can aggravate cerebral vasodilatation and is, of course, devastating if it results in inadequate oxygen delivery to neural tissue. Fluid restriction to one-half to two-thirds of maintenance prevents brain edema, which is aggravated by overzealous hydration. It is, however, important not to allow hypovolemia and hypotension to occur.

Hyperventilation

More specific and effective therapies directed at lowering ICP begin with implementation of hyperventilation. Because of the exquisite sensitivity of the cerebral vasculature to changes in $Paco_2$ and the rapidity with which it can be changed, hyperventilation is one of the most rapidly effective methods of acute control of ICP. An optimal level of $Paco_2$ is probably between 25 and 30 mm Hg. Lower levels may compromise oxygen delivery by shifting the oxyhemoglobin dissociation curve to a higher affinity state, as well as by causing excessive cerebral vasoconstriction with reduced flow. Areas of normal brain will vasoconstrict in response to lowered $Paco_2$ and may shunt blood toward abnormal ischemic areas that suffer from vasomotor paralysis (a reverse steal). It is important to make sure that ICP is not adversely affected by the maneuvers used to lower $Paco_2$, i.e., increases in mean airway pressure and positive pressure ventilation. Controversy continues concerning how long hyperventilation is effective. After 24 hours or more, the pH of CSF is reset by a lowering of bicarbonate levels, and cerebral vasoconstriction should theoretically disappear. A return of ICP toward its previously elevated level is usually observed despite continued hyperventilation. Although its mechanism is obscure, there is no doubt that in certain circumstances an effective therapeutic benefit from hyperventilation persists beyond this time period. A rapid return of $Paco_2$ to its normal level after prolonged hyperventilation results in vasodilatation and elevated ICP. Hyperventilation must be weaned slowly when no longer needed. It must be noted that there is an unpredictable subset of patients who do not respond to hyperventilation or who may get worse when it is implemented. Calculation of cerebral perfusion pressure following changes in $Paco_2$ will identify this subset and help guide therapy. Despite clear evidence that hyperventilation lowers ICP, there is some doubt about whether it has any effect on overall outcome of patients with acute brain insults.

Cerebrospinal Fluid Drainage

Removal of CSF through a ventriculostomy is the other rapidly effective way to lower ICP. The presence of a ventriculostomy is, of course, necessary. There are few contraindications to such a maneuver, although at times it could lead to some intracranial shifts and brain distortion. If too much fluid is removed, the ventricle collapses against the catheter and obstructs it. Not only may further fluid drainage be impossible, but the catheter's usefulness in measuring ICP may be lost. Ventriculostomies are usually drained against a gravity gradient of 10 to 25 cm H_2O to prevent collapse of the ventricle.

Diuretics

Osmotic Agents. Osmotic agents are the next step in treatment. Their use is widespread because of their proven effectiveness. Many agents have been used in the past. Urea was abandoned in the 1960s because of its inherent toxicity as well as its distribution into brain tissue, which led to later rebound elevation of ICP. Mannitol has emerged as the most commonly used osmotic agent, although some controversy persists about the dosages required and the mechanisms involved. Osmotic agents create a gradient across an intact blood brain barrier and decrease brain water, thus lowering ICP. Recent work suggests that mannitol lowers viscosity and has a consequent effect of lowering cerebral vascular resistance, countered by an autoregulatory response of vasoconstriction, which is responsible for the lowered ICP. Doses between 0.25 and 2.0 g/kg are effective. There are advocates of high- and low-dose therapy. Higher doses work slightly faster and perhaps longer, but have more complications. Use of a high dose often requires that another large dose be given if needed again. Maximum clinical effect is seen 30 minutes to 2 hours later in most cases and lasts for 2 to 10 hours, usually averaging 4 to 6 hours. Complications associated with osmotic agents are primarily the resultant hyperosmolarity and fluid shifts. Renal failure can occur when serum osmolarity exceeds 350 to 360 mOsm. Transient hypervolemia can result in congestive failure in susceptible individuals. Late diuresis may lead to hypovolemia and hypotension. Electrolyte disturbances are common with large doses and long-term therapy. Hypernatremia, hypocalcemia, and hypokalemia may require treatment. Perturbations are minimized when serum osmolarity is kept below 320 mOsm. Hemolysis and rhabdomyolysis have been reported, but only when excessive doses were given in desperate situations and extremely high osmolalities were achieved. Recent work has shown identical ICP effects from doses of mannitol of 0.25 up to 1.0 g/kg. Serum osmolarity changes of no more than 10 mOsm were seen with the smaller dosage, compared to more drastic changes with the higher doses. Rebound elevation of ICP has not been a problem clinically with mannitol.

Loop Diuretics. The loop diuretics furosemide and ethacrynic acid have been helpful in ICP treatment. They have effects on their own and also have synergistic effects when used with mannitol. Their action seems to be mediated through a reduction in sodium and water from edematous areas of brain as well as a decrease in the rate of CSF production. They often have a rapid effect on ICP that is unexplained by their presumed mechanism of action. Dosages range from 0.5 to 1.0 mg/kg. Complications are hypovolemia, hypotension, and the expected electrolyte disturbances, most notably hypokalemia.

Pharmacologic Measures

Lidocaine. Lidocaine deserves mention as a drug that can exert rapid control of ICP. Doses of 1.0 and 1.5 mg/kg IV may lower ICP but have action for only a short time. Lidocaine is most helpful when a brief stimulation might be expected to have a significant effect on ICP, as in endotracheal intubation and suctioning.

Steroids. Steroid therapy for the treatment of elevated ICP remains a controversial subject. Questions remain concerning whether steroids are effective and, if so, when and how they work. Unquestionably, steroids are helpful in decreasing edema surrounding gliomas and metastatic tumors, and decreases in ICP can be demonstrated. CSF production decreases in patients with pseudotumor cerebri. These mechanisms are not valid for acute neurologic problems such as stroke, hemorrhage, or traumatic injury. Some investigators have shown improved intracranial compliance with steroid treatment although possible mechanisms of action remain unclear. In a prospective trial of treatment of head injury with steroids, survival was improved without an associated improvement in meaningful neurologic outcome. Dexamethasone is the most frequently used steroid. Initial boluses of 10 to 20 mg are followed by 4 to 8 mg IV every 4 to 6 hours. Doses are tapered after 3 to 4 days. H_2-blockers and antacids are routinely given to decrease the risk of gastrointestinal hemorrhage, a risk more likely due to the concomitant neurologic problem than to the steroid usage. Hyperglycemia is aggravated and should be treated if extreme. Steroids will aggravate the susceptibility to infection and high rate of catabolism that accompany the stress of surgery or trauma.

Barbiturates. Barbiturates are extremely effective in the control of ICP. Thiopental rapidly lowers ICP and is helpful in situations of acute increases, such as with intubation, suctioning, and other short procedures. Boluses of 0.5 to 5.0 mg/kg are used. The mechanism of action to diminish ICP is unclear. Possible explanations include lowered cerebral metabolic rate with resultant decreased cerebral blood flow, blockage of the generation of oxygen-free radicals, and a direct vasoconstricting effect on the cerebral vasculature. Controversy begins when one considers the use of barbiturate for long-term therapy of elevated ICP or in situations where elevated ICP is refractory to all other interventions. Pentobarbital can be given in a bolus of 5 to 10 mg/kg and followed by a continuous infusion of 1 to 5 mg/kg/hr. Profound hypotension is not unusual because of myocardial depressant effects, and volume and inotropic support are commonly required. Most studies have failed to show any improvement in outcome in situations where barbiturates have been invoked for refractory elevated ICP control. Neurologic function is difficult to monitor clinically or electrophysiologically during barbiturate therapy.

Cardiovascular Complications

Hypotension

The cardiovascular system may have dramatic effects on the brain, just as the brain may have profound effects on the cardiovascular system. The output of the cardiovascular system as manifested by mean arterial blood pressure represents one of the main determinants of cerebral perfusion. Under normal conditions, the mean arterial pressure (MAP) should never be allowed to drop below 50 to 70 mm Hg, which represents the lower limits of cerebral autoregulation. Mean pressure must be kept even higher in chronically hypertensive patients who have shifted cerebral autoregulation as well as in patients who have elevated ICP. Cardiovascular instability is not an uncommon postoperative problem in the neurosurgical patient population. Hypotension needs to be treated aggressively when present. Fluid resuscitation is the best initial treatment in most patients, since hypovolemia is commonly present. Isotonic crystalloid or colloid may be used. Blood loss due to traumatic or intraoperative losses must be replaced. Osmotic and loop diuretics enlisted in the treatment of elevated ICP or in the facilitation of surgical exposure contribute to blood volume depletion. Diabetes insipidus, although unusual, needs to be considered. Hypothermia, residual anesthetic effects, and the use of myocardial depressant drugs may aggravate hypotension. Vasodilatation from fever or correction of postoperative hypothermia may reveal an underlying fluid deficiency. Although rare in patients other than those with atherosclerotic cerebrovascular disease, the occurrence of myocardial infarction leading to hypotension must be kept in mind. Inotropic and vasopressor support is the second step to be used for treatment of hypotension after fluid resuscitation has been shown to be ineffective. Cerebral vessels are minimally responsive to alpha-adrenergic drugs which, therefore, do not have deleterious effects on cerebral blood flow.

Hypertension

Pathophysiology

Hypertension is extremely common postoperatively. By exceeding the limits of cerebral autoregulation (>150 mm Hg mean), high blood pressure contributes to neurologic problems by leading to the breakdown of the blood-brain barrier, interstitial edema, and aggravation of elevated ICP. In addition, hypertension can lead to catastrophic intracranial hemorrhage in susceptible patients. Factors which can lead to hypertension postoperatively should be ruled out or treated accordingly prior to pharmacologic manipulation of blood pressure. These include hypothermia with concomitant vasoconstriction, hypoventilation with hypercarbia, fluid overload, hypoxia, emergence from anesthesia with pain, and Cushing reflex secondary to high ICP.

Treatment

Side Effects. Inherent in the treatment of hypertension is an understanding of the potential side effects of various drugs and the factors controlling ICP and net cerebral blood flow. Vasodilators lead to an increase in cerebral blood volume and may thus increase ICP with a resultant decrease in net global or regional blood flow. In addition, they may allow higher blood pressure to be experienced downstream and lead to an aggravation of cerebral edema in susceptible areas. There is no ideal drug to lower blood pressure in patients with cerebral insult.

Specific Agents. Sodium nitroprusside (Nipride, Nitropress) is commonly utilized for rapid blood pressure control. It is a potent, immediate-acting peripheral vasodilator with an onset of action between 0.5 and 5 minutes. It is given by continuous infusion and its use necessitates intra-arterial pressure monitoring. Doses range from 0.3 to 8 μg/kg/min. Tachyphylaxis may occur at high doses after long-standing use and may indicate impending toxicity. Cyanide is a metabolic by-product, and metabolic acidosis is a sign of toxicity. Trimethaphan camsylate is another rapidly acting drug given by infusion in doses of 0.3 to 6 mg/min of a 0.1% solution. It has ganglionic blocking actions and may possess direct peripheral vasodilating activity as well. Tachyphylaxis may be a problem and unreactive pupils often result, possibly clouding the clinical examination. Hydralazine is a direct vasodilator having greatest effect on arterial smooth muscle. Its onset of action is between 10 and 80 minutes following an initial parenteral dose of 5 to 20 mg. All of these drugs, with the exception of trimethaphan, lower cerebral vascular resistance and may potentially elevate ICP.

Methyldopa (Aldomet) and clonidine (Catapres) are effective antihypertensive agents that work via central alpha-adrenergic stimulation. The net result is a decrease in sympathetic outflow from the central nervous system. Methyldopa can be given parenterally, 250 to 500 mg IV every 6 hours, and has an onset of action of 3 to 4 hours. Clonidine exerts control of blood pressure elevations within 30 to 60 minutes following a 0.1-mg oral dose. Withdrawal of this drug may result in significant rebound hypertension, which may be avoided with the use of transdermal clonidine patches. Both methyldopa and clonidine may have central nervous system (CNS) side effects of sedation.

Nifedipine (Procardia) is a calcium-channel blocking drug that has become popular in the treatment of acute hypertension. It has actions on myocardial and vascular smooth muscle and results in a decreased systemic vascular resistance. It can be given orally or sublingually in 10-mg doses. Onset of action is between 10 and 30 minutes, with a duration of up to a few hours. Doses may be repeated as needed if hypertension persists. Cerebral vasodilatation may occur.

Labetalol (Normodyne, Trandate) is an antihypertensive drug that has unique properties of selective alpha-1-adrenergic and nonselective beta-adrenergic blockade. It results in a dose-related fall in blood pressure without reflex tachycardia and usually without a significant drop in heart rate. Intravenous doses of 0.15 mg/kg are given over 2 to 3 minutes and may be repeated as needed every 10 minutes. The usual maximum dose is 300 mg, after which additional drugs should be utilized. Labetalol may also be given as a continuous infusion beginning with 2 mg/min, and titrating the rate as necessary. Beta-blocking drugs should be avoided in patients with congestive heart failure, bronchospasm, heart block, or bradycardia. Esmolol (Brevibloc) is a new beta-blocking drug with rapid onset and termination of action. It is given by infusion in the ICU where continuous invasive arterial pressure monitoring is utilized.

Choice of Agents. The side effects of these drugs may often preclude their use, but more often their beneficial effects to normalize the hypertensive situation is more important. The potential benefit of calcium-channel blockers in ischemic brain protection, for example, may lead to the choice of nifedipine despite its tendency to elevate ICP. Similarly, the need for rapid and variable control of blood pressure may justify the use of nitroprusside despite the potential cerebral vasodilating effects of this agent. Close clinical monitoring of the neurologic status and the continuous determination of cerebral perfusion pressure remain the only ways to determine whether beneficial effects of these drugs outweigh their side effects. At present, we are often unable to make these determinations owing to inadequacies of our monitoring techniques to determine regional cerebral conditions.

Electrocardiographic Changes and Arrhythmias

Electrocardiographic (ECG) changes in neurologic patients are frequently observed. They are often related to hypokalemia from diuretic therapy, respiratory alkalosis, or concurrent cardiac diseases. However, intracranial pathology is a common cause for these abnormalities. Acute ECG changes such as T-wave inversion, S-T elevation, peaked

P waves, tall T waves, and prolonged Q-T intervals are seen after acute head injury and subarachnoid hemorrhage. These changes are similar to those seen with myocardial ischemia. Virtually any type of cardiac arrhythmia may be seen in these patients. Mechanisms to explain these observations may include hypothalamic dysfunction or elevated blood catecholamine levels with effects on myocardial and coronary arterial alpha-receptors. Close electrocardiographic monitoring is required in case there should be deterioration into a malignant arrhythmia that would require urgent treatment.

Respiratory Complications

Problems related to the respiratory system are important in all surgical patients, and particularly so in those with neurologic abnormalities or recent intracranial surgery. Respiratory failure occurs in up to 25% of patients with isolated head injuries, with most of those who die from these injuries having evidence of pulmonary abnormalities. Elective neurosurgical procedures in the elderly result in a high incidence of pulmonary complications which contribute to mortality. Respiratory problems contribute more morbidity and mortality to neurologically injured and postoperative neurosurgical patients than any other interrelated system. The importance is compounded by the frequency of diminished levels of consciousness in this patient group and by the exquisite sensitivity of the central nervous system to hypoxia, hypercarbia, and hypocarbia.

Protective Airway Reflexes

A patent and protected airway is of primary importance. The normal airway has four types of protective reflexes: pharyngeal, laryngeal, tracheal, and carinal. The pharyngeal reflex, mediated by cranial nerves IX and X, consists of the gag and swallowing reflexes. The laryngeal reflex controls the apposition of the vocal cords and closure of the glottis with laryngeal stimulation. Both its afferent and efferent fibers course via the vagus nerve, as do those mediating the following two reflexes. The tracheal and carinal reflexes lead to coughing with irritation of the airways. As the level of consciousness becomes depressed, these reflexes are lost, beginning with the pharyngeal reflex. Recovering patients show return of these reflexes in reverse order beginning with carinal and tracheal reflexes. Prevention of obstruction and aspiration caused by impairment of these reflexes is the most common indication for airway management in the neurosurgical patient.

Control of Breathing

Neural control of breathing resides in the brain stem, which receives information from peripheral and central receptors as well as cortical modulation from above. Chemical sensors in the carotid and aortic bodies respond to changes in PO_2, pH, and $Paco_2$, and transmit impulses via nerves IX and X to the medullary respiratory nuclei. Peripheral receptors are most important for hypoxic conditions, whereas the central receptors are more important for changes in $Paco_2$ and pH. Central receptors are located near the ventral surface of the medulla and are in direct contact with CSF. The mechanical receptors in the airways and lung tissue send signals to the brain stem and are responsible for initiating reflexes of sneezing, coughing, and other changes in respiratory rate and volume. Three respiratory centers in the medulla and pons control automatic respiration, and these are affected by voluntary cortical control from higher levels. Such actions as deep breathing and sighing are due to this higher cortical control.

Pathologic conditions can affect the different parts of the hierarchy of respiration and produce abnormal respiratory patterns. Cheyne-Stokes respiration is associated with destructive bilateral lesions in the cerebral hemispheres or basal ganglia. This type of respiration consists of periodic breathing in which hyperpnea alternates with apnea. Patients with this pattern of breathing are comatose and have a grave prognosis. These is also a Cheyne-Stokes variant in which apneic periods are not present, and this may be found in patients with unilateral lesions who are usually not comatose. Central neurogenic hyperventilation may be found with pontine lesions and mimics the response to systemic hypoxia and acidosis. This pattern is frequent in conditions of transtentorial herniation with midbrain compression. Apneustic breathing or cluster breathing is characterized by a series of ratchet-like steps followed by a long breath hold before the breakthrough of rapid breathing. This is characteristic of a pontine lesion. Ataxic or grossly irregular breathing occurs with medullary lesions or medullary compression, as might exist with an expanding posterior fossa mass. The pattern is unpredictable and occasional episodes of apnea are not unusual. The outcome is usually fatal in this situation. Although certain breathing patterns are clearly related to abnormalities at different levels of the hierarchy of neural control, often one cannot correlate a particular respiratory pattern with a specific lesion. An abnormal pattern of breathing often provides inadequate ventilation and is almost always indicative of a serious intracranial condition. Therefore, the institution of airway and ventilatory control is usually required.

Preexisting Disease

Preexisting or coexisting conditions may aggravate the pulmonary status of a neurosurgical patient. Preexisting conditions such as chronic obstructive pulmonary disease, asthma, heavy tobacco use, intercurrent infection, or severe restrictive airway disease have profound effects on respiratory care in the ICU. Residual anesthetic effects such as diffusion hypoxia, absorption atelectasis, decreased functional residual capacity (FRC), narcosis, sedation, and shivering will have bearing on airway and ventilatory management. Perioperative aspiration, particularly during the care of the head-injured patient, is not unusual and is reported in up to 25% of such patients. This may result in profound hypoxia and ventilatory difficulties and is known to have resulted in fatalities. The syndrome of neurogenic pulmonary edema has been studied extensively in the laboratory and many explanations for its etiology still remain. Although probably rare in clinical practice, it may be difficult to distinguish from other causes of acute pulmonary edema and respiratory insufficiency. Pulmonary edema is also aggravated by improper excessive fluid administration in the elderly patient and in the resuscitation of a trauma victim. Finally, there is often concomitant associated blunt or penetrating thoracic injury which may lead to pneumothorax, pulmonary contusion, or flail chest. These and other associated conditions such as disseminated intravascular coagulation (DIC) and fat embolism syndrome need to be evaluated and treated in the trauma patient.

Airway Management

Options and Indications

Establishment of airway control may be a life-saving maneuver. Obtunded or comatose patients will require airway protection. Posterior displacement of oropharyngeal soft tissue structures is probably the most common cause of upper airway obstruction in the neurosurgical patient. If this is the only problem, it may be satisfactorily remedied by an oral or nasopharyngeal airway. This, of course, requires that adequate ventilation is not a problem. Patients with more serious neurologic problems, such as those with posturing or Glasgow Coma Scale scores less than 7, require endotracheal intubation for airway control as well as treatment with ventilatory support. Patients with acute respiratory failure or those with problems requiring frequent tracheal suctioning also require endotracheal intubation.

Approaches to Intubation

Endotracheal intubation may be accomplished by either the nasal or oral route. Only rarely is an emergency tracheostomy or cricothyrotomy necessary to secure an airway. Such a situation might be a case of massive facial trauma, fractured larynx, or unstable cervical spine injury precluding oral or nasal tracheal intubation. Orotracheal intubation is accomplished with the aid of a laryngoscope, whereas nasotracheal intubation can be accomplished either blindly or under direct visualization, utilizing a laryngoscope. Blind placement of a nasotracheal tube usually requires that the patient be spontaneously breathing. There are several advantages and disadvantages of each technique. Oral intubation is more uncomfortable for an awake patient, and the tube is more difficult to secure in a patient who is moving significantly. Nasotracheal intubation, although more comfortable for an awake patient, carries the risks of sinusitis and otitis due to obstruction of the openings of the sinuses and eustachian tubes if continued for more than a few days. Nasal intubation in the presence of basilar skull fracture is relatively contraindicated. Nasal tubes may have to be smaller than their oral counterparts. They carry the risk of epistaxis and are therefore contraindicated if coagulopathy is present. Regardless of which tube is used, it is important that it be positioned so that the end is far enough above the carina to ensure ventilation of both lung fields. Cuff placement below the vocal cords is required to seal off the airway. When intubation is required for a prolonged period, tracheostomy may be performed. Usually it is preferable to delay tracheostomy for at least 2 weeks, at which time it may be easier to predict which patients will require long-term airway control. With modern techniques of endotracheal tube care, including low pressure cuffs, the incidence of permanent laryngeal and tracheal stenoses related to endotracheal intubation is small.

Blunting Responses to Intubation

While a description of techniques of intubation is beyond the scope of this chapter, the effects of intubation warrant mention. Laryngoscopy and intubation result in profound hemodynamic responses in many patients and although these may be taxing to the cardiovascular system, they can be catastrophic to a patient with intracranial abnormalities. In patients with diminished intracranial compliance, increases in blood pressure lead to large increases in ICP. Various maneuvers may be required to diminish these hemodynamic responses and ICP changes. Moderate to large doses of thiopental help blunt the responses to intubation but may be contraindicated if rapid intubation cannot be accomplished or if the patient is hemodynamically unstable. Lidocaine has also been shown to blunt intubation responses in patients with decreased intracranial compliance. The usual dose is 1.5 mg/kg IV. Narcotics blunt this response as well but may be contraindicated because of their respiratory depressant effects. It is not unusual for muscle relaxants to be required to accomplish laryngoscopy and intubation. Succinylcholine has been shown to elevate ICP and is best avoided. Relatively rapid-acting nondepolarizing muscle relaxants such as atracurium or vecuronium may be better choices for intubation in such patients. If succinylcholine is required, pretreatment with a nondepolarizing relaxant may blunt the ICP response to the succinylcholine. All these patients are at significant risk for aspiration, and therefore the use of cricoid pressure during intubation should not be forgotten.

Hyperventilation as a Therapeutic Measure

In addition to its use in acute respiratory failure, ventilatory support is commonly employed in the treatment of neurologically impaired patients. Hyperventilation will lead to an acute lowering of $Paco_2$, which will lead to an abrupt rise in the pH of brain extracellular fluid. This will then result in vasoconstriction of cerebral blood vessels with a 4% decrease in cerebral blood flow for every 1 mm Hg change in $Paco_2$ down to 25 mm Hg. The vasoconstriction and decrease in cerebral blood flow leads to a direct decrease in cerebral blood volume and thus a lowered ICP. In normal volunteers it has been shown that for every 1 mm Hg decrease in $Paco_2$ there is a drop in cerebral blood volume of 0.05 ml/100 g brain tissue. Hyperventilation to $Paco_2$ levels of less than 20 mm Hg may result in tissue hypoxia due to problems in unloading of hemoglobin at the tissue level. In addition, the increasing amounts of hyperventilation required to lower the $Paco_2$ to extreme levels may raise the mean airway pressure and thus have adverse effects on ICP. It is important to avoid hypoxemia, which leads to cerebral vasodilation as well as inadequate oxygen delivery. With prolonged hyperventilation, the brain responds to the altered extracellular fluid pH by decreasing CSF bicarbonate levels and normalizing the pH of CSF. The beneficial effect of hyperventilation may therefore be short-lived, although clinicians have at times noticed a definite benefit of hyperventilation beyond this 24- to 48-hour period. It is important to recognize that in patients being chronically hyperventilated, any decrease in ventilation may result in an increase in $Paco_2$ and cerebral vasodilatation and elevated ICP. Therefore, hyperventilation should be tapered over a period of 24 to 48 hours with close observation for changes in ICP.

Positive End-Expiratory Pressure and Intracranial Pressure

Respiratory Care Maneuvers

In a patient with reduced intracranial compliance and elevated ICP, certain respiratory care maneuvers may need to be modified in order to prevent problems. Tracheal suctioning will routinely stimulate tracheal and laryngeal reflexes leading to coughing or a Valsalva maneuver, and these will tend to raise ICP. It is therefore advantageous to blunt these responses. Pretreatment with either topical lidocaine in the airway or intravenous lidocaine will blunt ICP responses to suctioning, just as they do during endotracheal intubation. Systemic narcotics and barbiturates can also help blunt these responses.

Positive Airway Pressure

Pathophysiology. Positive pressure required for ventilatory support in the neurologic ICU has many adverse effects such as antidiuretic hormone production, decrease and redistribution of renal blood flow, and barotrauma. There are resultant hemodynamic disturbances and changes in ICP, however, which are unique to the neurologic patient and warrant discussion. Ordinarily, approximately 50% of the positive pressure applied to airways is transmitted to the pleural space. Alterations in intrapleural pressure may have profound effects on hemodynamic parameters, particularly venous return and central venous pressure. By diminishing the venous return, cardiac output and blood pressure are also diminished, and in the patient with elevated ICP this results in a decrease in cerebral perfusion pressure. In a small subset of patients, the increase in central venous pressure alone may be detrimental to cerebral perfusion pressure by means of transmission to the cranial vault. The significance of the changes in positive airway pressure will be determined for the large part by the compliance of the lungs and chest wall. In a patient with stiff lungs due to respiratory failure, the amount of pressure transmitted to the pleural space is actually smaller than in a patient with normal lungs. Paralysis of the chest wall results in a lesser increase in intrapleural pressure and may be particularly advantageous in situations where high degrees of positive pressure are required. Positive end-expiratory pressure (PEEP) is often necessary and will lead to an increase in mean airway pressure and transmitted intrapleural pressure. Experimental studies have verified that PEEP may have adverse effects on cerebral perfusion pressure. Pathophysiologic mechanisms involve diminished cardiac output or blood pressure and indirect effects of raising ICP through increases in cerebral venous pressure or blockage of CSF outflow.

Clinical Applications. The intracranial responses to the application of positive pressure in individual patients cannot be predicted. Most clinical studies, however, have failed to show detrimental effects in patients with baseline elevations of ICP. When PEEP is required at levels greater than 5 to 10 cm H_2O, it is best to be able to measure ICP simultaneously and therefore assure that cerebral perfusion pressure is not seriously diminished. Should cerebral perfusion pressure drop at a time when positive pressure and PEEP are required to support oxygenation, other maneuvers will be required. Vigorous volume expansion to restore preload to the heart is begun, and the use of inotropic drugs such as dopamine is considered. Additional measures to decrease ICP, if possible, would be helpful.

Patients with more compliant lungs and less compliant chest walls are expected to have the largest increases in intrapleural pressure and hence be susceptible to the greatest changes in cerebral perfusion pressure and ICP. Because of the unpredictability, it is important to measure cerebral perfusion pressure objectively during the institution of ventilatory support and when making changes in ventilatory parameters.

Respiratory Failure

The diagnosis of respiratory failure in the neurologic ICU is no different from that in any other critical care setting. The accompanying table (Table 18–1) shows criteria which define respiratory insufficiency. All of these are easily measurable in the ICU setting, although pulmonary artery catheterization is required to measure shunt and a capnometer or Douglas bag is needed to measure V_DD_T. Respiratory failure can occur as a result of central or peripheral problems in neurosurgical patients. Central problems of inadequate neurorespiratory drive have been discussed previously, as have peripheral causes such as airway obstruction. Hypoxia is often an indication for respiratory support.

Table 18-1 Criteria for Diagnosis of Respiratory Failure

Criteria	Volumes
Respiratory rate	>40/min or <8/min
Tidal volume	<3.5 ml/kg
Vital capacity	<15 ml/kg
Negative inspiratory force	<-20 cm H_2O
PaO_2	<60 mm Hg
$PaCO_2$	>50 mm Hg (if not chronic)
V_D/V_T	>0.5
Pulmonary shunt	>12%

There are five major conditions leading to hypoxia. Low administered oxygen concentration and alveolar hypoventilation are two obvious causes. Ventilation-perfusion mismatch or right-to-left shunt can be considered together. They are the cause of hypoxemia in atelectasis, adult respiratory distress syndrome (ARDS), and pneumonia. They have also been reported in patients with isolated head injuries with no other explanations for hypoxia. Finally, there is impairment to diffusion of oxygen across the alveolar membrane as is caused by pulmonary edema fluid. The latter is not a major cause of hypoxemia in most clinical settings.

Complications of Airway Management

Laryngeal Problems

Edema of the glottic area is the most common complication of endotracheal intubation. It may result from trauma during intubation, excessive movement of the tube, or local damage due to the presence of the tube. The anatomy of the larynx is such that an endotracheal tube touches its walls at the right and left vocal processes and at the cricoid cartilage. The area of contact is so small that even slight forces generate high local pressures, leading to mucosal ischemia. Motion of the tube with neck flexion or extension may contribute to laryngeal injury. In addition, longitudinal motion of the larynx with respiratory efforts aggravates local trauma caused by tube movement. Postextubation laryngeal edema may result in airway obstruction in rare cases, but commonly leads to stridor. Although it is uncommon for edema to require intervention, two options exist for treatment of symptomatic patients. Racemic epinephrine (0.5 ml of 2.25% solution in 3 ml of normal saline) may be administered as an aerosol every 1 to 4 hours. Steroids, either 10 mg of dexamethasone or 1 g of methylprednisolone, may be given in a single dose. Hoarseness and temporary inadequacy of glottic closure are not unusual following extubation. Long-term complications of laryngeal injury include hoarseness, granuloma formation, and laryngeal stenosis. Prevention relies on an adequately secured tube and the use of a small tube whenever possible.

Suctioning

As previously discussed, suctioning may have adverse effects on ICP. It may also result in hypoxia, hypercarbia, cardiac arrhythmias, and hypotension. Lung collapse may result from a large catheter placed within a narrow diameter airway. Mucosal damage relates directly to excessive force and frequency of suction catheter manipulations.

Obstruction of the Endotracheal Tube

Artificial airways are also susceptible to obstruction. The patient may bite on the tube, or movement may result in a kink. Other causes of obstruction are cuff herniation or overinflated cuff compressing the tube lumen, inspired secretions, blood clot, foreign body, or abutment of the tube bevel against the carina or endobronchial wall. Treatment of suspected tube obstruction requires suctioning to prove patency, cuff deflation, and repositioning. Lack of success necessitates tube removal, bag and mask ventilation, reintubation, and consideration of other problems such as pneumothorax.

Infection

Pneumonia is a common cause of respiratory failure and is a potentially life-threatening complication. Colonization of the pharynx and upper respiratory tract usually precedes pneumonia. The presence of an endotracheal tube or tracheostomy predisposes to infection by providing a means of access for bacteria to the upper respiratory tract while compromising native airway defenses. Pathogenic bacteria may be spread by health-care workers and are more likely to colonize the tissues of patients treated with broad-spectrum antibiotics. Contamination of respiratory care equipment, especially humidifiers, is another source of infection. Aspiration of small amounts of oropharyngeal secretions introduces infection to the susceptible host and unfortunately is all too common an occurrence in neurosurgical patients.

The diagnosis of pneumonia is often difficult. Concomitant stress and the presence of other medical and surgical illnesses may discount the reliability of fever and leukocytosis as a diagnostic tool. Pneumonia is suspected whenever a new infiltrate is seen on the chest film. Atelectasis is differentiated by its correction with aggressive pulmonary toilet. Some intensivists go so far as to recommend daily chest films in intubated patients to allow early diagnosis of pneumonia. Frequent Gram stains and cultures of tracheal secretions may suggest the causative organism, but accurate diagnosis may be enhanced with protected brush cultures obtained at bronchoscopy. Gram-negative bacilli are identified in 87% of patients, with gram-positive organisms isolated in 13%. Mortality from gram-negative pneumonias has been reported to be between 30 and 70%. Prevention is aided by steps to minimize aspiration and avoidance of unnecessary antibiotic use. Hand washing and meticulous respiratory care practices are essential.

Initiation of Ventilatory Therapy

Interrelationship with the Central Nervous System

When instituting ventilatory therapy, it is important to do so without adversely affecting the central nervous system. As mentioned above, the airway must be secured with care to minimize potential changes in ICP. When placing the patient on the ventilator, be careful that the positive pressure does not diminish venous return and cardiac output, thereby adversely affecting brain perfusion. Ventilator settings are selected to ensure adequate oxygenation and the desired degree of hyperventilation. They are confirmed within the first 10 to 15 minutes by an arterial blood gas sample.

Mechanical Ventilation

Three categories of ventilators are commonly available: time-cycled, pressure-cycled, and volume-cycled. High-frequency ventilation expands the number of available options to four.

Time- and pressure-cycled ventilators are rarely utilized in adult critical care. Volume-cycled ventilators deliver a preset quantity of gas before allowing exhalation to occur, unless a pressure limit is exceeded. This automatically compensates for any changes in compliance or resistance of the patient-ventilator system (within the range of the alarms and limits set).

Mechanical ventilation with volume-cycled ventilators can be characterized as full or partial support. Full support implies that a patient's normal alveolar ventilation will be provided by machine delivery of at least 8 breaths/min with a tidal volume of 10 to 15 ml/kg. Full support is possible with any of several modes: IMV (intermittent mandatory ventilation), SIMV (synchronized intermittent mandatory ventilation), CMV (controlled mechanical ventilation), assisted ventilation, and assist-control. Partial support is available only in IMV or SIMV modes.

CMV is insensitive to a patient's inspiratory efforts, and spontaneous breathing through the circuit is impossible. If a patient "fights" the ventilator, the work of breathing may be greatly increased. Rate is set by the operator and, since additional ventilation is not possible, there is a predisposition to hypo- or hyperventilation. CMV is therefore limited to a situation in which the patient is unconscious, paralyzed, or has severe CNS or neuromuscular dysfunction.

The assisted ventilation mode involves patient initiation of a breath by development of negative inspiratory pressure. The machine is thereby activated, delivering its preset volume. Patient work may be considerable because respiratory muscle function persists even after machine work begins. A potential advantage of this mode is that the patient may select his own level of ventilation. Protection from apnea or hypoventilation due to a lack of effort in a depressed or tired patient is afforded by a switch to assist-control mode. This latter mode offers a preset backup rate of breaths that is delivered if the patient fails to initiate a sufficient number of breaths spontaneously. While this theoretically may predispose to hyperventilation of the patient and respiratory alkalosis, this response has not been encountered frequently in clinical practice. A change to an IMV mode would correct such a problem if it were to occur.

IMV has become one of the most commonly applied ventilator modes. It is characterized by a preset number of machine-delivered breaths by a system that also allows spontaneous patient breathing. A demand valve is usually present that requires variable work of breathing in different ventilators. A valveless, high-flow circuit is ideal to eliminate any excess work of breathing. There are several theoretical advantages to IMV, including patient comfort with less need for sedation, decreased mean airway pressure (with less hemodynamic effects), and facilitated weaning, although these have not been proven clinically. Synchronized IMV prevents the machine delivered breath from being "stacked" on top of a patient-initiated breath. This is another concern of a theoretical nature that has not been found clinically to be a problem.

Finally, pressure support is another mode that has received recent attention and interest, especially with the availability of modern microprocessor-controlled ventilators. This mode combines features of assisted ventilation with continuous positive airway pressure (CPAP). Following initiation of a breath by the patient, the ventilator applies a preset degree of positive pressure to the airway. This augments the tidal volume and inspiratory flow rate. The actual volumes achieved are determined by the preset pressure and the compliance of the patient's lungs and chest wall. Overall work, however, is reduced. Patient comfort is supposedly enhanced as well.

PEEP is a commonly utilized adjunct to mechanical ventilation. Its main purpose is to increase FRC, which is diminished in many forms of respiratory failure. Optimization of FRC results in improved lung compliance, decreased pulmonary vascular resistance, decreased shunt, and improved oxygenation. CPAP is utilized for the same reasons as PEEP, but in situations where mechanical ventilation is not being performed. It may be delivered through a ventilator system or by mask. As discussed elsewhere, PEEP (and CPAP) may have adverse consequences on cardiac output and ICP.

Initial Ventilator Settings

For the typical patient requiring mechanical ventilation, initial settings using the 12/12 rule are sufficient. Total volume is set at 12 ml/kg and the rate is set at 12/min. Higher settings are of course required for deliberate hyperventilation. PaO_2 must be at least 60 to 65 mm Hg, although a value of 80 to 100 mm Hg allows a margin of safety should mucous plugging and atelectasis occur. FIO_2 should be minimized to prevent oxygen toxicity. An inspired concentration of 40 to 50% oxygen is probably safe for long periods of time. PEEP is a valuable tool to help lower FIO_2 but is not without risks, as has already been discussed. Peak and plateau airway pressures are measured and followed hourly, as they yield valuable information on changes in dynamic and static compliance, respectively (compliance is $\Delta V/\Delta P$).

Troubleshooting

If a ventilator malfunction occurs, the patient is removed from the ventilator and managed by hand ventilation with an Ambu bag until the difficulty is remedied. Causes of respiratory insufficiency in previously stable patients can often be determined by studying changes in dynamic and static compliance. Dynamic compliance is reduced in cases of chest wall rigidity or increases in airway resistance. Static compliance is affected by chest wall and lung compliance and not by airway resistance. If dynamic compliance is reduced without a simultaneous change in static compliance, a resistance problem, such as bronchospasm, retained secretions, or ventilator circuit obstruction is suggested. Symmetric decreases in both compliances may suggest pneumothorax, mainstem intubation, pulmonary edema, pneumonia, or atelectasis.

Weaning

Weaning of neurosurgical patients can be particularly difficult. Improvement in neurologic condition is a slow process and often precludes any consideration of weaning for quite some time. Tracheostomy is frequently required. Timing of weaning depends on variables other than the resolution of pulmonary failure. Neurologic status must be improved to a point where hyperventilation is no longer required and such that protective airway reflexes have returned. Traditional tests of weaning parameters may have to be altered owing to the inability of patients to cooperate with voluntary respiratory maneuvers. Traditional tests for weaning and extubation include negative inspiratory force greater than 20 to 25 cm H_2O, vital capacity greater than 10 ml/kg, and minute ventilation less than 10 L/min, with maintenance of $PaCO_2$ less than 40 mm Hg. If cooperation is possible, maximum minute ventilation should exceed twice the resting minute ventilation. During the actual weaning trial, if respiratory rate exceeds 30, the patient is likely to fail weaning at that time.

Weaning techniques consist of T-tube trials or IMV weaning protocols. T-tube techniques involve discontinuation of ventilatory therapy with subsequent measurement of serial blood gases. These have the advantage of no added resistance except the endotracheal tube or tracheostomy, but CPAP cannot be given. Failure to maintain satisfactory arterial blood gas values (ABGs) requires reinstitution of ventilatory therapy and weaning at a later time. IMV methods utilize progressively decreasing ventilator rates while allowing the patient to gradually increase his burden of ventilatory work. Serial ABGs aid in the assessment of a successful weaning trial. Pressure support ventilation is a relatively new ventilatory method. It is a technique whereby the patient's spontaneous inspiratory efforts are augmented by application of a preset positive pressure by the ventilator. Further study is needed before specific indications can be made concerning its use during weaning.

When extubation is contemplated, all equipment for reintubation must be close at hand. Reintubation may be required because of laryngeal or glottic edema, progressive tiring of muscles of respiration, or cerebral decompensation. A recently extubated patient is at risk for aspiration for several hours because of the effects of intubation on glottic function. Regardless of neurologic status, patients must be kept strictly NPO and observed closely for respiratory difficulties following extubation. Patients ventilated for more than a few days often require at least several hours to wean. Progressive respiratory muscle weakness accompanies prolonged periods of ventilatory support. More elaborate weaning protocols to gradually rebuild respiratory muscular strength may be needed.

Seizures

Incidence

Seizures are not uncommon in patients with neurologic disease. Postoperative seizures in the neurosurgical population occur in about 13% of previously normal patients. Epileptic patients have an incidence of postoperative seizures approaching 35%. Half of these seizures occur in the first 24 hours. Involvement of cortical sensory and motor areas increases the risk. Recognition is important to allow early termination of the seizure in order to reduce the potential complications. Morbidity and mortality are both related to the duration of seizure activity.

Definition and Etiology

Seizures are defined as paroxysmal excessive neuronal discharges that result in abnormal cerebral electrical activity and behavior. They can be classified as partial (focal) or generalized. The former are more often associated with underlying neurologic abnormalities, but the latter are more dangerous. The etiology of seizures is multifactorial and incompletely understood. Several instigating factors include head injury, tumor, cerebral vascular disease, CNS infection, and metabolic, drug, and toxic causes. Trauma leads to mechanical disruption of brain tissue in the presence of extravascular blood, both of which increase the likelihood of epileptic activity. Brain tumors, especially those near or in the cerebral cortices, lead to seizures by mechanisms of ischemia, local mechanical forces, and edema formation. Cerebrovascular disease leading to ischemic stroke or hemorrhage is highly associated with seizure activity. Local infection can result in epileptogenic foci. Electrolyte abnormalities, particularly hyponatremia, hypernatremia, hypocalcemia, and hypomagnesemia, can lead to seizures. Hypoglycemia and hypoxia, in addition to the preceding chemical abnormalities, produce refractory seizures if they are not corrected. Ethanol withdrawal is yet another possible etiology. Failure to control a seizure can lead to neurologic functional loss by several mechanisms. Hypertension accompanying a seizure results in breakdown of the blood-brain barrier with resulting cerebral edema formation. Respiratory insufficiency, which is a common occurrence in the seizing patient, results in dangerous hypoxia as well as hypercarbia, which aggravates cerebral vasodilatation. Local increases in cerebral metabolic rate due to the seizure activity may exceed the increase of blood flow possible in damaged or diseased areas of the brain. ICP elevations often result from seizure activity.

Status Epilepticus

Acute seizures may deteriorate to status epilepticus. This is defined as frequently repeated or prolonged seizure activity that results in a fixed or lasting epileptic condition, usually longer than 30 minutes. Therapy must be aggressive if convulsions last longer than 5 to 10 minutes. A search for the etiology must accompany treatment. Routine laboratory tests may reveal an underlying metabolic abnormality. Blood should be sent for levels of electrolytes, blood urea nitrogen, glucose, calcium, magnesium, and serum osmolarity. Radiologic studies, i.e., CT scanning or magnetic resonance imaging, should be done as needed once the situation has been stabilized. Lumbar puncture should be performed if there is no mass effect and infection is suspected.

Treatment

Initial management includes airway protection and the assurance of adequate respiration and circulation. Glucose, once given empirically, is now withheld until hypoglycemia is quickly documented because of the potential adverse effects on ischemic brain tissue. Pharmacologic therapy is instituted next, usually with phenytoin (Dilantin) along with a rapidly acting drug to effect early control.

Phenytoin is an effective antiseizure drug. Its advantages lie in its long half-life and its low side-effect profile, especially the minimal sedative effects. An initial dose of 5 to 20 mg/kg is given, but at a maximal rate of 50 mg/min in order to prevent cardiovascular side effects, such as arrhythmia or hypotension. Cardiac standstill has also been reported. Antiepileptic effects may take up to 20 minutes to occur, and a loading dose often takes 20 to 25 minutes to administer safely. For these reasons, an additional drug (benzodiazepine or barbiturate) is often given to terminate the seizure rapidly while Dilantin is started.

Benzodiazepines have become the most popular drugs for short-term seizure control. They rapidly gain access to the CNS and can quickly terminate the epileptic episode. Diazepam (Valium) is given in a dose of 5 to 10 mg IV (0.3 mg/kg) over 1 to 2 minutes. It is effective for 20 to 30 minutes prior to redistribution out of the CNS, but this allows time for a longer-acting agent to reach a therapeutic level. Lorazepam (Ativan) 2 to 4 mg (0.05 mg/kg) is another effective benzodiazepine that exerts rapid control and has the advantage of a longer half-life. While having a relatively clean side-effect profile, these drugs are likely to cause transient hypoventilation, especially in the seizing patient, and may cause hypotension.

Barbiturates are useful for both rapid short-term control and long-term therapy of seizures. Sodium thiopental, given in an anesthetizing dose (1 to 4 mg/kg), will usually terminate the seizure. Respiratory depression, requiring ventilatory support and hypotension, often results. Phenobarbital is a long-lasting drug commonly used for epilepsy. The usual loading dose is 15 to 25 mg/kg. Cardiovascular depression can result but usually responds to slow administration of the drug and concomitant fluid therapy. Respiratory depression is common, especially when given in combination with benzodiazepines.

Lidocaine can have antiseizure effects in a dose of 50 to 100 mg. It may have short-term benefits in an acute situation. Large doses of lidocaine are, of course, epileptogenic themselves.

When all other therapies have failed, infusions of paraldehyde or the induction of general anesthesia may be utilized to curtail seizure activity.

Nonconvulsive Status Epilepticus

Nonconvulsive status epilepticus should be mentioned for completeness. It is not dramatic and obvious as are grand mal generalized seizures. Diagnosis can be difficult because clinical disturbances are subtle. Absence attacks, aphasia, confusional states, stupor, and behavioral disturbances may be manifestations of nonconvulsive status epilepticus. These conditions can only be confirmed as being epileptic in nature using EEG documentation. Therapy is necessary but should not be so aggressive as to risk respiratory or cardiovascular depression from rapid drug administration.

Complications of Coagulation

Hemorrhagic complications are of concern in a neurosurgical practice. Intracerebral hematomas may occur spontaneously because of an underlying defect or may follow coagulation difficulties resulting from a primary cerebral insult. There is a high incidence of coagulation abnormalities in patients with head injuries, and they correlate with the degree of trauma. Penetrating trauma is most likely to lead to problems, although mass lesions, such as post-traumatic or spontaneous hematomas and brain tumors, have been implicated. Bleeding abnormalities can result in serious intraoperative hemorrhage, bleeding at ventriculostomy sites, and delayed or recurrent intracranial hematomas postoperatively. One must therefore have a high index of suspicion and follow patients closely with clinical and laboratory examinations of clotting function.

Disseminated Intravascular Coagulation

A multitude of clotting abnormalities have been reported despite previously normal coagulation function. Diminished platelet counts, abnormal platelet function, decreased fibrinogen levels, and decreases in levels of other clotting factors have all been variably reported. Up to 90% of head-injured patients have at least one abnormal coagulation test if studied within the first 2 hours. In the worst scenario, some of these patients develop DIC. It is characterized by uncontrollable activation of the coagulation system by intravascular thrombosis and simultaneous consumption of clotting factors along with fibrinogenolysis and fibrinolysis. It may be initiated by excessive activation of the intrinsic coagulation system by direct endothelial cell injury, activation of the extrinsic system by direct tissue injury, or by red cell and platelet destruction that results in the release of coagulant phospholipids. Diagnostic criteria for DIC include prolongation of the prothrombin and partial thromboplastin times, decreased fibrinogen and platelet levels, and elevated fibrin split products. Prolonged thrombin times as well as abnormal euglobulin clot lysis times are also present.

Other Abnormalities

Other mechanisms may result in coagulation abnormalities in the critically ill neurosurgical patient. Chronic or subacute malnutrition may result in vitamin K deficiency with prolongation of prothrombin time. Similarly, folate deficiency can lead to thrombocytopenia. Several other causes of decreased platelet counts may be implicated: dilution from massive transfusion, occult or overwhelming sepsis, ARDS, and drug reactions to heparin, phenytoin, or antibiotics. Large amounts of Hetastarch may lead to coagulation difficulties.

Intracranial Bleeding

The main concern over abnormal coagulation studies is the risk of intracranial bleeding. Clinical presentation of patients with intracranial hematoma is difficult to distinguish from other causes of brain dysfunction. A deteriorating level of consciousness, newly developed third-nerve palsy, or rapid increases in ICP are suggestive symptoms. Symptoms may be insidious in onset at times. CT scanning is the study of choice to determine the cause for observed changes. Delayed intracerebral hematomas are almost always lobar, often multiple, and are commonly found in areas of previous cerebral contusions. They may be found in patients who had previously normal CT scans.

Treatment

Treatment of clotting difficulties is occasionally unnecessary because spontaneous resolution may occur. In severe cases of head injury, treatment may be ineffective because the severe degree of coagulopathy reflects a devasting degree of brain damage that is invariably lethal. In viable patients, abnormalities must be corrected if persistent and associated with known bleeding or the need for intracranial surgery. Coagulation abnormalities are often latent, and one must have a high index of suspicion in order to detect subclinical coagulation disorders. When treatment is needed, fresh frozen plasma (15 ml/kg initially) is helpful to correct abnormalities reflected by prolongation of the prothrombin time. Cryoprecipitate (initial empiric treatment using 5 to 10 bags) may be helpful to treat DIC and its resultant consumption of factors including fibrinogen and factor VIII. Platelets (usually 5 to 10 packs) are used to treat thrombocytopenia. Platelets are not given through a 40-micron blood filter. Each unit can be expected to raise the platelet count by $10,000/\mu l$. The best and most effective treatment for DIC is correction of the underlying abnormality that led to its initiation. Heparin therapy is usually contraindicated in patients with acute neurosurgical disorders because of the grave consequences of hemorrhage and, therefore, cannot be used to manage DIC in this setting. Caution is required in the use of drugs that could aggravate a latent bleeding tendency in a patient with neurologic disease, i.e., aspirin, dipyridamole, nonsteroidal anti-inflammatory drugs, and low-dose heparin.

Complications of Metabolism

Patients who have a head injury or cerebral disease, or who have had a cerebral operation, have a metabolic response similar to that seen with other types of general body trauma. Aspects of this response include accelerated body protein catabolism, increased protein and urine nitrogen losses, increased blood sugar, decreased sodium and water excretion, increased urinary potassium losses, and an overall decrease in body weight. These responses are mediated primarily through the hormonal secretions of the brain, pituitary, and adrenal glands. They are compounded by the effects of various treatments, and the result is often disarray of fluid, electrolyte, and nutritional balance.

Volume Status

Water Intoxication

Neurologic patients are susceptible to excessive hydration. Due to stress responses of surgery, including endogenous antidiuretic hormone secretion, excesses of administered fluid may result in overhydration. Ventilated patients have a noticeable decrease in insensible fluid loss and, in fact, gain excess free water (250 to 500 ml/day) from humidified gases. Hypotonic fluid administration then leads to dilutional hyponatremia that can be particularly hazardous, as it aggravates cerebral swelling. Warning symptoms occur when serum sodium levels reach 120 to 125 mEq/L and are related to the rapidity of change. Nausea, vomiting, apathy, and disorientation are early signs, with stupor and convulsions being the more feared late complications. The best treatment is, of course, prevention by judicious fluid administration.

Dehydration

Dehydration is also common in this patient group. Patients with impaired consciousness do not have a normal thirst mechanism to regulate fluid balance. Excessive fluid losses are common as a result of diarrhea, deliberate use of loop and osmotic diuretics, and the occasional presence of diabetes insipidus. Hypernatremia may result in symptoms of delirium, muscle twitching, and hyporeactive reflexes. Its correction requires judicious administration of fluid to avoid rapid and dangerous changes in serum osmolarity. Isotonic fluid is utilized if concomitant dehydration is present.

Diabetes Insipidus

Diabetes insipidus represents a lack of vasopressin secretion. It occurs with trauma to the posterior pituitary gland or hypothalamus. It is characterized by polyuria (>3 L/day), polydipsia, hypernatremia, elevated serum osmolarity (320 to 330 mOsm), and dilute urine with urine-to-sodium osmolarity ratios less than 1. Differential diagnosis involves ruling out a solute diuresis as is present with glycosuria, osmotic diuretics, loop diuretics, or mineralocorticoid deficiency. Clinical tests involve simultaneous measurements of urine and serum osmolarity. Treatment is instituted when excessive urine output makes fluid management difficult or if one is unable to keep up with fluid resuscitation. Exogenous vasopressin is available in three preparations. Aqueous vasopressin (5 to 10 IU, IM, or IV) is given every 4 to 6 hours. Vasopressin-tannate-in-oil (5 IU IM) may be used every 1 to 3 days as needed. The use of the synthetic drug desmopressin (DDAVP) has become popular in this setting. Intranasal doses of 10 to 20 μg or IV doses of 1 to 2 μg may be administered as needed every 8 to 24 hours.

Syndrome of Inappropriate Antidiuretic Hormone Secretion

The syndrome of inappropriate antidiuretic hormone secretion (SIADH) results from excessive vasopressin secretion. It occurs in various CNS conditions, such as meningitis, encephalitis, head injury, brain abscess, tumor, Guillain-Barré syndrome, and subarachnoid hemorrhage. It may result in severe water intoxication. There is continued renal excretion of sodium, and urine osmolarity is quite high. Normal renal and adrenal function is present. Serum osmolarity and sodium concentrations fall and result in symptoms. Treatment involves restriction of fluids to 600 to 800 ml/day, usually using $D_5 1/2$ NS or NS. Coma or seizures usually warrant more aggressive treatment with hypertonic saline and furosemide. Demeclocycline (300 to 600 mg twice per day) inhibits vasopressin and may be helpful at times to aid pharmacologically in the treatment of this problem. This syndrome usually occurs within 3 to 15 days after a traumatic CNS injury, and may last up to 2 weeks.

Glucose

Hyperglycemia

Hyperglycemia commonly will require therapy in the neurologic ICU. Many factors lead to elevated serum glucose levels in addition to the possible presence of latent diabetes mellitus. Stress leads to growth hormone and steroid secretion, both of which directly elevate serum glucose levels. It also results in catecholamine secretion, which inhibits the release of insulin. Exogenous glucocorticoid use is common. Exogenous glucose from maintenance or hyperalimentation fluids may be excessive. Early sepsis is associated with elevated glucose levels as well. The net results can be hyperglycemia and high osmolarity with intracellular dehydration and resultant cerebral depression. Glycosuria can make electrolyte management more difficult. Neuronal dysfunction caused by excessive lactate production during ischemia is another potentially adverse effect of maladjusted glucose homeostasis. The goal of treatment is to keep serum glucose between 100 and 200 mg/dl.

Nonketotic Hyperosmolar Coma

Nonketotic hyperosmolar coma (NHHC) is the extreme example of an abnormality resulting from excessive serum glucose levels. It is characterized by extreme hyperglycemia and serum osmolarities greater than 330 mOsm. Total body dehydration is present with severe intracellular dehydration resulting in CNS dysfunction. In addition to the above-mentioned diabetogenic factors, this condition is aggravated by prolonged mannitol use, hyperosmolar feedings, inadequate fluid replacement, and possibly by hypothalamic injury. If untreated, it may lead to arrhythmias, renal failure, stroke, systemic thrombotic complications, and death. Treatment is initiated with hydration and usually an insulin infusion. Electrolyte abnormalities such as hypokalemia and hypophosphatemia are treated as indicated.

Hormonal Insufficiency

Hormonal insufficiency may occur in patients with various neurologic conditions. Posterior pituitary problems have been discussed. Anterior pituitary insufficiency has been reported as a sequela to head injury and skull fracture but is, in fact, rare. It may of course be seen following intracranial surgery in the region of the pituitary gland. Late developments such as amenorrhea, galactorrhea, and regression of secondary sexual characteristics would not be of concern in the acute care setting. Hypothyroidism may require treatment, although the earliest likely intervention would be at 5 days because of the slow uptake of thyroxine under normal conditions. Hypocortisolism is a potential problem but one that is more commonly related to suppression of pituitary function by exogenous steroid use rather than by primary pituitary insufficiency itself. High doses of steroids are commonly used for therapeutic purposes in neurologic disease. When their use is not indicated for therapeutic reasons, one must not forget to administer steroids to cover stress in patients with potentially suppressed adrenocortical responses. Various tests may be employed to evaluate the responsiveness of the hypothalamic-pituitary-adrenal axis, but they are beyond the scope of this discussion.

Nutrition

Metabolic Stress Response

Concern with the nutritional management of acutely ill patients has been routine in the surgical ICU, and neurosurgical patients are no exception. Trauma, surgical stress, and infection increase the resting energy expenditures of neurosurgical patients by 25 to 120% in various studies. The period of hypermetabolism, which usually lasts 5 to 10 days after a systemic injury, has been reported to persist throughout the duration of coma in the neurologically impaired patient. There is an obligatory nitrogen loss that reflects accelerated gluconeogenesis at the expense of body protein stores. Protein-calorie malnutrition, which can result from inattention to the hypermetabolism and nitrogen losses, can lead to impaired cell-mediated immunity and decreased pulmonary function. These defects could potentially lead to more frequent episodes of sepsis, prolonged ventilatory dependency, and other complications. Indeed, in a recent study in which head-injured patients received early aggressive nutritional therapy, there was an increased survival compared with historical controls.

Parenteral Hyperalimentation

Nutritional therapy should be instituted early in the postoperative or post-traumatic period. Negative nitrogen balance cannot always be reversed but can always be minimized. If early use of the gastrointestinal tract is not expected to be possible, parenteral hyperalimentation should be implemented. This must be started slowly and with careful monitoring of fluid and electrolyte balance in all patients, but particularly in patients at risk for cerebral edema and elevated ICP. Guidelines for the initiation of parenteral nutrition and its potential complications can be found in many surgical texts and patient care manuals. Of particular concern in the neurosurgical population is avoidance of hyperglycemia and its associated glucosuria, dehydration, and hyperosmolar nonketotic coma. In addition, the likelihood of occult catheter sepsis must be kept in mind.

Enteral Alimentation

When abdominal injuries do not preclude its use, the gastrointestinal tract provides the most effective means of alimentation. Frequent aspiration of the stomach to measure residual volumes will rule out gastric paresis. Should residuals be high, metoclopramide can be utilized to enhance emptying, or the stomach could be bypassed entirely by the use of a nasojejunal tube positioned with radiographic guidance. Gastric aspiration is a dreaded complication that can often be avoided by careful use of the gastrointestinal tract. A multitude of enteral formulas are available for use. They should be chosen to provide adequate protein and calorie intake (usually a calorie-to-nitrogen ratio of

150:1). Diarrhea should be avoided. Slow implementation of feedings and judicious use of Lomotil or Imodium will control most tendencies toward loose stools. Again, one must take care to avoid hyperosmolar conditions aggravated by high-density feedings with inadequate free water intake.

Other Complications

Deep Venous Thrombosis and Pulmonary Embolism

Neurosurgical patients are at high risk for the complications of deep venous thrombosis (DVT) and pulmonary embolus. If extremely sensitive diagnostic criteria are utilized, as many as 40 to 50% of patients can be shown to have calf thrombi. This incidence approaches that of orthopedic surgical cases. Intraoperative venous stasis and long periods of postoperative immobilization are the greatest risk factors. Clinical symptoms and signs of DVT are frequently lacking. Diagnosis cannot be made by clinical examination with any reliability. Doppler venous studies and impedance plethysmography represent accurate noninvasive methods to make the diagnosis. Simple auscultation with a portable Doppler device over the femoral or popliteal veins can detect a high proportion of cases when performed by an experienced observer. Venography remains the gold standard for diagnosis. Treatment requires anticoagulation, which is often contraindicated in the postoperative surgical patient. In such situations, measures must be taken to prevent pulmonary emboli. Vena caval interruption with a caval filter is undertaken for cases of ileofemoral thrombosis, and expectant observation may be elected for cases of isolated calf thrombi. Prevention is, of course, the best form of management, although, once again, drugs such as subcutaneous heparin are often contraindicated. Intermittent compression boots are helpful for long procedures, especially for patients at higher risk such as those with the additional risk factors of obesity or previous venous disease. Mortality from pulmonary embolus in the hospitalized patient may exceed 20% and is higher if left untreated. The possibility of pulmonary embolus must always be entertained in the neurosurgical patient with acute respiratory problems, despite other explanations. A normal scintigraphic perfusion scan can rule out the diagnosis. Questionable scans require simultaneous performance of a ventilation scan with pulmonary angiography held back to clarify confusion following these noninvasive tests.

Upper Gastrointestinal Hemorrhage

Gastrointestinal hemorrhage following neurologic injury used to be common. Gastric stress ulceration, initially described as Cushing's ulcers, has decreased in incidence owing to the widespread prophylactic treatment of susceptible patients. There is a large stimulus for gastric acid secretion following head injury and other forms of stress. Large amounts of H_2-blockers and/or antacids may be required to neutralize gastric pH. Actual measurements are helpful to verify the adequacy of treatment, with a goal being a pH greater than 4. Sepsis is another potent stimulus for gastric acid secretion. Occult sepsis may be diagnosed by the recognized failure of a previously successful regimen to control gastric pH. Sucralfate (Carafate) has been shown to speed healing of gastrointestinal ulcers and has actions that should provide effective prophylaxis as well. It may find increased clinical usage because of its lack of effects on gastric acidity. Acid decreases bacterial counts and thereby may decrease the incidence and severity of nosocomial pneumonias that result from aspirated gastric contents.

Brain Death

The unfortunate reality in neurointensive care is that some patients suffer devastating irreversible brain damage, often incompatible with life. Criteria have been developed to define neurologic death so that unnecessary means to prolong vital functions are not continued. This has become even more important in the modern era of organ transplantation plagued by a dearth of donor organs. Initial brain death criteria were developed in 1968 by a committee from Harvard Medical School. These criteria have been modified and adapted with experience to yield criteria that facilitate more practical delineation of the brain death state. Brain death is widely accepted by the lay public as well as the medical and legal communities.

Brain death is determined by clinical diagnosis, aided by laboratory examinations. Cerebral unresponsiveness is a prerequisite and is manifested by a lack of evidence of withdrawal or posturing to a painful stimulus. Spinal reflexes do not indicate cerebral responsiveness. Pupils must be unresponsive to light. Oval pupils represent persistent midbrain activity. Eye movements must be absent by "doll's eye" testing as well as ice water irrigation. Corneal, cough, and gag reflexes must be similarly absent. Apnea must be documented 5 minutes after removal from the ventilator, preferably with a documented $Paco_2$ greater than 50 mm Hg. An apnea test is performed after preoxygenation and while insufflating 8 to 12 L/min of oxygen by catheter at the carinal level or via the endotracheal tube.

Laboratory studies that can be utilized include EEG and blood-flow studies. EEG recordings should show complete electrocerebral silence, including a lack of change with painful, auditory, and visual stimulation. Hypothermia does not preclude the use of EEG unless body temperature is below 32.3°C (90°F). Barbiturate levels should be below 1 mg/dl, and other CNS depressants should not be present. Contrast angiography or radionuclide flow studies can demonstrate a lack of cerebral blood flow, which, of course, represents a situation of irreversible brain damage. Laboratory studies alone cannot be used to make the diagnosis, and their use is not always required to supplement clinical examinations.

Confirmation of brain death usually requires a repeat examination after 24 hours, but this can be shortened to 6 to 12 hours given a clinical situation in which improvement is not expected because of the mechanism of injury. A neurologist or neurosurgeon should be involved in the decision-making process or be called upon to confirm the diagnosis. For ethical and medicolegal reasons, a transplant surgeon must not be involved in both the determination of brain death and the subsequent transplantation operation.

Subarachnoid Hemorrhage

Subarachnoid hemorrhage (SAH) is a common reason for admission to a neurologic ICU. The majority of the nontraumatic cases involve rupture of a saccular aneurysm at the branch point of a large artery at the base of the brain. Other causes include trauma, arteriovenous malformation, mycotic aneurysm, hypertensive crisis, or other anatomic variants. Mortality and morbidity following SAH are extremely high. The most important aspect of management is accurate diagnosis. Characteristic symptoms and signs include meningismus, coma, nausea and vomiting, and generalized headache. The cardinal symptom remains unusually severe headache of sudden onset. Accurate diagnosis allows for identification of subsets of patients who may be at risk for the development of other complications.

While specific symptom complexes may suggest the presence and location of a ruptured aneurysm, more accurate radiographic or invasive tests are required. CT scanning is the initial test of choice and should be obtained without use of contrast. Blood is frequently seen in the basal cisterns. Contrast scanning may then allow actual definition of an aneurysm. Lumbar puncture is helpful in patients with negative CT scans to demonstrate small bleeds or warning leaks that would otherwise be missed. Angiography is the gold standard diagnostic test for identification of lesions that lead to SAH. It is not without risk and is generally delayed until surgery is planned. The timing of surgery remains controversial, with some clinicians advocating early surgery at 48 to 96 hours and others delaying surgery until approximately 2 weeks following the hemorrhage.

Complications

Patients with SAH are susceptible to a multitude of complications. Several of these, which have been discussed in general terms, are electrocardiographic changes: pulmonary edema; fluid and electrolyte disturbances, such as diabetes insipidus and SIADH; gastrointestinal hemorrhage; and DVT. There are four complications specific to SAH that need to be prevented or treated: rebleeding, hydrocephalus, vasospasm, and mass effects.

Rebleeding

The incidence of rebleeding may approach 30%. Its peak incidence is usually in the first 24 hours and diminishes over the next 2 weeks. Unless surgically obliterated, a persistent aneurysm always remains at risk for rupture with rebleeding. Prevention of rebleeding begins with control of transmural "bursting" pressure (MAP − ICP). This involves the control of blood pressure surges. Patients are nursed in quiet rooms without excessive stimulation. Sedatives and analgesics are used liberally. Antihypertensives are used as needed early in the course of treatment unless hypertensive, hypervolemic therapy is indicated for vasospasm.

Attempts to prevent lysis of clot around the aneurysm remain another source of controversy. Epsilon-aminocaproic acid has been studied with conflicting results. It is an antifibrinolytic drug which, while preventing a rebleeding episode, may result in thrombotic and ischemic complications at other sites. At present, most authorities agree that its use cannot be definitively recommended. It does, however, remain in widespread use and is given as a continuous infusion of 30 to 36 g/day beginning at the time of admission and continuing until the time of surgery.

Hydrocephalus

Hydrocephalus, usually of the communicating variety, occurs not infrequently after aneurysmal rupture. Its peak incidence ranges from 4 to 20 days after the event. Mild drowsiness, urinary incontinence, and the inability to move the eyes above the equator are the usual clinical signs. Unfortunately, not all patients have detectable neurologic symptoms or signs, and the diagnosis can be missed. Hydrocephalus may be transient and not require therapy. Therapeutic options when needed include repeated lumbar puncture or ventriculoperitoneal shunting. Sudden decreases in ICP due to removal of CSF could theoretically increase transmural pressure across an untreated aneurysm and lead to rerupture. Therefore, hydrocephalus is treated after definitive aneurysm therapy whenever possible.

Vasospasm

Vasospasm remains the most devastating complication of SAH other than the neurologic damage associated with the initial or recurrent hemorrhage. The incidence of vasospasm may be as high as 80%. Clinically significant vasospasm, defined as that leading to deterioration of neurologic function, occurs in only 30% of patients. Onset is delayed, with a peak incidence between the fourth and fourteenth days. It usually follows a period of neurologic improvement and stabilization. The stems of major cerebral vessels and the circle of Willis are affected initially, although vasospasm may then proceed distally. Spasm may be diffuse, segmental, or localized. Prediction of vasospasm is often possible with documentation of blood clots in the basal cisterns by CT scans performed 2 to 4 days following SAH. Specific criteria concerning the amount and location of blood clots allow identification of a high-risk group of patients. Vasospasm has also been correlated with the presence of elevated ICP. The cause of vasospasm remains unknown, although several mechanisms have been proposed. Elucidation of the exact mechanisms may lead to more effective treatment in the future.

Mild vasospasm undoubtedly occurs without neurologic symptoms in many patients. The occurrence of clinically significant vasospasm is heralded by the onset of new symptoms after stabilization of the initial clinical situation. Common presentations include increasing headaches, increasing nuchal rigidity, increasing lethargy, deteriorating neurologic status, and low-grade fever. Focal changes on EEG may also suggest the diagnosis. Elevated CSF lactate correlates with the presence of vasospasm with ischemia. Cerebral angiography has always been required to prove the presence of vasospasm. Recent work has suggested that noninvasive transcranial Doppler techniques may ultimately replace angiography as a diagnostic tool.

Effective treatment of existing vasospasm and the prevention of likely vasospasm remain goals of modern neurologic intensive care. A variety of treatments with theoretical potential have proved clinically ineffective. Aminophylline and isoproterenol have failed to work despite having actions that lead to elevated cyclic AMP, which causes cerebral vasodilatation. Aminophylline may actually cause cerebral vasoconstriction by direct purinergic receptor effects. Nitroprusside may relieve spasm, but also leads to increases in cerebral blood volume and elevated ICP, and thus has not been helpful. Calcium-channel blockers have yet to show beneficial effects. Much work at present involves trials of nitroglycerin and the newer calcium-channel blockers. Barbiturate coma has failed to improve outcome. The most commonly accepted form of therapy for symptomatic vasospasm remains volume expansion and blood pressure elevation in an attempt to increase cerebral perfusion pressure. Phenylephrine and dopamine are commonly used, the latter in doses of 3 to 6 μg/kg/min. Systolic blood pressure should be kept below 170 to 180 mm Hg. Volume expansion involves administration of whole blood, packed cells, plasma, albumin, or dextran. Even this apparently straightforward technique may not be effective and has at times resulted in pulmonary edema or aneurysmal rebleeding.

Mass Effects and Edema

Intracerebral hematomas as well as epidural and subdural collections can result from bleeding of a ruptured aneurysm. Direct damage occurs locally and accompanies global damage, which may occur as a result of the elevated ICP and mass effects. There are many other reasons for cerebral swelling and edema, including irritation of parenchyma by blood clot surrounding the intracerebral hematoma, vasospasm or iatrogenic vascular compromise during surgery leading to ischemic brain tissue, operative retraction of brain, and elevated ICP associated with the acute hemorrhage. Such swelling and edema reveals or aggravates the problems related to the original blood collection.

Suggested Reading

Aidinis SJ, et al. Intracranial responses to PEEP. Anesthesiology 1976; 45:275.

Ausman JI, et al. Current management of cerebral aneurysms: is it based on facts or myths? Surg Neurol 1985; 24:625.

Bedford RF, et al. Lidocaine or thiopental for rapid control of intracranial hypertension. Anesth Analg 1980; 59:435.

Bishop MJ, et al. Laryngeal effects of prolonged intubation. Anesth Analg 1984; 63:335.

Clifton GL, et al. The metabolic response to severe head injury. J Neurosurg 1984; 60:687.

Cooper KR, et al. Safe use of PEEP in patients with severe head injury. J Neurosurg 1985; 63:552.

Delgado-Escheta AV, et al. Management of status epilepticus. N Engl J Med 1982; 306:1337.

Flitter MA. Techniques of intracranial pressure monitoring. Clin Neurosurg 1981; 28:547.

Frost EAM. Respiratory problems associated with head trauma. Neurosurgery 1977; 1:300.

Frost EAM. The physiopathology of respiration in neurosurgical patients. J Neurosurg 1979; 50:699.

Gudeman SK, et al. Gastric secretory and mucosal injury response to severe head trauma. Neurosurgery 1983; 12:175.

Havill JH. Prolonged hyperventilation and intracranial pressure. Crit Care Med 1984; 12:72

Heffner JE, Sahn SA. Controlled hyperventilation in patients with intracranial hypertension: Application and management. Arch Intern Med 1983; 143:765.

Kassell NF, et al. Cerebral vasospasm following aneurysmal subarachnoid hemorrhage. Stroke 1985; 16:562.

Malik AB. Mechanisms of neurogenic pulmonary edema. Circ Res 1985; 57:1.

Matjasko J, Pitts L. Controversies in severe head injury management. In: Clinical controversies in neuroanesthesia and neurosurgery. Orlando: Grune & Stratton, 1986.

McLaurin RL, King LR. Recognition and treatment of metabolic disorders after head injury. Clin Neurosurg 1972; 19:281.

Muizelaar JP, et al. Effect of mannitol on ICP and CBF and correlation with pressure autoregulation in severely head-injured patients. J Neurosurg 1984; 61:700.

Pierson DJ. Weaning from mechanical ventilation. In: Pierson DJ, ed. Respiratory intensive care. Dallas: Daedalus Enterprises, 1986.

Rapp RP, et al. The favorable effect of early parenteral feeding on survival in head-injured patients. J Neurosurg 1983; 58:906.

Robertson CS, et al. Treatment of hypertension associated with head injury. J Neurosurg 1983; 59:455.

Ropper AH, Kennedy SK, eds. Neurological and neurosurgical intensive care, 2nd ed. Rockville, MD: Aspen, 1988.

Ropper AH, et al. Head position, intracranial pressure, and compliance. Neurology 1982; 32:1288.

Rosner MJ, Coley IB. Cerebral perfusion pressure, intracranial pressure, and head elevation. J Neurosurg 1986; 65:636.

Segal BJ, et al. Mechanical ventilation. In: MacDonnell KF, Fahey PJ, Segal MS, eds. Respiratory intensive care. Boston: Little, Brown, 1987.

Shapiro HM. Intracranial hypertension: therapeutic and anesthetic considerations. Anesthesiology 1975; 43:445.

Shucart WA, Jackson I. Management of diabetes insipidus in neurosurgical patients. J Neurosurg 1976; 44:65.

Simon RP. Physiologic consequences of status epilepticus. Epilepsia 1985; 26(Suppl 1):S58.

Swann KW, Black P McL. Deep vein thrombosis and pulmonary emboli in neurosurgical patients: a review. J Neurosurg 1984; 61:1055.

Wirth FP, Ratcheson RA, eds. Neurosurgical critical care. Vol I. Concepts in neurosurgery. Baltimore: Williams & Wilkins, 1987.

Zwillich CW, et al. Complications of assisted ventilation. A prospective study of 354 consecutive episodes. Am J Med 1974; 57:161.

Index